HYPERTENSION MANAGEMENT

CLINICAL PATHWAYS, GUIDELINES, AND PATIENT EDUCATION

HEALTH & ADMINISTRATION DEVELOPMENT GROUP

Jo Gulledge
Executive Director

Shawn Beard
Research Editor

AN ASPEN PUBLICATION®
Aspen Publishers, Inc.
Gaithersburg, Maryland
1999

ASPEN CHRONIC DISEASE MANAGEMENT SERIES

Library of Congress Cataloging-in-Publication Data

Hypertension management: clinical pathways, guidelines, and patient education / Health & Administration Development Group; Jo Gulledge, executive director; Shawn Beard, research editor.
p. cm. — (Aspen chronic disease management series)
Includes index.
ISBN: 0-8342-1702-3
1. Hypertension Handbooks, manuals, etc.
I. Gulledge, Jo. II. Beard, Shawn. III. Health and Administration Development Group (Aspen Publishers) IV. Series.
[DNLM] 1. Hypertension—therapy. 2. Hypertension—diagnosis. 3. Critical Pathways. 4. Patient Education. WG 340 M998 1999]
RC685.H8H7885 1999
616.1'32—dc21
DNLM/DLC
for Library of Congress 99-31851
CIP

Editorial Services: Marsha Davies

Orders· (800) 638-8437
Customer Service: (800) 234-1660

About Aspen Publishers • For more than 35 years, Aspen has been a leading professional publisher in a variety of disciplines. Aspen's vast information resources are available in both print and electronic formats. We are committed to providing the highest quality information available in the most appropriate format for our customers. Visit Aspen's Internet site for more information resources, directories, articles, and a searchable version of Aspen's full catalog, including the most recent publications: **http://www.aspenpublishers.com**
Aspen Publishers, Inc. • The hallmark of quality in publishing
Member of the worldwide Wolters Kluwer group

Library of Congress Catalog Card Number: 99-31851
ISBN: 0-8342-1702-3

Printed in the United States of America

1 2 3 4 5

Table of Contents

Editorial Board

Claire B. Rossé, RN, BS, MBA
Founder and CEO
FutureHealth Corporation
Timonium, Maryland

Rachel Stipe, RN, BS, CPHQ
Quality Improvement/Reimbursement Specialist
Spectracare, Inc.
Louisville, Kentucky

Maura J. Sughrue, MD
Medical Director
Fairfax Family Practice Centers
Fairfax, Virginia

Warren E. Todd, MBA
Vice President, Business Development
Hastings Healthcare Group
Pennington, New Jersey

Marcus D. Wilson, PharmD
President
Health Core, Inc.
Newark, Delaware

Introduction

Disease management is based on the understanding that a small proportion of the population—individuals with chronic conditions—consumes the vast majority of health care resources. Focusing on chronic illnesses, disease management programs strive to reduce costly hospitalizations through continual, rather than episodic, care. The logic is straightforward: providing a continuum of care dramatically reduces the incidence of acute episodes requiring inpatient treatment.

Because of disease management's emphasis on continual care, effective education of patients, families, and other informal caregivers is a vital component. Providers form partnerships with patients and families, teaching them to take daily responsibility for managing disease.

Hypertension, or high blood pressure, is one of several chronic disease states affecting millions of Americans. Without proper management, hypertension can lead to coronary artery disease, congestive heart failure, or stroke. Because of its prevalence and gravity, it is imperative to create a disease-management program that aids clinicians in diagnosing and effectively treating the disease.

Hypertension Management provides comprehensive, detailed guide-lines on all aspects of managing hypertension from the initial diagnosis in the clinical examination to the treatment strategy, which may include drug therapy, nonpharmacologic intervention, lifestyle modification, and/or nutrition counseling. *Hypertension Management* couples these clinical guidelines with patient education handouts, which teach patients to comply with interventions, while also learning the principles of demand management: recognizing and prioritizing their health care needs. Through education, patients know when professional interventions are required and use resources accordingly.

To ensure quick access to the information clinicians need most, *Hypertension Management* is divided into two parts.

Part I, "Managing Hypertension: Clinical Pathways and Guidelines," addresses the essentials of administering hypertension management programs, with information on developing and implementing clinical guidelines/pathways, measuring and managing outcomes, and monitoring and improving patient satisfaction. While the guidelines originate from nationally recognized sources, their purpose is to serve as a starting point for providers and payers pursuing disease management. They are meant to be adapted to meet the needs of specific populations and to be further refined for individual patients.

Part II, "Self-Management of Hypertension: Patient Education," recognizes the patient education component of disease management. Consisting entirely of large-print patient handouts, including Spanish-language patient information sheets, this section is designed for clinicians across the care continuum to distribute freely to patients. The educational materials encourage patients and their families to become active partners in managing chronic conditions.

Hypertension Management is not intended to add new information to the abundant literature relevant to disease management, but rather to extract from hundreds of publications the most sound and useful information available. The goal is to provide this information in such a manner that is concise, practical, and pertinent. To that end, *Hypertension Management* distills the traditional narrative text and presents it in a quick-read format.

Shawn K. Beard
Research Editor
Health & Administration Development Group

ix

Acknowledgments

Creating a reference volume such as *Hypertension Management* demands tremendous effort during the development period—shaping the manual's focus, collecting and evaluating materials, and ensuring that the format is practical and easy to use.

Foremost among the people who help us fulfill these responsibilities are the editorial board members. By answering queries, providing contacts, and reviewing materials, they play an instrumental role in the development of a high quality resource.

I am grateful to all the health care facilities, organizations, individual professionals, and others who generously shared their clinical guidelines, pathways, and patient education materials with us—special thanks to Janet Yozura, RD, Clinical Nutrition Manager, Youville Hospital and Rehabilitation Center, Cambridge, Massachusetts and Nutrition Screening Initiative, Washington, D.C.

In addition, this project never could have progressed from a bare-bones idea to a comprehensive resource without the untiring support of Rosemarie Cooper, Administrative Assistant; the skill of Marsha Davies, Editorial Services; and the guidance of Jo Gulledge, Executive Director, Health & Administration Development Group.

Shawn Beard
Research Editor
Health & Administration Development Group

Tracking Form

POLICY

Patient education documentation

PURPOSE

To provide interdisciplinary documentation of patient/family education

PROCEDURE

1. On admission, stamp the Tracking Form with patient's Addressograph plate and place in front of chart.
2. Within first three days of admission, have licensed nursing/therapy staff identify patient/family educational needs.
3. Read and follow directions 1–3 on the Tracking Form.
4. Fill out specific sections of the Tracking Form.

- **Document:** List of materials from manual by chapter.
- **Initial/Date Given:** As material is given, initial and date in the space provided.
- **Primary Caregiver:** Indicate who is receiving education information (the caregiver or the patient).
- **Comments:** Write comments regarding when material was reviewed (provide date/initials), with whom, and any required special needs.
- **Demonstrates Understanding of Activity:** Initial and date when primary caregiver has demonstrated understanding of activity (must be completed before discharge).
- **Other Classes Attended:** List other education opportunities (classes attended and additional handouts) not already listed.
5. Sign full name, with initials and title, on back of form.

Place Facility Logo Here	A D D R E S S O G R A P H

Hypertension Management

DIRECTIONS:
1. Highlight APPROPRIATE patient education materials.
2. Initial and date when material was given/reviewed/completed.
3. Use comments column for:
   a. Charting dates reviewed.
   b. Special patient/family needs.
   c. Receiver of education.

DOCUMENT	Init/Date Given	Primary Caregiver	COMMENTS Init/Dates Material Reviewed • Special Needs • Who Received Education	Init/Date States &/or Demonstrates Understanding of Activity
5. Diagnosis and Management of Hypertension				
Your High Blood Pressure				
What Is High Blood Pressure?				
Testing for High Blood Pressure				
Using Home Blood Pressure Monitoring Devices				
Record Your Blood Pressure				
High Blood Pressure—What You and Your Family Should Know				
Presión alta—Lo que usted y su familia deben saber				
Taking Action To Control High Blood Pressure				
Tips for Reaching Your Blood Pressure Goal				
High Blood Pressure Glossary				
Healthy Heart IQ				
6. Preventing Hypertension				
Prevent High Blood Pressure				
What Else Might Prevent High Blood Pressure?				
¡Póngase en acción—Prevenga la presión alta!				
High Blood Pressure Prevention IQ				
7. Exercise and Hypertension				
Exercise and High Blood Pressure				
A Sample Walking Program				
Check Your Target Heart Rate				
8. Nutrition and Hypertension				
Losing Weight				

DOCUMENT	Init/Date Given	Primary Caregiver	COMMENTS Init/Dates Material Reviewed • Special Needs • Who Received Education	Init/Date States &/or Demonstrates Understanding of Activity
Hypertension and Your Diet				
Choose Low-Salt Foods				
Cut Down on Salt and Sodium				
¡Coma menos sal y sodio!				
No Added Salt Diet				
The DASH Diet				
Reading Nutrition Labels				
Using Spices Instead of Salt				
Sodium in Foods				
Sodium Intake Information				
Contract for a Sodium-Modified Diet				
Menu Ideas for People with High Blood Pressure				
Alcohol and High Blood Pressure				
Heart Healthy Eating Self-Contract				
9. Medications for Hypertension				
Types of Medications for High Blood Pressure				
Generic Names of High Blood Pressure Medicines				
How To Take Diuretics				
How To Take Beta Blocker Medicines				

OTHER CLASSES ATTENDED/HANDOUTS GIVEN	INIT	SIGNATURE

PART I

Managing Hypertension: Clinical Pathways and Guidelines

1. Hypertension and Disease Management*

Hypertension is a common medical finding. Yet, the specific diagnostic workup and treatment of hypertension are dependent on a number of medical and demographic factors.

Since hypertension can have diverse etiologies and treatment regimens, no "one-fits-all" strategy to deal with the disease will work. However, because it is a common disease usually requiring lifelong treatment, it is worth the effort to design disease-management programs to help practitioners with diagnostic strategies and therapeutic decisions.

FACTORS TO CONSIDER

In addition to differences in strategies based on the age of the patient, many other factors may influence the workup and treatment plan. For example, the socioeconomic background of the patient will influence the treatment plan. Is the patient likely to be noncompliant with medication or lifestyle changes? Can the patient easily be contacted for follow-up? Perhaps the patient does not have a telephone.

HOME MONITORING

An important strategy for monitoring home blood pressure, which is often different than office blood pressure, is to teach the patient to take and record blood pressure frequently. Home blood pressure monitoring is an indispensable ally in the care of patients who require frequent blood pressure monitoring and drug changes.

Nurses or other practitioners such as pharmacists can modify treatment regimens over the telephone if the patient is capable of accurate blood pressure measurements. Careful assessment of the patient's ability to obtain accurate meas-

urements is necessary. Not all patients will be able to take their own blood pressure reliably, but many of these patients will have family members who can assist in obtaining blood pressures and other vital signs such as pulse rate and weight.

COMORBIDITIES

Comorbid conditions also play a role in diagnostic and therapeutic decision making. If the patient has congestive heart failure or diabetes mellitus, angiotensin-converting enzyme (ACE) inhibitors may assume a greater therapeutic role. If the patient has a history of asthma, beta-blockers may be contraindicated. In contrast, patients who suffer from angina without congestive heart failure may find double benefit from beta-blockers. Patients with benign prostatic hypertrophy could find a double benefit from alpha-blockers.

FACTORING IN THE COST

While there may be many patients who would benefit from more expensive therapy with ACE inhibitors or calcium channel blockers, many more patients who currently receive these drugs may achieve equal benefit from nonpharmacologic lifestyle changes or less expensive therapy with diuretics or beta-blockers.

Older patients may be more compliant with lifestyle changes than younger patients. Weight loss, dietary restriction, and exercise may help lower blood pressure in compliant individuals, and may obviate the use of antihypertensive medications. In instances where blood pressure is not normalized with nonpharmacologic treatment, the number of medications necessary to control blood pressure may be reduced.

Lifestyle changes offer the added benefit of an increased sense of well-being, and potentially decreased risk for other vascular complications. Stroke and coronary artery disease are associated with hypertension, and a reduction in the incidence of these crippling comorbid diseases has obvious medical and economic benefit.

---

*Source: "Disease State Management," *Pharmacy Cost Control News*, Vol. 2:11, Aspen Publishers, Inc., © 1995.

FACTS ABOUT HYPERTENSION

DEFINITION

Systolic blood pressure >140 mm Hg
Diastolic blood pressure >90 mm Hg
Elevated systolic pressure associated with greater health risk
   in the elderly

PREVALENCE

50 million Americans (1 in 4)

SUBGROUPS AT RISK

African-Americans, elderly, less well educated, lower
   socioeconomic groups, residents of southeastern US
Most frequent diagnosis in ambulatory care settings

RISK FACTORS

Excess calories, sodium, alcohol; inadequate calcium,
   potassium; smoking, inactivity Obesity, Diabetes Mellitus,
   Dyslipidemias

ADVERSE HEALTH OUTCOMES

Coronary Artery Disease, Left Ventricular Hypertrophy,
   Congestive Heart Failure, Renal Disease, Cerebrovascular
   Disease, Stroke, Peripheral Vascular Disease, Retinal
   Hemorrhage

COSTS

Approximately $15 billion, percent spent on drugs greater
   than that spent for treatment of all other cardiovascular
   system diseases combined

Noncompliance a major contributor to costs
Expenditures for treatment with diet, lifestyle modifications,
   and drugs lower than for treatment with drugs alone

TREATMENT OPTIONS

Lifestyle Modifications (nutrition education and counseling,
   weight reduction, smoking cessation, exercise)
Lifestyle Modifications plus Single Drug Therapy
Lifestyle Modifications plus Multiple Drug Therapy

NUTRITION INTERVENTION

Reduce caloric intake (if overweight)
Limit alcohol
Reduce sodium intake (if black or elderly)
Maintain adequate intakes of dietary potassium, calcium,
   magnesium
Reduce fat and cholesterol intakes

LIFESTYLE MODIFICATIONS

Stop Smoking
Increase activity/exercise regularly

IMPACT

Prevention/reduction in blood pressure elevation
Elimination/reduction in dose/number of medications needed
   to control blood pressure
Prevention/reduction in target organ damage
Prevention/reduction in incidence of diseases associated with
   elevated blood pressure
Reduction in health care costs
Improved quality of life

Source: Reprinted with permission by The Nutrition Screening Initiative, a project of The American Academy of Family Physicians, The American Dietetic Association, and The National Council on Aging, Inc., and funded in part by a grant from Ross Products Division, Abbott Laboratories Inc.

2. Guidelines for Managing Hypertension

TRENDS IN THE AWARENESS, TREATMENT, AND CONTROL OF
HIGH BLOOD PRESSURE IN ADULTS: UNITED STATES, 1976–1994**

	NHANES II (1976–80)	NHANES III (Phase 1) 1988–1991	NHANES III (Phase 2) 1991–1994
Awareness	51%	73%	68.4%
Treatment	31%	55%	53.6%
Control[†]	10%	29%	27.4%

**Data are for adults age 18 to 74 with systolic blood pressure (SBP) of 140 mm Hg or greater, with diastolic blood pressure (DBP) of 90 mm Hg or greater, or taking antihypertensive medication.
[†]SBP below 140 mm Hg and DBP below 90 mm Hg.
Source: Burt V et al. and unpublished National Health and Nutrition Examination Survey (NHANES) III, phase 2, data provided by the Centers for Disease Control and Prevention, National Center for Health Statistics.

LIST OF ABBREVIATIONS

ACE	angiotensin-converting enzyme
CAD	coronary artery disease
CHF	congestive heart failure
CVD	cardiovascular disease
DBP	diastolic blood pressure
EWPHE	European Working Party on High Blood Pressure in the Elderly
HDFP	Hypertension Detection and Follow-Up Program
ISA	intrinsic sympathomimetic activity
ISH	isolated systolic hypertension
JNC V	*Fifth Report of the Joint National Committee on Detection, Evaluation, and Treatment of High Blood Pressure*
mg/dL	milligrams per deciliter
mm Hg	millimeters of mercury
MRC	Medical Research Council
NHANES	National Health and Nutrition Examination Survey
SBP	systolic blood pressure
SHEP	Systolic Hypertension in the Elderly Program
STOP-Hypertension	Swedish Trial in Old Patients with Hypertension

Source: *Working Group Report on Hypertension in the Elderly*, National Heart, Lung, and Blood Institute, NIH Publication 94-3527, July 1994.

STRATEGIES EFFICACIOUS IN THE PREVENTION/TREATMENT OF HYPERTENSION

Desired Outcome: Normalization of Blood Pressure (SBP <140 mm Hg, DBP <90 mm Hg)

Screening Alert/Indicator	Strategy/Strategies	Expected Outcome(s)	Provider(s)
Excessive Body Weight • BMI >27 • Weight above the norm on standard Ht/Wt tables • Excessive waist/hip ratio • Elevated blood pressure • Inappropriate weight gain • Elevated blood sugar • Elevated blood lipids	• Reduce caloric intake • Reduce fat intake • Reduce sweets intake • Increase intake of fruit, vegetables, grains • Moderate alcohol intake • Increase activity	Maintenance of a reasonable weight • BMI 22–27 • Weight in desirable range on standard Ht/Wt Tables • Waist/Hip Ratio <1.0 males/ <0.8 females • Normalization of blood pressure • Normalization of blood sugar • Normalization of serum lipids	• General nutrition education: Family Member, MD, RN, Pharmacist, SW • Complex diet/lifestyle modifications: RD
Hyperlipidemias • Total Cholesterol < 200mg/dl • HDL Cholesterol < 35mg/dl • LDL Cholesterol < 130mg/dl • Triglycerides < 200mg/dl	• Reduce total fat intake to < 30% of daily calories • Reduce saturated fat intake to < 10% • Reduce cholesterol intake to < 300 mg/day • Increase intake of complex carbohydrates • Moderate alcohol intake	Normalization of blood lipid levels • Total Cholesterol < 200mg/dl • HDL Cholesterol < 35mg/dl • LDL Cholesterol < 130mg/dl • Triglycerides < 200 mg/dl	• General lipid education: Family Member, MD, RN, Pharmacist, SW • Complex diet/lifestyle modifications: RD
Excessive Sodium Consumption • Elevated blood pressure • Fluid retention	• Limit salt added to food • Limit salt used in cooking • Limit consumption of salt preserved foods	Optimize sodium intake • Sodium intake—3g per day • Normalize blood pressure • Minimize fluid retention	• General nutrition education: Family Member, MD, RN, Pharmacist, SW • When sodium intake should be < 2g per day: RD
Excessive Alcohol Consumption • < 1–2 drinks per day	• Decrease intake of alcoholic beverages • Enroll in alcohol rehabilita- tion program if alcohol abuse is diagnosed	Optimize alcohol intake • Not more than 1–2 drinks daily	• General education regarding alcohol: Family Member, MD, RD, RN, Pharmacist, SW • Complex lifestyle modification: SW, Addictionologist, Behaviorist

Other Beneficial Lifestyle Modifications	Strategy/Strategies	Expected Outcome(s)	Provider(s)
Inadequate Physical Activity • Diminished capacity for self- care • Diminished muscle strength • Diminished flexibility	• 30 minutes sustained aerobic activity a minimum of 3 times per week • Strength training • Flexibility training	Maintenance of age/physical status appropriate activity	• General physical education: Family Member, MD, RD, RN, Pharmacist, SW • Complex physical training requirements: MD, Physical Therapist, Occupational Therapist, Exercise Physiolo- gist, Rehabilitation Specialist
Cigarette Smoking	• Encourage quitting • Prescribe drugs, patches to facilitate quitting • Encourage participation in a smoking cessation program	Smoking Cessation	• General information regarding smoking cessation: Family Member, MD, RD, RN, Pharmacist, SW • Complex lifestyle modification: MD, SW, Addictionologist, Behaviorist

Source: Reprinted with permission by the Nutrition Screening Initiative, a project of the American Academy of Family Physicians, The American Dietetic Association, and The National Council on Aging, Inc., and funded in part by a grant from Ross Products Division, Abbott Laboratories Inc.

TREATMENT RECOMMENDATIONS

BLOOD PRESSURE MEASUREMENT

Patient should:
- Rest for 5 minutes before measurement.
- Refrain from smoking or ingesting caffeine for 30 minutes prior to measurement.
- Be seated with feet flat on floor, back and arm supported, arm at heart level.

Clinician should:
- Use the appropriate size cuff for the patient; the bladder should encircle at least 80 percent of the upper arm.
- Use calibrated or mercury manometer.
- Average two or more readings, separated by at least 2 minutes.

PRIMARY PREVENTION

Encourage patients to make healthy lifestyle choices:
- Quit smoking to reduce cardiovascular risk.
- Lose weight, if needed.
- Restrict sodium intake to no more than 100 mmol per day.
- Limit alcohol intake to no more than 1–2 drinks per day.
- Get at least 30–45 minutes of aerobic activity on most days.
- Maintain adequate potassium intake—about 90 mmol per day.
- Maintain adequate intakes of calcium and magnesium for general health.

GOAL

Set a clear goal of therapy based on patient's risk. Control blood pressure to below:
- 140/90 mm Hg for patients with uncomplicated hypertension; set a lower goal for those with target organ damage or clinical cardiovascular disease.
- 130/85 mm Hg for patients with diabetes.
- 125/75 mm Hg for patients with renal insufficiency with proteinuria greater than 1 gram per 24 hours.

TREATMENT

Begin with lifestyle modifications (see primary prevention box) for all patients. Be supportive!
- Add pharmacologic therapy if blood pressure remains uncontrolled.
- Start with a diuretic or beta-blocker unless there are compelling indications to use other agents. Use low dose and titrate upward. Consider low dose combinations.
- If no response, try a drug from another class or add a second agent from a different class (diuretic if not already used).

ADHERENCE

- Encourage lifestyle modifications. Be supportive!
- Educate patient and family about disease. Involve them in measurement and treatment.
- Maintain communications with patient.
- Discuss how to integrate treatment into daily activities.
- Keep care inexpensive and simple.
- Favor once-daily, long-acting formulations.
- Use combination tablets, when needed.
- Consider using generic formulas or larger tablets that can be divided. This may be less expensive.
- Be willing to stop unsuccessful therapy and try a different approach.
- Consider using nurse case management.

continues

Treatment Recommendations continued

- Determine blood pressure stage.
- Determine risk group by major risk factors and TOD/CCD.
- Determine treatment recommendations (by using the table below).
- Determine goal blood pressure.
- Refer to specific treatment recommendations.

Major Risk Factors
- Smoking
- Dyslipidemia
- Diabetes mellitus
- Age > 60 years
- Gender :
  - Men
  - Postmenopausal women
- Family history :
  - Women < age 65
  - Men < age 55

TOD/CCD (Target Organ Damage/ Clinical Cardiovascular Disease)
Heart diseases
- LVH
- Angina/prior MI
- Prior CABG
- Heart failure
Stroke or TIA
Nephropathy
Peripheral arterial disease
Hypertensive retinopathy

Blood pressure stages (mm Hg)	Risk Group A No major risk factors No TOD/CCD	Risk Group B At least one major risk factor, not including diabetes No TOD/CCD	Risk Group C TOD/CCD and/or diabetes, with or without other risk factors
High-normal (130-139/85-89)	Lifestyle modification	Lifestyle modification	Drug therapy for those with heart failure, renal insufficiency or diabetes Lifestyle modification
Stage 1 (140-159/90-99)	Lifestyle modification (up to 12 months)	Lifestyle modification (up to 6 months) For patients with multiple risk factors, clinicians should consider drugs as initial therapy plus lifestyle modifications.	Drug therapy Lifestyle modification
Stages 2 and 3 (≥160/≥100)	Drug therapy Lifestyle modification	Drug therapy Lifestyle modification	Drug therapy Lifestyle modification

Example: A patient with diabetes and a blood pressure of 142/94 mm Hg plus left ventricular hypertrophy should be classified as having stage 1 hypertension with target organ disease (left ventricular hypertrophy) and with another major risk factor (diabetes). This patient would be categorized as **Stage 1, Risk Group C**, and recommended for immediate initiation of pharmacologic treatment.

Goal Blood Pressure

<140/90 mm Hg	Uncomplicated hypertension, Risk Group A, Risk Group B, Risk Group C except for the following:
<130/85 mm Hg	Diabetes; renal failure; heart failure
<125/75 mm Hg	Renal failure with proteinuria > 1 gram/24 hours

SPECIFIC TREATMENT RECOMMENDATIONS

Lifestyle modification should be definitive therapy for some patients and adjunctive therapy for all patients recommended for pharmacologic therapy.

INITIAL DRUG CHOICES

- Start with a low dose of a long-acting once-daily drug, and **titrate dose**
- Low-dose combinations may be appropriate

Uncomplicated Hypertension	Compelling Indications		Specific Indications for the Following Drugs:
Diuretics Beta-blockers	Diabetes type 1 (IDDM)	start with ACE inhibitor if proteinuria is present	(See Table 9 in JNC VI for specific indications) ACE inhibitors
	Heart failure	start with ACE inhibitor or diuretic	Angiotensin II receptor blockers Alpha-blockers
	Myocardial infarction	beta-blocker (non-ISA) after MI; ACE inhibitor for LV dysfunction after MI	Alpha-beta-blockers Beta-blockers
	Isolated systolic hypertension (older patients)	diuretics (preferred) or calcium antagonists (long-acting DHP)	Calcium antagonists Diuretics

Source: "JNC VI Risk Stratification and Treatment Recommendations," *The Sixth Report of the Joint National Committee on Prevention, Detection, Evaluation, and Treatment of High Blood Pressure*, NIH Publication No. 96-1060, National Institutes of Health.

BLOOD PRESSURE MEASUREMENT AND CLINICAL EVALUATION*

Hypertension is defined as systolic blood pressure (SBP) of 140 mm Hg or greater, diastolic blood pressure (DBP) of 90 mm Hg or greater, or taking antihypertensive medication. The objective of identifying and treating high blood pressure is to reduce the risk of cardiovascular disease and associated morbidity and mortality. To that end, it is useful to provide a classification of adult blood pressure for the purpose of identifying high-risk individuals and to provide guidelines for follow-up and treatment.

The positive relationship between SBP and DBP and cardiovascular risk has long been recognized. This relationship is strong, continuous, graded, consistent, independent, predictive, and etiologically significant for those with and without coronary heart disease. Therefore, although classification of adult blood pressure is somewhat arbitrary, it is useful to clinicians who must make treatment decisions based on a constellation of factors including the actual level of blood pressure. The exhibit "Classification of Blood Pressure for Adults Age 18 and Older" provides criteria for individuals who are not taking antihypertensive medication and who have no acute illness. This classification is based on

the average of two or more blood pressure readings (taken in accordance with the following recommendations) at each of two or more visits after an initial screening visit. When SBP and DBP fall into different categories, the higher category should be selected to classify the individual's blood pressure. The classification is slightly modified from the *Fifth Report of the Joint National Committee on Detection, Evaluation, and Treatment of High Blood Pressure (JNC V)* in that stage 3 and stage 4 hypertension are now combined because of the relative infrequency of stage 4 hypertension.

Detection and Confirmation

Hypertension detection begins with proper blood pressure measurements, which should be obtained at each health care encounter. Repeated blood pressure measurements will determine whether initial elevations persist and require prompt attention or have returned to normal and need only periodic surveillance. Blood pressure should be measured in a standardized fashion using equipment that meets certification criteria. The following techniques are recommended:

- Patients should be seated in a chair with their backs supported and their arms bared and supported at heart level. Patients should refrain from smoking or ingesting caffeine during the 30 minutes preceding the measurement.
- Under special circumstances, measuring blood pressure in the supine and standing positions may be indicated.
- Measurement should begin after at least five minutes of rest.

---

*Source: Joint National Committee on Detection, Evaluation, and Treatment of High Blood Pressure, "The Sixth Report of the Joint Committee on Detection, Evaluation, and Treatment of High Blood Pressure," National Heart, Lung, and Blood Institute, NIH Publication No. 98-4080, November 1997.

CLASSIFICATION OF BLOOD PRESSURE FOR ADULTS AGE 18 AND OLDER*

Category	Systolic (mm Hg)		Diastolic (mm Hg)
Optimal†	<120	and	<80
Normal	<130	and	<85
High normal	130–139	or	85–89
Hypertension‡			
Stage 1	140–159	or	90–99
Stage 2	160–179	or	100–109
Stage 3	≥180	or	≥110

*Not taking antihypertensive drugs and not acutely ill. When systolic and diastolic blood pressures fall into different categories, the higher category should be selected to classify the individual's blood pressure status. For example, 160/92 mm Hg should be classified as stage 2 hypertension, and 174/120 mm Hg should be classified as stage 3 hypertension. Isolated systolic hypertension is defined as SBP of 140 mm Hg or greater and DBP below 90 mm Hg and staged appropriately (e.g., 170/82 mm Hg is defined as stage 2 isolated systolic hypertension). In addition to classifying stages of hypertension on the basis of average blood pressure levels, clinicians should specify presence or absence of target organ disease and additional risk factors. This specificity is important for risk classification and treatment (see the exhibit "Risk Stratification and Treatment").

†Optimal blood pressure with respect to cardiovascular risk is below 120/80 mm Hg. However, unusually low readings should be evaluated for clinical significance.

‡Based on the average of two or more readings taken at each of two or more visits after an initial screening.

Source: Joint National Committee on Detection, Evaluation, and Treatment of High Blood Pressure, "The Sixth Report of the Joint Committee on Detection, Evaluation, and Treatment of High Blood Pressure," National Heart, Lung, and Blood Institute, NIH Publication No. 98-4080, November 1997.

- The appropriate cuff size must be used to ensure accurate measurement. The bladder within the cuff should encircle at least 80 percent of the arm. Many adults will require a large adult cuff.
- Measurements should be taken with a mercury sphygmomanometer; otherwise, a recently calibrated aneroid manometer or a validated electronic device can be used.
- Both SBP and DBP should be recorded. The first appearance of sound (phase 1) is used to define SBP. The disappearance of sound (phase 5) is used to define DBP.
- Two or more readings separated by two minutes should be averaged. If the first two readings differ by more than 5 mm Hg, additional readings should be obtained and averaged.

Clinicians should explain to patients the meaning of their blood pressure readings and advise them of the need for periodic remeasurement. The "Recommendations for Follow-Up" exhibit provides follow-up recommendations based on the initial set of blood pressure measurements. More information regarding blood pressure measurement may be found in the American Heart Association's *Recommendations for Human Blood Pressure Determination by Sphygmomanometers* and the American Society of Hypertension's *Recommendations for Routine Blood Pressure Measurement by Indirect Cuff Sphygmomanometry*.

Self-Measurement of Blood Pressure

Measurement of blood pressure outside the clinician's office may provide valuable information for the initial evaluation of patients with hypertension and for monitoring the response to treatment. Self-measurement has four general advantages: (1) distinguishing sustained hypertension from "white-coat hypertension," a condition noted in patients whose blood pressure is consistently elevated in the physician's office or clinic but normal at other times; (2) assessing response to antihypertensive medication; (3) improving patient adherence to treatment; and (4) potentially reducing costs. The blood pressure of persons with hypertension tends to be higher when measured in the clinic than outside of the office. There is no universally agreed on upper limit of normal home blood pressure, but readings of 135/85 mm Hg or greater should be considered elevated.

Choice of Monitors for Personal Use

Although the mercury sphygmomanometer is still the most accurate device for clinical use, it is generally not practical for home use. Therefore, either validated electronic devices or aneroid sphygmomanometers that have proven to be accurate according to standard testing are recommended for use along with appropriate sized cuffs. Finger monitors are inaccurate. Periodically, the accuracy of the patient's device should be checked by comparing readings with simultaneously recorded auscultatory readings taken with a mercury device. Independent evaluations of the instruments available to patients are published from time to time.

Ambulatory Blood Pressure Monitoring

A variety of commercially available monitors that are reliable, convenient, easy to use, and accurate are now available. These monitors typically are programmed to take

---

RECOMMENDATIONS FOR FOLLOW-UP BASED ON INITIAL BLOOD PRESSURE MEASUREMENTS FOR ADULTS

Initial Blood Pressure (mm Hg)*		Follow-up Recommended†
Systolic	**Diastolic**	
<130	<85	Recheck in 2 years
130–139	85–89	Recheck in 1 year‡
140–159	90–99	Confirm within 2 months‡
160–179	100–109	Evaluate or refer to source of care within 1 month
≥180	≥110	Evaluate or refer to source of care immediately or within 1 week depending on clinical situation

*If systolic and diastolic categories are different, follow recommendations for shorter time follow-up (e.g., 160/86 mm Hg should be evaluated or referred to source of care within one month).

†Modify the scheduling of follow-up according to reliable information about past blood pressure measurements, other cardiovascular risk factors, and target organ disease.

‡Provide advice about lifestyle modifications.

Source: Joint National Committee on Detection, Evaluation, and Treatment of High Blood Pressure, "The Sixth Report of the Joint Committee on Detection, Evaluation, and Treatment of High Blood Pressure," National Heart, Lung, and Blood Institute, NIH Publication No. 98-4080, November 1997.

readings every 15 to 30 minutes throughout the day and night while patients go about their normal daily activities. The readings can then be downloaded onto a personal computer for analysis. Normal blood pressure values taken by ambulatory measurement (1) are lower than clinic readings taken while patients are awake (below 135/85 mm Hg); (2) are even lower while patients are asleep (below 120/75 mm Hg); and (3) provide measures of SBP and DBP load. In the majority of individuals, blood pressure falls by 10 to 20 percent during the night; this change is more closely related to patterns of sleep and wakefulness than to time of day, as illustrated by the blood pressure rhythm following the inverted cycle of activity in night-shift workers.

Among persons with hypertension, an extensive and very consistent body of evidence indicates that ambulatory blood pressure correlates more closely than clinic blood pressure with a variety of measures of target organ damage such as left ventricular hypertrophy. Prospective data relating ambulatory blood pressure to prognosis suggest that, in patients in whom an elevated clinic pressure is the only abnormality, ambulatory monitoring may identify a group at relatively low risk of morbidity.

Ambulatory blood pressure monitoring is most clinically helpful and most commonly used in patients with suspected "white-coat hypertension," but it is also helpful in patients with apparent drug resistance, hypotensive symptoms with antihypertensive medications, episodic hypertension, and autonomic dysfunction. However, this procedure should not be used indiscriminately such as in the routine evaluation of patients with suspected hypertension.

Evaluation

Evaluation of patients with documented hypertension has three objectives: (1) to identify known causes of high blood pressure; (2) to assess the presence or absence of target organ damage and cardiovascular disease, the extent of the disease, and the response to therapy; and (3) to identify other cardiovascular risk factors or concomitant disorders that may define prognosis and guide treatment. Data for evaluation are acquired through medical history, physical examination, laboratory tests, and other diagnostic procedures.

Medical History

A medical history should include the following:

- known duration and levels of elevated blood pressure
- patient history or symptoms of coronary heart disease (CHD), heart failure, cerebrovascular disease, peripheral vascular disease, renal disease, diabetes mellitus, dyslipidemia, other comorbid conditions, gout, or sexual dysfunction

- family history of high blood pressure, premature CHD, stroke, diabetes, dyslipidemia, or renal disease
- symptoms suggesting causes of hypertension
- history of recent changes in weight, leisure-time physical activity, and smoking or other tobacco use
- dietary assessment including intake of sodium, alcohol, saturated fat, and caffeine
- history of all prescribed and over-the-counter medications, herbal remedies, and illicit drugs, some of which may raise blood pressure or interfere with the effectiveness of antihypertensive drugs
- results and adverse effects of previous antihypertensive therapy
- psychosocial and environmental factors (e.g., family situation, employment status and working conditions, educational level) that may influence hypertension control

Physical Examination

The initial physical examination should include the following:

- two or more blood pressure measurements separated by two minutes with the patient either supine or seated and after standing for at least two minutes in accordance with the recommended techniques mentioned earlier
- verification in the contralateral arm (if values are different, the higher value should be used)
- measurement of height, weight, and waist circumference
- funduscopic examination for hypertensive retinopathy (i.e., arteriolar narrowing, focal arteriolar constrictions, arteriovenous crossing changes, hemorrhages and exudates, disc edema)
- examination of the neck for carotid bruits, distended veins, or an enlarged thyroid gland
- examination of the heart for abnormalities in rate and rhythm, increased size, precordial heave, clicks, murmurs, and third and fourth heart sounds
- examination of the lungs for rales and evidence for bronchospasm
- examination of the abdomen for bruits, enlarged kidneys, masses, and abnormal aortic pulsation
- examination of the extremities for diminished or absent peripheral arterial pulsations, bruits, and edema
- neurological assessment

Laboratory Tests and Other Diagnostic Procedures

Routine laboratory tests recommended before initiating therapy are tests to determine the presence of target organ damage and other risk factors. These routine tests include urinalysis, complete blood cell count, blood chemistry (potassium, sodium, creatinine, fasting glucose, total cholesterol, and high-density lipoprotein [HDL] cholesterol), and 12-lead electrocardiogram.

Optional tests include creatinine clearance, microalbuminuria, 24-hour urinary protein, blood calcium, uric acid, fasting triglycerides, low-density lipoprotein (LDL) cholesterol, glycosolated hemoglobin, thyroid-stimulating hormone, and limited echocardiography (to determine the presence of left ventricular hypertrophy). More complete assessment of cardiac anatomy and function by standard echocardiography, examination of structural alterations in arteries by ultrasonography, measurement of ankle/arm index, and plasma renin activity/urinary sodium determination may be useful in assessing cardiovascular status in selected patients.

Identifiable Causes of Hypertension

Additional diagnostic procedures may be indicated to seek causes of hypertension, particularly in patients (1) whose age, history, physical examination, severity of hypertension, or initial laboratory findings suggest such causes; (2) whose blood pressures are responding poorly to drug therapy; (3) with well-controlled hypertension whose blood pressures begin to increase; (4) with stage 3 hypertension; and (5) with sudden onset of hypertension. For example, labile hypertension or paroxysms of hypertension accompanied by headache, palpitations, pallor, and perspiration suggest pheochromocytoma. Abdominal bruits, particularly those that lateralize to the renal areas or have a diastolic component, suggest renovascular disease. Abdominal or flank masses may be polycystic kidneys. Delayed or absent femoral arterial pulses and decreased blood pressure in the lower extremities may indicate aortic coarctation. And truncal obesity with purple striae suggests Cushing's syndrome. Examples of clues from the laboratory tests include unprovoked hypokalemia (primary aldosteronism), hypercalcemia (hyperparathyroidism), and elevated creatinine or abnormal urinalysis (renal parenchymal disease). Appropriate investigations should be conducted when there is a high index of suspicion of an identifiable cause.

Genetics of Hypertension

Blood pressure levels are correlated among family members, a fact attributable to common genetic background, shared environment, or lifestyle habits. High blood pressure appears to be a complex trait that does not follow the classic Mendelian rules of inheritance attributable to a single gene locus. The currently documented exceptions are a few rare forms of hypertension, such as those related to a single mutation involving a chimeric 11-beta-hydroxylase/aldosterone synthase gene. High blood pressure appears to be a polygenic and multifactorial disorder in which several genes interact with each other and with the environment. Potential candidate genes suggested by recent experimental data include those that affect various components of the renin-angiotensin-aldosterone system, the kallikrein-kinin system, and the sympathetic nervous system.

Risk Stratification

The risk of cardiovascular disease in patients with hypertension is determined not only by the level of blood pressure but also by the presence or absence of target organ damage or other risk factors such as smoking, dyslipidemia, and diabetes, as shown in the exhibit "Components of Cardiovascular Risk Stratification." These factors independently modify the risk for subsequent cardiovascular disease, and their presence or absence is determined during the routine evaluation of patients with hypertension (i.e., history, physical examination, laboratory tests). Based on this assessment and the level of blood pressure, the patient's risk group can be determined, as shown in the exhibit "Risk Stratification and Treatment." This empiric classification stratifies patients with hypertension into risk groups for therapeutic decisions.

COMPONENTS OF CARDIOVASCULAR RISK STRATIFICATION IN PATIENTS WITH HYPERTENSION*

Major Risk Factors

Smoking
Dyslipidemia
Diabetes mellitus
Age older than 60 years
Sex (men and postmenopausal women)
Family history of cardiovascular disease: women under age 65 or men under age 55

Target Organ Damage/Clinical Cardiovascular Disease

Heart diseases

- Left ventricular hypertrophy
- Angina/prior myocardial infarction
- Prior coronary revascularization
- Heart failure

Stroke or transient ischemic attack
Nephropathy
Peripheral arterial disease
Retinopathy

*See "Risk Stratification and Treatment" exhibit.

Source: Joint National Committee on Detection, Evaluation, and Treatment of High Blood Pressure, "The Sixth Report of the Joint Committee on Detection, Evaluation, and Treatment of High Blood Pressure," National Heart, Lung, and Blood Institute, NIH Publication No. 98-4080, November 1997.

RISK STRATIFICATION AND TREATMENT*

Blood Pressure Stages (mm Hg)	Risk Group A (No Risk Factors, No TOD/CCD)[†]	Risk Group B (At Least One Risk Factor, Not Including Diabetes; No TOD/CCD)	Risk Group C (TOD/CCD and/or Diabetes, with or without Other Risk Factors)
High normal (130–139/85–89)	Lifestyle modification	Lifestyle modification	Drug therapy[‡]
Stage 1 (140–159/90–99)	Lifestyle modification (up to 12 months)	Lifestyle modification[§] (up to 6 months)	Drug therapy
Stages 2 and 3 (≥160/≥100)	Drug therapy	Drug therapy	Drug therapy

For example, a patient with diabetes and a blood pressure of 142/94 mm Hg plus left ventricular hypertrophy should be classified as having stage 1 hypertension with target organ disease (left ventricular hypertrophy) and with another major risk factor (diabetes). This patient would be categorized as Stage 1, Risk Group C, and recommended for immediate initiation of pharmacological treatment.

*Lifestyle modification should be adjunctive therapy for all patients recommended for pharmacological therapy.
†TOD/CCD indicates target organ disease/clinical cardiovascular disease.
‡For those with heart failure, renal insufficiency, or diabetes.
§For patients with multiple risk factors, clinicians should consider drugs as initial therapy plus lifestyle modifications.

Source: Joint National Committee on Detection, Evaluation, and Treatment of High Blood Pressure, "The Sixth Report of the Joint Committee on Detection, Evaluation, and Treatment of High Blood Pressure," National Heart, Lung, and Blood Institute, NIH Publication No. 98-4080, November 1997.

The World Health Organization Expert Committee on Hypertension Control recently recommended a similar approach. Obesity and physical inactivity are also predictors of cardiovascular risk and interact with other risk factors, but they are of less significance in the selection of antihypertensive drugs.

Risk Group A

Risk group A includes patients with high-normal blood pressure or stage 1, 2, or 3 hypertension who do not have clinical cardiovascular disease, target organ damage, or other risk factors. Persons with stage 1 hypertension in risk group A are candidates for a longer trial (up to one year) of vigorous lifestyle modification with vigilant blood pressure monitoring. If goal blood pressure is not achieved, pharmacological therapy should be added. For those with stage 2 or stage 3 hypertension, drug therapy is warranted.

Risk Group B

Risk group B includes patients with hypertension who do not have clinical cardiovascular disease or target organ damage but have one or more of the risk factors shown in the exhibit "Components of Cardiovascular Risk Stratification" but not diabetes mellitus. This group contains the large majority of patients with high blood pressure. If multiple risk factors are present, clinicians should consider antihypertensive drugs as initial therapy. Lifestyle modification and management of reversible risk factors should be strongly recommended.

Risk Group C

Risk group C includes patients with hypertension who have clinically manifest cardiovascular disease or target organ damage, as delineated in the exhibit "Components of Cardiovascular Risk Stratification." It is the clinical opinion of the *JNC VI* executive committee that some patients who have high-normal blood pressure as well as renal insufficiency, heart failure, or diabetes mellitus should be considered for prompt pharmacologic therapy. Appropriate lifestyle modifications always should be recommended as adjunct treatment.

This classification (blood pressure stage and risk grouping) is directly linked to treatment and treatment goals. It provides practicing clinicians with a simple method of identifying risk strata for individual patients (by history, physical examination, and routine laboratory testing) as well as guidelines for treatment of those patients. From these findings, an assessment of absolute risk can be made. Tables, formulas, computer software programs, and World Wide Web sites are available for calculating cardiovascular risk in individual patients by means of data from epidemiological studies.

PREVENTION AND TREATMENT OF HIGH BLOOD PRESSURE*

Potential for Primary Prevention of Hypertension

Before the active treatment of established hypertension is considered, the even greater need for prevention of disease should be recognized. Without primary prevention, the hypertension problem would never be solved and would rely solely on detection of existing high blood pressure. Primary prevention provides an attractive opportunity to interrupt and prevent the continuing costly cycle of managing hypertension and its complications. Primary prevention reflects a number of realities:

- A significant portion of cardiovascular disease occurs in people whose blood pressure is above the optimal level (120/80 mm Hg) but not so high as to be diagnosed or treated as hypertension. A populationwide approach to lowering blood pressure can reduce this considerable burden of risk.
- Active treatment of established hypertension, as carefully as can be provided, poses financial costs and potential adverse effects.
- Most patients with established hypertension do not make sufficient lifestyle changes, do not take medication, or do not take enough medication to achieve control.
- Even if adequately treated according to current standards, patients with hypertension may not lower their risk to that of persons with normal blood pressure.
- Blood pressure rise and high blood pressure are not inevitable consequences of aging.

An effective populationwide strategy to prevent blood pressure rise with age and to reduce overall blood pressure levels, even by a little, could affect overall cardiovascular morbidity and mortality as much as or more than treating only those with established disease.

Such a populationwide approach has been promulgated. It is based on lifestyle modifications that have been shown to prevent or delay the expected rise in blood pressure in susceptible people. A recent study demonstrated that a diet rich in fruits, vegetables, and low-fat dairy foods, and with reduced saturated and total fats, significantly lowers blood pressure.

Lifestyle modifications could have an even greater impact on disease prevention and should be recommended to the entire population. Modifications that can be provided to the entire population without requiring individuals to ac-

tively participate, such as a reduction in the amount of sodium chloride added to processed foods, may be even more effective.

Goal

The goal of prevention and management of hypertension is to reduce morbidity and mortality by the least intrusive means possible. This may be accomplished by achieving and maintaining SBP below 140 mm Hg and DBP below 90 mm Hg, while controlling other modifiable risk factors for cardiovascular disease. Treatment to lower levels may be useful, particularly to prevent stroke, preserve renal function, and prevent or slow heart failure progression. The goal may be achieved by lifestyle modification alone or with pharmacological treatment.

Lifestyle Modifications

Lifestyle modifications (see "Lifestyle Modifications" exhibit) may prevent hypertension, have been shown to be effective in lowering blood pressure, and can reduce other cardiovascular risk factors at little cost and with minimal risk. Patients should be strongly encouraged to adopt these lifestyle modifications, particularly if they have additional risk factors for premature cardiovascular disease, such as dyslipidemia or diabetes mellitus. Even when lifestyle modifications alone are not adequate in controlling hypertension, they may reduce the number and dosage of antihypertensive medications needed to manage the condition. Achieving and maintaining lifestyle changes is difficult, but a systematic team approach utilizing health care professionals and community resources when possible can provide the necessary education, support, and follow-up.

Weight Reduction

Excess body weight—body mass index (weight in kilograms divided by height, in meters, squared) of 27 or greater—is correlated closely with increased blood pressure. Excess fat in the upper part of the body (visceral or abdominal), as evidenced by a waist circumference of 34 inches (85 cm) or greater in women or 39 inches (98 cm) or greater in men, also has been associated with the risk for hypertension, dyslipidemia, diabetes, and coronary heart disease mortality.

Weight reduction of as little as 10 pounds (4.5 kg) reduces blood pressure in a large proportion of overweight persons with hypertension. In overweight patients with hypertension, weight reduction enhances the blood-pressure–lowering effect of concurrent antihypertensive agents and can significantly reduce concomitant cardiovascular risk factors, such as diabetes and dyslipidemia.

Therefore, all patients with hypertension who are above their desirable weight should be placed on an individualized,

---

*Source: Joint National Committee on Detection, Evaluation, and Treatment of High Blood Pressure, "The Sixth Report of the Joint Committee on Detection, Evaluation, and Treatment of High Blood Pressure," National Heart, Lung, and Blood Institute, NIH Publication No. 98-4080, November 1997.

LIFESTYLE MODIFICATIONS FOR HYPERTENSION PREVENTION AND MANAGEMENT

- Lose weight if overweight.
- Limit alcohol intake to no more than 1 oz (30 mL) ethanol (e.g., 24 oz [720 mL] beer, 10 oz [300 mL] wine, or 2 oz [60 mL] 100-proof whiskey) per day or 0.5 oz (15 mL) ethanol per day for women and lighter weight people.
- Increase aerobic physical activity (30 to 45 minutes most days of the week).
- Reduce sodium intake to no more than 100 mmol per day (2.4 g sodium or 6 g sodium chloride).
- Maintain adequate intake of dietary potassium (approximately 90 mmol per day).
- Maintain adequate intake of dietary calcium and magnesium for general health.
- Stop smoking and reduce intake of dietary saturated fat and cholesterol for overall cardiovascular health.

monitored weight reduction program involving caloric restriction and increased physical activity. Recidivism is common and can be discouraging, but persistence may be rewarded by reduction of multiple cardiovascular risk factors and a step-down in antihypertensive drug therapy. Anorectic agents should be used with caution because many can raise blood pressure and some may increase the risk for valvular heart disease and pulmonary hypertension.

Moderation of Alcohol Intake

Excessive alcohol intake is an important risk factor for high blood pressure, can cause resistance to antihypertensive therapy, and is a risk factor for stroke. A detailed history of current alcohol consumption should be elicited from patients. Those who drink beverages containing alcohol should be counseled to limit their daily intake to no more than 1 ounce (30 mL) of ethanol—for example, 24 ounces (720 mL) of beer, 10 ounces (300 mL) of wine, or 2 ounces (60 mL) of 100-proof whiskey. Because women absorb more ethanol than men and lighter weight people are more susceptible than heavier people to the effects of alcohol, these groups should be counseled to limit their intake to no more than 0.5 ounce (15 mL) of ethanol per day. Such amounts do not raise blood pressure and have been associated with a lower risk for CHD. Significant hypertension may develop during abrupt withdrawal from heavy alcohol consumption but recedes a few days after alcohol consumption is reduced.

Physical Activity

Regular aerobic physical activity—adequate to achieve at least a moderate level of physical fitness—can enhance weight loss and functional health status and reduce the risk for cardiovascular disease and all-cause mortality. When compared with their more active and fit peers, sedentary individuals with normal blood pressure have a 20 percent to 50 percent increased risk of developing hypertension.

Blood pressure can be lowered with moderately intense physical activity (40 percent to 60 percent of maximum oxygen consumption), such as 30 to 45 minutes of brisk walking most days of the week. Most people can safely increase their level of physical activity without an extensive medical evaluation. Patients with cardiac or other serious health problems need a more thorough evaluation, often including a cardiac stress test, and may need referral to a specialist or medically supervised exercise program.

Moderation of Dietary Sodium

Intake of sodium, in the form of sodium chloride or table salt, is linked to levels of blood pressure. Individual response of blood pressure to variation in sodium intake differs widely; as groups, African Americans, older people, and patients with hypertension or diabetes are more sensitive to changes in dietary sodium chloride than are others in the general population.

Epidemiological data demonstrate a positive association between sodium intake and level of blood pressure. Meta-analysis of clinical trials reveals that a reduction of 75 to 100 mmol in daily sodium intake lowers blood pressure over periods of several weeks to a few years. These effects are greater for older persons and those with elevated pressures. An analysis of 17 published randomized controlled trials involving patients age 45 or older with hypertension found an average decrease of 6.3/2.2 mm Hg with a urinary sodium reduction of 95 mmol per day. Although concern about severe sodium restriction has been raised in one observational study, there is no evidence that lower levels of sodium intake, as achieved in intervention trials, present any safety hazards.

Moreover, a variety of controlled and observational studies suggest that a diet with moderately reduced intake of sodium may be associated with other favorable effects such as less need for antihypertensive medication, reduced diuretic-induced potassium wastage, regression of left ventricular hypertrophy, and protection from osteoporosis and renal stones through a reduction in urinary calcium excretion.

Seventy-five percent of sodium intake is from processed food. Because the average American consumption of sodium is in excess of 150 mmol per day, moderate sodium reduction to a level of no more than 100 mmol per day (approximately 6 grams of sodium chloride or 2.4 grams of sodium per day) is recommended and achievable. With appropriate counseling, patients and their families can learn to read food labels and select foods lower in sodium. Such items are becoming more readily available in supermarkets and restaurants.

Potassium Intake

High dietary potassium intake may protect against developing hypertension and improve blood pressure control in patients with hypertension. Inadequate potassium intake may increase blood pressure. Therefore, an adequate intake of potassium (approximately 50 to 90 mmol per day), preferably from food sources such as fresh fruits and vegetables, should be maintained. If hypokalemia occurs during diuretic therapy, additional potassium may be needed from potassium-containing salt substitutes, potassium supplements, or potassium-sparing diuretics. These agents must be used with caution in patients susceptible to hyperkalemia, including those with renal insufficiency or those receiving angiotensin-converting enzyme (ACE) inhibitors or angiotensin II receptor blockers.

Calcium Intake

In most epidemiological studies, low dietary calcium intake is associated with an increased prevalence of hypertension. An increased calcium intake may lower blood pressure in some patients with hypertension, but the overall effect is minimal. Although it is important to maintain an adequate intake of calcium for general health, there is currently no rationale for recommending calcium supplements to lower blood pressure.

Magnesium Intake

Although evidence suggests an association between lower dietary magnesium intake and higher blood pressure, no convincing data currently justify recommending an increased magnesium intake in an effort to lower blood pressure.

Other Dietary Factors

Dietary fats. Dyslipidemia is a major independent risk factor for coronary artery disease; therefore, dietary therapy and, if necessary, drug therapy for dyslipidemia are important adjuncts to antihypertensive treatment. In randomized controlled studies, diets varying in total fat and proportions of saturated to unsaturated fats have had little, if any, effect on blood pressure. Large amounts of omega-3 fatty acids may lower blood pressure; however, some patients experience abdominal discomfort. One study found no significant effect in preventing hypertension.

Caffeine. Caffeine may raise blood pressure acutely. Tolerance to this pressor effect develops rapidly, and no direct relationship between caffeine intake and elevated blood pressure has been found in most epidemiological surveys.

Other factors. Although recent epidemiological studies have shown an inverse relationship between dietary protein and blood pressure, no consistent effects have been demonstrated. Furthermore, controlled trials of varying proportions of carbohydrate, garlic, or onion in the diet have demonstrated no consistent effects on blood pressure.

Relaxation and Biofeedback

Emotional stress can raise blood pressure acutely. The role of stress management techniques in treating patients with elevated blood pressure is uncertain. Relaxation therapies and biofeedback have been studied in multiple controlled trials with little effect beyond that seen in the control groups. A study of African Americans showed significant decreases in SBP and DBP at three months. However, the available literature does not support the use of relaxation therapies for definitive therapy or prevention of hypertension. One study found no effect of stress management on prevention of hypertension.

Tobacco Avoidance for Overall Cardiovascular Risk Reduction

Cigarette smoking is a powerful risk factor for cardiovascular disease, and avoidance of tobacco in any form is essential. A significant rise in blood pressure accompanies the smoking of each cigarette. Those who continue to smoke may not receive the full degree of protection against cardiovascular disease from antihypertensive therapy. The cardiovascular benefits of discontinuing tobacco use can be seen within a year in all age groups. Smoking cessation information is available from voluntary health organizations and federal agencies. Smokers must be told repeatedly and unambiguously to stop smoking. The lower amounts of nicotine contained in smoking cessation aids usually will not raise blood pressure; therefore, they may be used with appropriate counseling and behavior interventions. Actions to avoid or minimize weight gain after quitting smoking are often needed.

Implementation of lifestyle modifications should not delay the start of an effective antihypertensive drug regimen in those at higher risk (see "Risk Stratification and Treatment" exhibit).

Pharmacological Treatment

The decision to initiate pharmacological treatment requires consideration of several factors: the degree of blood pressure elevation, the presence of target organ damage, and the presence of clinical cardiovascular disease or other risk factors (see exhibits "Components of Cardiovascular Risk Stratification" and "Risk Stratification and Treatment").

Efficacy

Reducing blood pressure with drugs clearly decreases cardiovascular morbidity and mortality. Protection has been demonstrated for stroke, coronary events, heart failure, progression of renal disease, progression to more severe hypertension, and all-cause mortality. Among older persons, treatment of hypertension has been associated with an even more significant reduction in CHD.

These results have been obtained in patients in various countries regardless of sex, age, race, blood pressure level, or socioeconomic status. Therefore, these findings can be generalized with confidence to the entire adult population with high blood pressure.

Drug Therapy Considerations

Most antihypertensive drugs currently available in the United States are listed in the exhibits "Oral Antihypertensive Drugs" and "Combination Drugs for Hypertension." For most patients, a low dose of the initial drug choice should be used at first and slowly titrated upward at a schedule dependent on the patient's age, needs, and responses. The optimal formulation should provide 24-hour efficacy with a once-daily dose, with at least 50 percent of the peak effect remaining at the end of the 24 hours. Long-acting formulations that provide 24-hour efficacy are preferred over short-acting agents for many reasons: (1) adherence is better with once-daily dosing; (2) for some agents, fewer tablets incur lower

ORAL ANTIHYPERTENSIVE DRUGS*

Drug	Trade Name	Usual Dose Range, Total mg/day (Frequency per Day)	Selected Side Effects and Comments
Diuretics (partial list)			Short-term: increases cholesterol and glucose levels; biochemical abnormalities: decreases potassium, sodium, and magnesium levels, increases uric acid and calcium levels; rare: blood dyscrasias, photosensitivity, pancreatitis, hyponatremia
Chlorthalidone (G)	Hygroton	12.5–50 (1)	
Hydrochlorothiazide (G)	Hydrodiuril, Microzide, Esidrix	12.5–50 (1)	
Indapamide	Lozol	1.25–5 (1)	(Less or no hypercholesterolemia)
Metolazone	Mykrox	0.5–1.0 (1)	
	Zaroxolyn	2.5–10 (1)	
Loop diuretics			
Bumetanide (G)	Bumex	0.5–4 (2–3)	(Short duration of action, no hypercalcemia)
Ethacrynic acid	Edecrin	25–100 (2–3)	(Only nonsulfonamide diuretic, ototoxicity)
Furosemide (G)	Lasix	40–240 (2–3)	(Short duration of action, no hypercalcemia)
Torsemide	Demadex	5–100 (1–2)	
Potassium-sparing agents			Hyperkalemia
Amiloride hydrochloride (G)	Midamor	5–10 (1)	
Spironolactone (G)	Aldactone	25–100 (1)	(Gynecomastia)
Triamterene (G)	Dyrenium	25–100 (1)	
Adrenergic inhibitors			
Peripheral agents			
Guanadrel	Hylorel	10–75 (2)	(Postural hypotension, diarrhea)
Guanethidine monosulfate	Ismelin	10–150 (1)	(Postural hypotension, diarrhea)
Reserpine (G)†	Serpasil	0.05–0.25 (1)	(Nasal congestion, sedation, depression, activation of peptic ulcer)

continues

Oral Antihypertensive Drugs continued

Drug	Trade Name	Usual Dose Range, Total mg/day (Frequency per Day)	Selected Side Effects and Comments
Central α-agonists			Sedation, dry mouth, bradycardia, withdrawal hypertension
Clonidine hydrochloride (G)	Catapres	0.2–1.2 (2–3)	(More withdrawal)
Guanabenz acetate (G)	Wytensin	8–32 (2)	
Guanfacine hydrochloride (G)	Tenex	1–3 (1)	(Less withdrawal)
Methyldopa (G)	Aldomet	500–3,000 (2)	(Hepatic and "autoimmune" disorders)
α-blockers			Postural hypotension
Doxazosin mesylate	Cardura	1–16 (1)	
Prazosin hydrochloride (G)	Minipress	2–30 (2–3)	
Terazosin hydrochloride	Hytrin	1–20 (1)	β-blockers
			Bronchospasm, bradycardia, heart failure, may mask insulin-induced hypoglycemia; less serious; impaired peripheral circulation, insomnia, fatigue, decreased exercise tolerance, hypertriglyceridemia (except agents with intrinsic sympathomimetic activity)
Acebutolol[‡§]	Sectral	200–800 (1)	
Atenolol (G)[§]	Tenormin	25–100 (1–2)	
Betaxolol[§]	Kerlone	5–20 (1)	
Bisoprolol fumarate[§]	Zebeta	2.5–10 (1)	
Carteolol hydrochloride[‡]	Cartrol	2.5–10 (1)	
Metoprolol succinate[§]	Toprol-XL	50–300 (1)	
Metoprolol tartrate (G)[§]	Lopressor	50–300 (2)	
Nadolol (G)	Corgard	40–320 (1)	
Penbutolol sulfate[‡]	Levatol	10–20 (1)	
Pindolol (G)[‡]	Visken	10–60 (2)	
Propranolol hydrochloride (G)	Inderal	40–480 (2)	
	Inderal LA	40–480 (1)	
Timolol maleate (G)	Blocadren	20–60 (2)	
Combined alpha- and beta-blockers			Postural hypotension, bronchospasm
Carvedilol	Coreg	12.5–50 (2)	
Labetalol hydrochloride (G)	Normodyne, Trandate	200–1,200 (2)	
Direct vasodilators			
Hydralazine hydrochloride (G)	Apresoline	50–300 (2)	(Lupus syndrome)
Minoxidil (G)	Loniten	5–100 (1)	(Hirsutism)
Calcium antagonists			
Nondihydropyridines			Conduction defects, worsening of systolic dysfunction, gingival hyperplasia
Diltiazem hydrochloride	Cardizem SR	120–360 (2)	(Nausea, headache)
	Cardizem CD, Dilacor XR, Tiazac	120–360 (1)	
Mibefradil dihydrochloride (T-channel calcium antagonist)	Posicor	50–100 (1)	(No worsening of systolic dysfunction; contraindicated with terfenadine [Seldane], astemizole [Hismanal], and cisapride [Propulsid])

continues

Oral Antihypertensive Drugs continued

Drug	Trade Name	Usual Dose Range, Total mg/day (Frequency per Day)	Selected Side Effects and Comments
Verapamil hydrochloride	Isoptin SR, Calan SR	90–480 (2)	(Constipation)
	Verelan, Covera HS	120–480 (1)	
Dihydropyridines			Edema of the ankle, flushing, headache, gingival hypertrophy
Amlodipine besylate	Norvasc	2.5–10 (1)	
Felodipine	Plendil	2.5–20 (1)	
Isradipine	DynaCirc	5–20 (2)	
	DynaCirc CR	5–20 (1)	
Nicardipine	Cardene SR	60–90 (2)	
Nifedipine	Procardia XL	30–120 (1)	
	Adalat CC		
Nisoldipine	Sular	20–60 (1)	
ACE inhibitors			Common: cough; rare: angioedema, hyperkalemia, rash, loss of taste, leukopenia
Benazepril hydrochloride	Lotensin	5–40 (1–2)	
Captopril (G)	Capoten	25–150 (2–3)	
Enalapril maleate	Vasotec	5–40 (1–2)	
Fosinopril sodium	Monopril	10–40 (1–2)	
Lisinopril	Prinivil, Zestril	5–40 (1)	
Moexipril	Univasc	7.5–15 (2)	
Quinapril hydrochloride	Accupril	5–80 (1–2)	
Ramipril	Altace	1.25–20 (1–2)	
Trandolapril	Mavik	1–4 (1)	
Angiotensin II receptor blockers			Angioedema (very rare), hyperkalemia
Irbesartan	Avapro	150–300 (1)	
Losartan potassium	Cozaar	25–100 (1–2)	
Valsartan	Diovan	80–320 (1)	

*These dosages may vary from those listed in the *Physicians' Desk Reference* (51st edition), which may be consulted for additional information. The listing of side effects is not all-inclusive, and side effects are for the class of drugs except where noted for individual drugs (in parentheses); clinicians are urged to refer to the package insert for a more detailed listing. ACE indicates angiotensin-converting enzyme; (G), generic available.

†Also acts centrally.

‡Has intrinsic sympathomimetic activity.

§Cardioselective.

Source: Joint National Committee on Detection, Evaluation, and Treatment of High Blood Pressure, "The Sixth Report of the Joint Committee on Detection, Evaluation, and Treatment of High Blood Pressure," National Heart, Lung, and Blood Institute, NIH Publication No. 98-4080, November 1997.

COMBINATION DRUGS FOR HYPERTENSION*

Drug	Trade Name
β-adrenergic blockers and diuretics	
Atenolol, 50 or 100 mg/chlorthalidone, 25 mg	Tenoretic
Bisoprolol fumarate, 2.5, 5, or 10 mg/hydrochlorothiazide, 6.25 mg	Ziac†
Metoprolol tartrate, 50 or 100 mg/hydrochlorothiazide, 25 or 50 mg	Lopressor HCT
Nadolol, 40 or 80 mg/bendroflumethiazide, 5 mg	Corzide
Propranolol hydrochloride, 40 or 80 mg/hydrochlorothiazide 25 mg	Inderide
Propranolol hydrochloride (extended release), 80, 120, or 160 mg/hydrochlorothiazide, 50 mg	Inderide LA
Timolol maleate, 10 mg/hydrochlorothiazide, 25 mg	Timolide
ACE inhibitors and diuretics	
Benazepril hydrochloride, 5, 10, or 20 mg/hydrochlorothiazide, 6.25, 12.5, or 25 mg	Lotensin HCT
Captopril, 25 or 50 mg/hydrochlorothiazide, 15 or 25 mg	Capozide*
Enalapril maleate, 5 or 10 mg/hydrochlorothiazide, 12.5 or 25 mg	Vaseretic
Lisinopril, 10 or 20 mg/hydrochlorothiazide, 12.5 or 25 mg	Prinzide, Zestoretic
Angiotensin II receptor antagonists and diuretics	
Losartan potassium, 50 mg/hydrochlorothiazide, 12.5 mg	Hyzaar
Calcium antagonists and ACE inhibitors	
Amlodipine besylate, 2.5 or 5 mg/benazepril hydrochloride, 10 or 20 mg	Lotrel
Diltiazem hydrochloride, 180 mg/enalapril maleate, 5 mg	Teczem
Felodipine, 5 mg/enalapril maleate, 5 mg	Lexxel
Verapamil hydrochloride (extended release), 180 or 240 mg/trandolapril, 1, 2, or 4 mg	Tarka
Other combinations	
Triamterene, 37.5, 50, or 75 mg/hydrochlorothiazide, 25 or 50 mg	Dyazide, Maxide
Spironolactone, 25 or 50 mg/hydrochlorothiazide, 25 or 50 mg	Aldactazide
Amiloride hydrochloride, 5 mg/hydrochlorothiazide, 50 mg	Moduretic
Guanethidine monosulfate, 10 mg/hydrochlorothiazide, 25 mg	Esimil
Hydralazine hydrochloride, 25, 50, or 100 mg/hydrochlorothiazide, 25 or 50 mg	Apresazide
Methyldopa, 250 or 500 mg/hydrochlorothiazide, 15, 25, 30, or 50 mg	Aldoril
Reserpine, 0.125 mg/hydrochlorothiazide, 25 or 50 mg	Hydropres
Reserpine, 0.10 mg/hydralazine hydrochloride, 25 mg/hydrochlorothiazide, 15 mg	Ser-Ap-Es
Clonidine hydrochloride, 0.1, 0.2, or 0.3 mg/chlorthalidone, 15 mg	Combipres
Methyldopa, 250 mg/chlorothiazide, 150 or 250 mg	Aldochlor
Reserpine, 0.125 or 0.25 mg/chlorthalidone, 25 or 50 mg	Demi-Regroton
Reserpine, 0.125 or 0.25 mg/chlorothiazide, 250 or 500 mg	Diupres
Prazosin hydrochloride, 1, 2, or 5 mg/polythiazide, 0.5 mg	Minizide

*ACE indicates angiotensin-converting enzyme.
†Approved for initial therapy.

Source: Joint National Committee on Detection, Evaluation, and Treatment of High Blood Pressure, "The Sixth Report of the Joint Committee on Detection, Evaluation, and Treatment of High Blood Pressure," National Heart, Lung, and Blood Institute, NIH Publication No. 98-4080, November 1997.

cost; (3) control of hypertension is persistent and smooth rather than intermittent; and (4) protection is provided against the risk for sudden death, heart attack, and stroke that may be caused by an abrupt increase of blood pressure after arising from overnight sleep. Agents with a duration of action beyond 24 hours are attractive because many patients inadvertently miss at least one dose of medication each week. Nonetheless, twice-daily dosing may offer similar control at possibly lower cost.

Newly developed formulations provide additional medication choices. For example, combinations of low doses of two agents from different classes have been shown to provide additional antihypertensive efficacy, thereby minimizing the likelihood of dose-dependent adverse effects (see exhibit "Combination Drugs for Hypertension"). Very low doses of a diuretic (e.g., 6.25 mg of hydrochlorothiazide) can potentiate the effect of the other agent without producing adverse metabolic effects. Low-dose combinations with an ACE inhibitor and a nondihydropyridine calcium antagonist may reduce proteinuria more than either drug alone. Combinations of a dihydropyridine calcium antagonist and an ACE inhibitor induce less pedal edema than the calcium antagonist alone. In some instances, drugs with similar modes of action may provide additive effects, such as metolazone and a loop diuretic in renal failure.

ACE inhibitors have been shown to provide beneficial effects in a variety of hypertension-related processes including heart failure from systolic dysfunction and nephropathy. The recently introduced angiotensin II receptor blockers produce hemodynamic effects similar to those of ACE inhibitors while avoiding the most common adverse effect, dry cough. However, in the absence of data documenting equal long-term cardiac and renal protection in patients with these conditions, angiotensin II receptor blockers should be used primarily in patients in whom ACE inhibitors are indicated but who are unable to tolerate them.

Some antihypertensive agents—such as direct-acting smooth-muscle vasodilators, central a$_2$-agonists, and peripheral adrenergic antagonists—are not well suited for initial monotherapy because they produce annoying adverse effects in many patients. Reserpine has a uniquely prolonged therapeutic effect and is better tolerated in low doses (0.05 to 0.10 mg per day); however, patients and their families still should be warned about the possibility of depression. The direct-acting smooth-muscle vasodilators (e.g., hydralazine hydrochloride, minoxidil) often induce reflex sympathetic stimulation of the cardiovascular system and fluid retention.

Immediate-release nifedipine has precipitated ischemic events and, in large doses, may increase coronary mortality in patients who had a myocardial infarction. Therefore, this agent should be used only with great caution, if at all. There have been inconsistent reports regarding adverse health effects of short-acting or immediate-release formulations of nifedipine, diltiazem hydrochloride, and verapamil hydrochloride. Randomized controlled trials are now in progress with long-acting types and formulations of calcium antagonists approved for treatment of hypertension. In the meantime, specific recommendations are provided in the exhibits "Considerations for Individualizing Antihypertensive Drug Therapy," "Parenteral Drugs for Treatment of Hypertensive Emergencies," and "Algorithm for the Treatment of Hypertension."

Special Considerations

Special considerations in the selection of initial therapy include demographic characteristics, concomitant diseases that may be beneficially or adversely affected by the antihypertensive agent chosen (see "Considerations" exhibit), quality of life, cost, and use of other drugs that may lead to drug interactions (see "Selected Drug Interactions" exhibit). When choosing a certain drug for its favorable effect on comorbidity, clinicians should be aware that reduction of long-term cardiovascular morbidity and mortality may not have been demonstrated.

Demographics. Neither sex nor age usually affects responsiveness to various agents. In general, hypertension in African Americans is more responsive to monotherapy with diuretics and calcium antagonists than to beta-blockers or ACE inhibitors. However, if a beta-blocker or ACE inhibitor is needed for other therapeutic benefits, differences in efficacy usually can be overcome with reduction of salt intake, higher doses of the drug, or addition of a diuretic.

Concomitant diseases and therapies. Antihypertensive drugs may worsen some diseases and improve others (see "Considerations" exhibit). Selection of an antihypertensive agent that also treats a coexisting disease will simplify therapeutic regimens and reduce costs.

Quality of life. Although antihypertensive drugs may cause adverse effects in some patients (see exhibit "Oral Antihypertensive Drugs"), quality of life is maintained and possibly improved by any of the agents recommended for initial therapy.

Physiological and biochemical measurements. Some clinicians have found certain physiological and biochemical measurements (e.g., body weight, heart rate, plasma renin activity, hemodynamic measurements) to be helpful in choosing specific therapy.

Economic considerations. The cost of therapy may be a barrier to controlling high blood pressure and should be an important consideration in selecting antihypertensive medication. Generic formulations are acceptable. Nongeneric newer drugs are usually more expensive than diuretics or beta-blockers. If newer agents eventually prove to be equally

CONSIDERATIONS FOR INDIVIDUALIZING ANTIHYPERTENSIVE DRUG THERAPY*

Indication	Drug Therapy
Compelling Indications Unless Contraindicated	
Diabetes mellitus (Type I) with proteinuria	ACE I
Heart failure	ACE I, diuretics
Isolated systolic hypertension (older patients)	Diuretics (preferred), CA (long-acting DHP)
Myocardial infarction	Beta-blockers (non-ISA), ACE I (with systolic dysfunction)
May Have Favorable Effects on Comorbid Conditions[†]	
Angina	Beta-blockers, CA
Atrial tachycardia and fibrillation	Beta-blockers, CA (non-DHP)
Cyclosporine-induced hypertension (caution with the dose of cyclosporine)	CA
Diabetes mellitus (Type I and II) with proteinuria	ACE I (preferred), CA
Diabetes mellitus (Type II)	Low-dose diuretics
Dyslipidemia	Alpha-blockers
Essential tremor	Beta-blockers (non-CS)
Heart failure	Carvedilol, losartan potassium
Hyperthyroidism	Beta-blockers
Migraine	Beta-blockers (non-CS), CA (non-DHP)
Myocardial infarction	Diltiazem hydrochloride, verapamil hydrochloride
Osteoporosis	Thiazides
Preoperative hypertension	Beta-blockers
Prostatism (BPH)	Alpha-blockers
Renal insufficiency (caution in renovascular hypertension and creatinine ≥265.2 mmol/L [3 mg/dL])	ACE I
May Have Unfavorable Effects on Comorbid Conditions[†‡]	
Bronchospastic disease	Beta-blockers[§]
Depression	Beta-blockers, central alpha-agonists, reserpine[§]
Diabetes mellitus (Types I and II)	Beta-blockers, high-dose diuretics
Dyslipidemia	Beta-blockers (non-ISA), diuretics (high-dose)
Gout	Diuretics
2° or 3° heart block	Beta-blockers[§], CA (non-DHP)[§]
Heart failure	Beta-blockers (except carvedilol), CA (except amlodipine besylate, felodipine)
Liver disease	Labetalol hydrochloride, methyldopa[§]
Peripheral vascular disease	Beta-blockers
Pregnancy	ACE I[§], angiotensin II receptor blockers[§]
Renal insufficiency	Potassium-sparing agents
Renovascular disease	ACE I, angiotensin II receptor blockers

*For initial drug therapy recommendations, see the exhibit "Algorithm for the Treatment of Hypertension." For references, see *Physicians' Desk Reference* (51st edition) and Kaplan and Gifford. ACE I indicates angiotensin-converting enzyme inhibitors; BPH, benign prostatic hyperplasia; CA, calcium antagonists; DHP, dihydropyridine; ISA, intrinsic sympathomimetic activity; MI, myocardial infarction; and non-CS, noncardioselective.

[†]Conditions and drugs are listed in alphabetical order.

[‡]These drugs may be used with special monitoring unless contraindicated.

[§]Contraindicated.

Source: Joint National Committee on Detection, Evaluation, and Treatment of High Blood Pressure, "The Sixth Report of the Joint Committee on Detection, Evaluation, and Treatment of High Blood Pressure," National Heart, Lung, and Blood Institute, NIH Publication No. 98-4080, November 1997.

PARENTERAL DRUGS FOR TREATMENT OF HYPERTENSIVE EMERGENCIES*

Drug	Dose	Onset of Action	Duration of Action	Adverse Effects[†]	Special Indications
Vasodilators					
Sodium nitroprusside	0.25–10 μg/kg per min as IV infusion[‡] (maximal dose for 10 min only)	Immediate	1–2 min	Nausea, vomiting, muscle twitching, sweating, thiocyanate and cyanide intoxication	Most hypertensive emergencies; caution with high intracranial pressure or azotemia
Nicardipine hydrochloride	5–15 mg/h IV	5–10 min	1–4 h	Tachycardia, headache, flushing, local phlebitis	Most hypertensive emergencies except acute heart failure; caution with coronary ischemia
Fenoldopam mesylate	0.1–0.3 μg/kg per min IV infusion	<5 min	30 min	Tachycardia, headache, nausea, flushing	Most hypertensive emergencies; caution with glaucoma
Nitroglycerin	5–100 μg/min as IV infusion[‡]	2–5 min	3–5 min	Headache, vomiting, methemoglobinemia, tolerance with prolonged use	Coronary ischemia
Enalaprilat	1.25–5 mg every 6 h IV	15–30 min	6 h	Precipitous fall in pressure in high-renin states; response variable	Acute left ventricular failure; avoid in acute myocardial infarction
Hydralazine hydrochloride	10–20 mg IV 10–50 mg IM	10–20 min 20–30 min	3–8 h	Tachycardia, flushing, headache, vomiting, aggravation of angina	Eclampsia
Diazoxide	50–100 mg IV bolus repeated, or 15–30 mg/min infusion	2–4 min	6–12 h	Nausea, flushing, tachycardia, chest pain	Now obsolete; when no intensive monitoring available
Adrenergic inhibitors					
Labetalol hydrochloride	20–80 mg IV bolus every 10 min, 0.5–2.0 mg/min IV infusion	5–10 min	3–6 h	Vomiting, scalp tingling, burning in throat, dizziness, nausea, heart block, orthostatic hypotension	Most hypertensive emergencies except acute heart failure
Esmolol hydrochloride	250–500 μg/kg/min for 1 min, then 50–100 μg/kg/min for 4 min; may repeat sequence	1–2 min	10–20 min	Hypotension, nausea	Aortic dissection, perioperative
Phentolamine	5–15 mg IV	1–2 min	3–10 min	Tachycardia, flushing, headache	Catecholamine excess

*These doses may vary from those in the *Physicians' Desk Reference* (51st edition). IV indicates intravenous; IM, intramuscular.
[†]Hypotension may occur with all agents.
[‡]Requires special delivery system.

Source: Joint National Committee on Detection, Evaluation, and Treatment of High Blood Pressure, "The Sixth Report of the Joint Committee on Detection, Evaluation, and Treatment of High Blood Pressure," National Heart, Lung, and Blood Institute, NIH Publication No. 98-4080, November 1997.

ALGORITHM FOR THE TREATMENT OF HYPERTENSION*

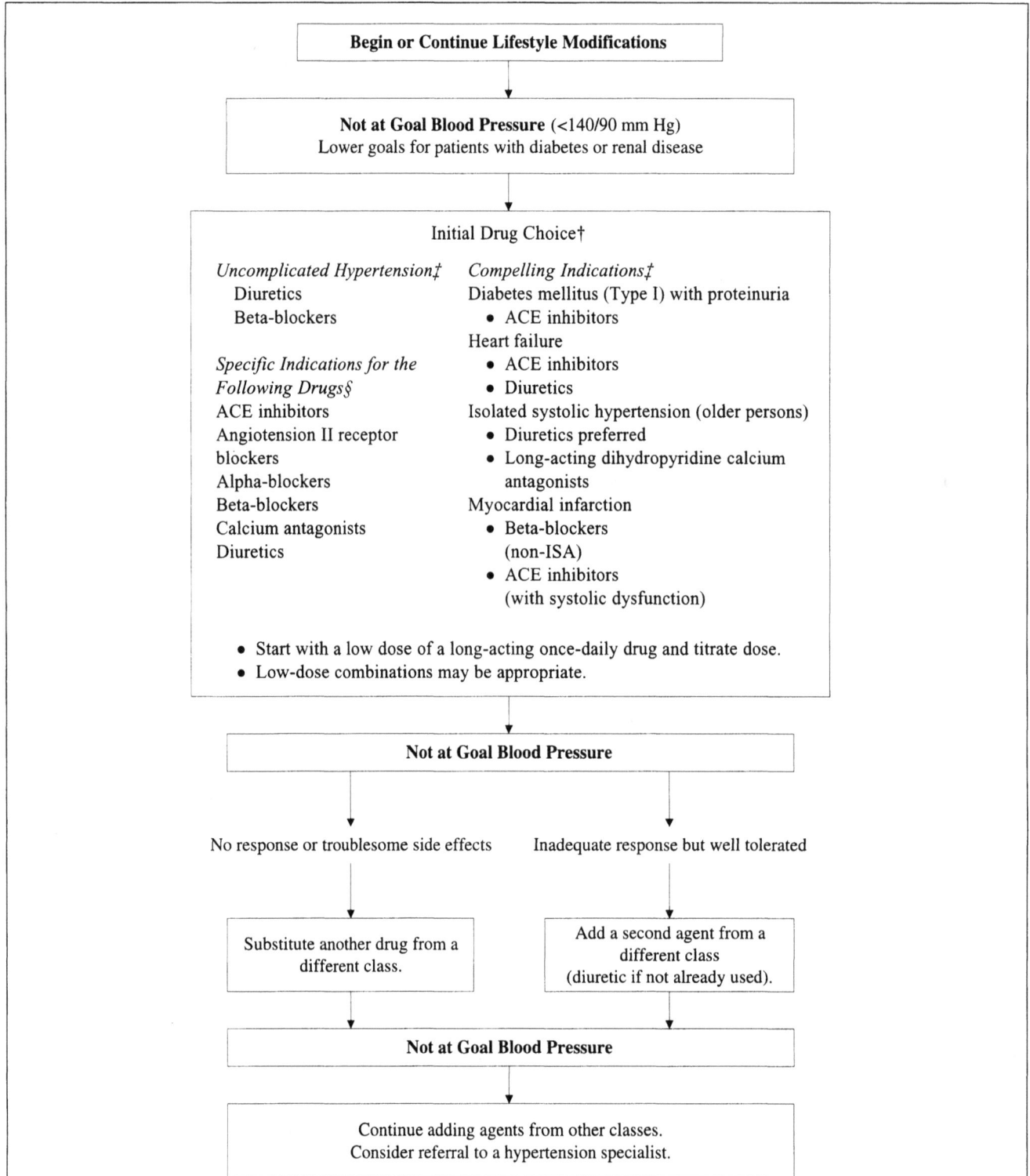

Begin or Continue Lifestyle Modifications

↓

Not at Goal Blood Pressure (<140/90 mm Hg)
Lower goals for patients with diabetes or renal disease

↓

Initial Drug Choice†

Uncomplicated Hypertension‡
Diuretics
Beta-blockers

*Specific Indications for the
Following Drugs§*
ACE inhibitors
Angiotension II receptor
blockers
Alpha-blockers
Beta-blockers
Calcium antagonists
Diuretics

Compelling Indications‡
Diabetes mellitus (Type I) with proteinuria
- ACE inhibitors
Heart failure
- ACE inhibitors
- Diuretics
Isolated systolic hypertension (older persons)
- Diuretics preferred
- Long-acting dihydropyridine calcium
  antagonists
Myocardial infarction
- Beta-blockers
  (non-ISA)
- ACE inhibitors
  (with systolic dysfunction)

- Start with a low dose of a long-acting once-daily drug and titrate dose.
- Low-dose combinations may be appropriate.

↓

Not at Goal Blood Pressure

↓ No response or troublesome side effects   ↓ Inadequate response but well tolerated

Substitute another drug from a
different class.

Add a second agent from a
different class
(diuretic if not already used).

↓

Not at Goal Blood Pressure

↓

Continue adding agents from other classes.
Consider referral to a hypertension specialist.

*ACE indicates angiotensin-converting enzyme; ISA, intrinsic sympathomimetic activity.
†Unless contraindicated.
‡Based on randomized controlled trials.
§See exhibit "Considerations for Individualizing Antihypertensive Drug Therapy."

Source: Joint National Committee on Detection, Evaluation, and Treatment of High Blood Pressure, "The Sixth Report of the Joint Committee on Detection, Evaluation, and Treatment of High Blood Pressure," National Heart, Lung, and Blood Institute, NIH Publication No. 98-4080, November 1997.

SELECTED DRUG INTERACTIONS WITH ANTIHYPERTENSIVE THERAPY*

Class of Agent	Increase Efficacy	Decrease Efficacy	Effect on Other Drugs
Diuretics	• Diuretics that act at different sites in the nephron (e.g., furosemide + thiazides)	• Resin-binding agents • NSAIDs • Steroids	• Diuretics raise serum lithium levels. • Potassium-sparing agents may exacerbate hyperkalemia due to ACE inhibitors.
Beta-blockers	• Cimetidine (hepatically metabolized beta-blockers) • Quinidine (hepatically metabolized beta-blockers) • Food (hepatically metabolized beta-blockers)	• NSAIDs • Withdrawal of clonidine • Agents that induce hepatic enzymes, including rifampin and phenobarbital	• Propranolol hydrochloride induces hepatic enzymes to increase clearance of drugs with similar metabolic pathways. • Beta-blockers may mask and prolong insulin-induced hypoglycemia. • Heart block may occur with nondihydropyridine calcium antagonists. • Sympathomimetics cause unopposed alpha-adrenoceptor–mediated vasoconstriction. • Beta-blockers increase angina: inducing potential of cocaine.
ACE inhibitors	• Chlorpromazine or clozapine	• NSAIDs • Antacids • Food decreases absorption (moexipril)	• ACE inhibitors may raise serum lithium levels. • ACE inhibitors may exacerbate hyperkalemic effect of potassium-sparing diuretics.
Calcium antagonists	• Grapefruit juice (some dihydropyridines) • Cimetidine or ranitidine (hepatically metabolized calcium antagonists)	• Agents that induce hepatic enzymes, including rifampin and phenobarbital	• Cyclosporine levels increase[†] with diltazem hydrochloride, verapamil hydrochloride, mibefradil dihydrochloride, or nicardipine hydrochloride (but not felodipine, isradipine, or nifedipine). • Nondihydropyridines increase levels of other drugs metabolized by the same hepatic enzyme system, including digoxin, quinidine, sulfonylureas, and theophylline. • Verapamil hydrochloride may lower serum lithium levels.
Alpha-blockers			• Prazosin may decrease clearance of verapamil hydrochloride.
Central alpha$_2$-agonists and peripheral neuronal blockers		• Tricyclic antidepressants (and probably phenothiazines) • Monoamine oxidase inhibitors • Sympathomimetics or phenothiazines antagonize guanethidine monosulfate or guanadrel sulfate • Iron salts may reduce methyldopa absorption	• Methyldopa may increase serum lithium levels. • Severity of clonidine hydrochloride withdrawal may be increased by beta-blockers. • Many agents used in anesthesia are potentiated by clonidine hydrochloride.

*For initial drug therapy recommendations, see the exhibit "Algorithm for the Treatment of Hypertension." See also *Physicians' Desk Reference* (51st edition) and *Cardiovascular Pharmacotherapeutics* (New York: McGraw Hill), 1997. NSAIDs indicate nonsteroidal anti-inflammatory drugs; ACE, angiotensin-converting enzyme.

[†]This is a clinically and economically beneficial drug–drug interaction because it both retards progression of accelerated atherosclerosis in heart transplant recipients and reduces the required daily dose of cyclosporine.

Source: Joint National Committee on Detection, Evaluation, and Treatment of High Blood Pressure, "The Sixth Report of the Joint Committee on Detection, Evaluation, and Treatment of High Blood Pressure," National Heart, Lung, and Blood Institute, NIH Publication No. 98-4080, November 1997.

effective, then cost should be considered in choosing them for initial therapy; if they prove to be more effective, then cost should be a secondary consideration. Treatment costs include not only the price of drugs but also the expense of routine or special laboratory tests, supplemental therapies, office visits, and time lost from work for visits to physicians' offices. The costs of medications may be reduced by using combination tablets and generic formulations. Patients should be advised to check prices at different sources. Some larger tablets can be divided, saving money when larger doses cost little more than smaller doses. Some sustained-release formulations should not be divided because cutting the tablet eliminates the sustained-release function.

Managed care. Because high blood pressure is so common, its management requires a major commitment from clinicians and managed care organizations. This commitment will need to expand even further because the majority of patients with hypertension do not have adequately controlled blood pressure. Additional demands will develop from the projected increase in the number of persons with hypertension due to the aging of the population. However, the cost of managing hypertension is lower overall than the sum of direct and indirect costs of treating hypertension-associated heart disease, stroke, and renal failure, especially because these adverse events often lead to expensive hospitalizations, surgical procedures, and use of high-cost technologies. Randomized controlled trials have demonstrated that reductions in these complications occur in a relatively short time and are sustained for years.

Managed care programs offer the opportunity for a coordinated approach to care, using various health care professionals and featuring an appropriate frequency of office visits, short waiting times, supportive patient counseling, and controlled formularies. The outcomes of the management of hypertension will need to be monitored, in keeping with the requirements of organizations that monitor quality, such as the Health Plan Employer Data and Information Set (HEDIS). These outcomes may be divided into three categories: immediate (e.g., blood pressure levels, percentage of adherence to therapy), intermediate (e.g., cardiac or renal function, health resource utilization), and long-term (e.g., morbidity and mortality, cost-effectiveness).

Hypertension specialists may play an important role in providing more cost-effective management of high blood pressure by adapting national guidelines for local implementation, providing guidance for new drugs and diagnostic methods, and managing patients with identifiable causes of hypertension, resistance to therapy, or complex concomitant conditions.

Drug interactions. As shown in the "Selected Drug Interactions" exhibit, some drug interactions may be helpful. For example, diuretics that act on different sites in the nephron,

such as furosemide and thiazides, increase natriuresis and diuresis, and certain calcium antagonists reduce the required amount of cyclosporine. Other interactions are deleterious: nonsteroidal anti-inflammatory drugs (NSAIDs) may blunt the action of diuretics, beta-blockers, and ACE inhibitors.

Dosage and Follow-up

Therapy for most patients (uncomplicated hypertension, stages 1 and 2) should begin with the lowest dosage listed in the exhibit "Oral Antihypertensive Drugs" to prevent adverse effects of too great or too abrupt a reduction in blood pressure. If blood pressure remains uncontrolled after one to two months, the next dosage level should be prescribed. It may take months to control hypertension adequately while avoiding adverse effects of therapy. Most antihypertensive medications can be given once daily, and this should be the goal to improve patient adherence. Home or office blood pressure measurement in the early morning, before patients have taken their daily dose, is useful to ensure that modulation of the surge in blood pressure after arising is adequate. Measurements in the late afternoon or evening help monitor control throughout the day. Treatment goals based on out-of-office measurements should be lower than those based on office recordings.

Initial Drug Therapy

When the decision has been made to begin antihypertensive therapy (see exhibit "Risk Stratification and Treatment") and if there are no indications for another type of drug, a diuretic or beta-blocker should be chosen because numerous randomized controlled trials have shown a reduction in morbidity and mortality with these agents.

As shown in the "Considerations" and "Algorithm" exhibits, there are compelling indications for specific agents in certain clinical conditions, based on outcomes data from RCTs. In other situations where outcomes data are not yet available, there are indications for other agents and the choice should be individualized, using the agent that most closely fits the patient's needs.

If the response to the initial drug choice is inadequate after reaching the full dose, two options for subsequent therapy should be considered (see the "Algorithm" exhibit):

- If the patient is tolerating the first choice well, add a second drug from another class.
- If the patient is having significant adverse effects or no response, substitute an agent from another class.

If a diuretic is not chosen as the first drug, it is usually indicated as a second-step agent because its addition will enhance the effects of other agents. If addition of a second agent controls blood pressure satisfactorily, an attempt to withdraw the first agent may be considered.

Before proceeding to each successive treatment step, clinicians should consider possible reasons for lack of responsiveness to therapy, including those listed in the exhibit "Causes of Inadequate Responsiveness to Therapy."

High-Risk Patients

Although similar general approaches are advocated for all patients with hypertension, modifications may be needed for those with stage 3 hypertension, those in risk group C, or those at especially high risk for a coronary event or stroke (see exhibit "Risk Stratification and Treatment"). Drug therapy should begin with minimal delay. Although some patients may respond adequately to a single drug, it is often necessary to add a second or third agent after a short interval if control is not achieved. The intervals between changes in the regimen should be decreased, and the maximum dose of some drugs may be increased. In some patients, it may be necessary to start treatment with more than one agent. Patients with average SBP of 200 mm Hg or greater and average DBP of 120 mm Hg or greater require more immediate therapy and, if symptomatic target organ damage is present, may require hospitalization.

Step-Down Therapy

An effort to decrease the dosage and number of antihypertensive drugs should be considered after hypertension has been controlled effectively for at least one year. The reduction should be made in a deliberate, slow, and progressive manner. Step-down therapy is more often successful in patients who also are making lifestyle modifications. Patients whose drugs have been discontinued should have scheduled follow-up visits because blood pressure usually rises again to hypertensive levels, sometimes months or years after discontinuance, especially in the absence of sustained improvements in lifestyle.

CAUSES OF INADEQUATE RESPONSIVENESS TO THERAPY

Pseudoresistance

"White-coat hypertension" or office elevations
Pseudohypertension in older patients
Use of regular cuff on very obese arm

Nonadherence to therapy

(See exhibit "General Guidelines To Improve Patient Adherence to Antihypertensive Therapy")

Volume overload

Excess salt intake
Progressive renal damage (nephrosclerosis)
Fluid retention from reduction of blood pressure
Inadequate diuretic therapy

Drug-related causes

Doses too low
Wrong type of diuretic
Inappropriate combinations
Rapid inactivation (e.g., hydralazine)
Drug actions and interactions

Sympathomimetics
Nasal decongestants
Appetite suppressants
Cocaine and other illicit drugs
Caffeine
Oral contraceptives
Adrenal steroids
Licorice (as may be found in chewing tobacco)
Cyclosporine, tacrolimus
Erythropoietin
Antidepressants
Nonsteroidal anti-inflammatory drugs

Associated conditions

Smoking
Increasing obesity
Sleep apnea
Insulin resistance/hyperinsulinemia
Ethanol intake of more than 1 oz (30 mL) per day
Anxiety-induced hyperventilation or panic attacks
Chronic pain
Intense vasoconstriction (arteritis)
Organic brain syndrome (e.g., memory deficit)

Source: Joint National Committee on Detection, Evaluation, and Treatment of High Blood Pressure, "The Sixth Report of the Joint Committee on Detection, Evaluation, and Treatment of High Blood Pressure," National Heart, Lung, and Blood Institute, NIH Publication No. 98-4080, November 1997.

J-Curve Hypothesis

Concerns have been raised that lowering DBP too much may increase the risk for coronary events by lowering diastolic perfusion pressure in the coronary circulation—the so-called J-curve hypothesis. The J-curve also has been detected in the placebo group of clinical trials of older persons with hypertension. The J-curve concern may be more relevant to patients with both hypertension and preexisting coronary disease and to those with pulse pressure greater than 60 mm Hg. On the other hand, data support a progressive reduction in both cerebrovascular disease and renal disease with even greater reductions in blood pressure. All available evidence supports the value of the reduction of DBP and SBP at all ages to the levels achieved in clinical trials—usually DBP to below 90 mm Hg and SBP to below 140 mm Hg in patients with isolated systolic hypertension. In trials of persons with isolated systolic hypertension, no increase in cardiovascular morbidity and mortality was observed, despite further reductions of DBP.

Considerations for Adherence to Therapy

Poor adherence to antihypertensive therapy remains a major therapeutic challenge, contributing to the lack of adequate control in more than two-thirds of patients with hypertension. As attempts to improve adherence are made, patients have the right and responsibility to be active and well-informed participants in their own care and to achieve maximal physical and emotional well-being. Health care professionals have the responsibility to provide patients with complete and accurate information about their health status, allowing patients to participate in their care and to achieve goal blood pressure.

Follow-up Visits

Achieving and maintaining target blood pressure often requires continuing encouragement for lifestyle modification and medication adjustment. Most patients should be seen within one to two months after the initiation of therapy to determine the adequacy of hypertension control, the degree of patient adherence, and the presence of adverse effects. Associated medical problems—including target organ damage, other major risk factors, and laboratory test abnormalities—also play a part in determining the frequency of patient follow-up. Visits to other members of the health care team may provide opportunities for more frequent follow-up. Once blood pressure is stabilized, follow-up at three- to six-month intervals (depending on patient status) is generally appropriate. In some patients, particularly older persons and those with orthostatic symptoms, monitoring should include blood pressure measurement in the seated position and, to recognize postural hypotension, after standing quietly for two to five minutes.

Strategies for Improving Adherence to Therapy and Control of High Blood Pressure

Various strategies may improve adherence significantly (see "General Guidelines" exhibit). The choice and application of specific strategies depend on individual patient characteristics, and health care providers are not expected to apply all of them at any one time or to all patients. In particular, pharmacists should be encouraged to monitor patients' use of medications, to provide information about potential adverse effects, and to avoid drug interactions. Nurse-managed clinics offer attractive opportunities to improve adherence and outcomes. The services of other members of the health care team, such as those who provide counseling in nutrition or exercise, should be used.

GENERAL GUIDELINES TO IMPROVE PATIENT ADHERENCE TO ANTIHYPERTENSIVE THERAPY

- Be aware of signs of patient nonadherence to antihypertensive therapy.
- Establish the goal of therapy: to reduce blood pressure to nonhypertensive levels with minimal or no adverse effects.
- Educate patients about the disease, and involve them and their families in its treatment. Have them measure blood pressure at home.
- Maintain contact with patients; consider telecommunication.
- Keep care inexpensive and simple.
- Encourage lifestyle modifications.
- Integrate pill-taking into routine activities of daily living.

- Prescribe medications according to pharmacological principles, favoring long-acting formulations.
- Be willing to stop unsuccessful therapy and try a different approach.
- Anticipate adverse effects, and adjust therapy to prevent, minimize, or ameliorate side effects.
- Continue to add effective and tolerated drugs, stepwise, in sufficient doses to achieve the goal of therapy.
- Encourage a positive attitude about achieving therapeutic goals.
- Consider using nurse case management.

Source: Joint National Committee on Detection, Evaluation, and Treatment of High Blood Pressure, "The Sixth Report of the Joint Committee on Detection, Evaluation, and Treatment of High Blood Pressure," National Heart, Lung, and Blood Institute, NIH Publication No. 98-4080, November 1997.

Resistant Hypertension

Hypertension should be considered resistant if blood pressure cannot be reduced to below 140/90 mm Hg in patients who are adhering to an adequate and appropriate triple-drug regimen that includes a diuretic, with all three drugs prescribed in near maximal doses. For older patients with isolated systolic hypertension, resistance is defined as failure of an adequate triple-drug regimen to reduce SBP to below 160 mm Hg.

Of the various causes of true resistance listed in the "Causes of Inadequate Responsiveness" exhibit, one of the most common is volume overload due to inadequate diuretic therapy. Frequently, a cause for resistance can be recognized and overcome. However, if goal blood pressure cannot be achieved without intolerable adverse effects, even suboptimal reduction of blood pressure contributes to decreased morbidity and mortality. Patients who have resistant hypertension or who are unable to tolerate antihypertensive therapy may benefit from referral to a hypertension specialist.

Hypertensive Crises: Emergencies and Urgencies

Hypertensive emergencies are those rare situations that require immediate blood pressure reduction (not necessarily to normal ranges) to prevent or limit target organ damage. Examples include hypertensive encephalopathy, intracranial hemorrhage, unstable angina pectoris, acute myocardial infarction, acute left ventricular failure with pulmonary edema, dissecting aortic aneurysm, or eclampsia. Hypertensive urgencies are those situations in which it is desirable to reduce blood pressure within a few hours. Examples include upper levels of stage 3 hypertension, hypertension with optic disk edema, progressive target organ complications, and severe perioperative hypertension. Elevated blood pressure alone, in the absence of symptoms or new or progressive target organ damage, rarely requires emergency therapy.

Parenteral drugs for hypertensive emergencies are listed in the "Parenteral Drugs" exhibit. Most hypertensive emergencies are treated initially with parenteral administration of an appropriate agent. Hypertensive urgencies can be managed with oral doses of drugs with relatively fast onset of action. The choices include loop diuretics, beta-blockers, ACE inhibitors, alpha$_2$-agonists, and calcium antagonists.

The initial goal of therapy in hypertensive emergencies is to reduce mean arterial blood pressure by no more than 25 percent (within minutes to two hours), then toward 160/100 mm Hg within two to six hours, avoiding excessive falls in pressure that may precipitate renal, cerebral, or coronary ischemia. Although sublingual administration of fast-acting nifedipine has been widely used for this purpose, several serious adverse effects have been reported with its use, and the inability to control the rate or degree of fall in blood pressure makes this agent unacceptable. The routine use of sublingual nifedipine whenever blood pressure rises beyond a predetermined level in postoperative or nursing home patients is also inappropriate. Rather, the proximate causes of the elevated blood pressure, such as pain or a distended urinary bladder, should be addressed. Blood pressure should be monitored over 15- to 30-minute intervals; if it remains greater than 180/120 mm Hg, one of the previously mentioned oral agents may be given. If such high levels of blood pressure are frequent, adequate doses of long-acting agents should be provided.

DESIGN OF NONPHARMACOLOGIC INTERVENTION TRIALS IN PREVENTION OF HYPERTENSION

| Study | Sample Size | Demographic Characteristics | | | Duration of Follow-Up Blood Pressure | Intervention |
		Mean Age	% Male	% White		
Primary Prevention of Hypertension Trial	201	38	87	82	5 years	Multifactorial (reduced calorie, sodium, and alcohol intake, and increased physical activity)
Hypertension Prevention Trial	252	38	68	80	3 years	Reduced calorie intake
	392	39	62	84		Reduced sodium intake
	255	39	62	82		Reduced calorie and sodium intake
	391	38	63	85		Reduced sodium and increased potassium intake
Trials of Hypertension Prevention	564	43	72	79	18 months	Weight loss (reduced calorie intake and increased physical activity)
	744	43	72	77	18 months	Reduced sodium intake
	562	43	71	84	18 months	Stress management
	471	43	68	85	6 months	Calcium supplementation
	461	43	68	85	6 months	Magnesium supplementation
	351	43	72	87	6 months	Potassium supplementation
	350	43	70	86	6 months	Fish oil supplementation

Source: Gail C. Frank-Spohrer, *Community Nutrition: Applying Epidemiology to Contemporary Practice,* Aspen Publishers, Inc., © 1996. Adapted from *Working Group Report on Primary Prevention of Hypertension,* p. 10, National High Blood Pressure Education Program, National Institutes of Health, Publication No. 93-2669, May 1993.

EFFECT OF NONPHARMACOLOGIC INTERVENTIONS ON BLOOD PRESSURE AND RISK OF HYPERTENSION IN PERSONS WITH HIGH NORMAL BLOOD PRESSURE

| Study | Average Initial Blood Pressure (mm Hg) | | Average Net Change in Blood Pressure (mm Hg) | | Effect: Relative Risk of Increased Blood Pressure (95% CI) |
	Systolic	Diastolic	Systolic	Diastolic	
Primary Prevention of Hypertension Trial	122.6	82.5	-1.3	-1.02	0.46
Hypertension Prevention Trial	125.0	83.2	-2.4	-1.8	0.77
	123.9	82.8	0.2	0.1	0.79
	124.5	82.9	-1.0	-1.3	0.95
	124.0	82.6	-1.2	-0.7	0.77
Trials of Hypertension Prevention Phase I	124.4	83.8	-2.9	-2.3	0.49/(0.29,0.83)
	125.0	83.8	-1.7	-0.9	0.76/(0.49,1.18)
	124.6	83.7	-0.5	-0.8	1.07/(0.65,1.76)
	125.7	84.0	-0.5	0.2	0.91/(0.43,1.96)
	125.1	83.9	-0.2	-0.1	0.63/(0.27,1.50)
	121.6	80.9	0.1	-0.4	0.87/(0.34,2.21)
	122.7	81.1	-0.2	-0.6	1.11/(0.46,2.67)

Source: Gail C. Frank-Spohrer, *Community Nutrition: Applying Epidemiology to Contemporary Practice,* Aspen Publishers, Inc., © 1996. Adapted from *Working Group Report on Primary Prevention of Hypertension,* p. 10, National High Blood Pressure Education Program, National Institutes of Health, Publication No. 93-2669, May 1993.

SPECIAL POPULATIONS AND SITUATIONS*

Hypertension in Racial and Ethnic Minorities

The United States is a diverse nation composed of individuals from many cultures. The 1990 census reported that the U.S. population was 0.8 percent American Indians, Aleuts, and Inuits; 2.9 percent Asians and Pacific Islanders; 9.0 percent persons of Hispanic origin; 12.1 percent African Americans; and 80.3 percent whites. (These self-reported categories are not mutually exclusive; thus, the total is greater than 100 percent.) In the past decade, the country has experienced a marked increase in minority populations and the number of immigrants. This trend is expected to continue.

As immigrant populations acculturate, their risk for cardiovascular disease changes. The prevalence of hypertension differs among racial and ethnic groups compared with the general population. For example, American Indians have the same prevalence as, or a higher prevalence than, the general population; among Hispanics, blood pressure is generally the same as or lower than that of non-Hispanic whites, despite a high prevalence of obesity and Type II diabetes mellitus. It also appears that South Asians are more responsive to various antihypertensive medications than whites. Evidence shows that hypertension awareness, treatment, and control in some groups, especially those with generally lower socioeconomic status, require more focused hypertension education and intervention programs.

The prevalence of hypertension in African Americans is among the highest in the world. Compared with whites, hypertension develops earlier in life and average blood pressures are much higher in African Americans. African Americans have higher rates of stage 3 hypertension than whites, causing a greater burden of hypertension complications. This earlier onset, higher prevalence, and greater rate of stage 3 hypertension in African Americans is accompanied by an 80 percent higher stroke mortality rate, a 50 percent higher heart disease mortality rate, and a 320 percent greater rate of hypertension-related end-stage renal disease than seen in the general population.

Available evidence indicates that, compared with whites, African Americans receiving adequate treatment will achieve similar overall declines in blood pressure and may experience a lower incidence of cardiovascular disease. However, African Americans often do not receive treatment until blood pressure has been elevated for a long time and target organ damage is present. This also may account for the higher incidence of hypertension-related morbidity and mortality, including end-stage renal disease, in the African American population.

Because of the high prevalence of cardiovascular risk factors in African Americans—such as obesity, cigarette smoking, and Type II diabetes—as well as increased responsiveness to reduced salt intake, lifestyle modifications are particularly important.

In African Americans, as well as in whites, diuretics have been proven in controlled trials to reduce hypertensive morbidity and mortality; thus, diuretics should be the agent of first choice in the absence of conditions that prohibit their use. Calcium antagonists and alpha-beta-blockers are also effective in lowering blood pressure. Monotherapy with beta-blockers or ACE inhibitors is less effective, but the addition of diuretics markedly improves response. However, these agents are indicated regardless of ethnicity when patients have other specific indications (e.g., beta-blockers for angina or post–myocardial infarction, ACE inhibitors for diabetic nephropathy or left ventricular systolic dysfunction).

Because of their greater prevalence of stage 3 hypertension, many African-American patients require multidrug therapy. Every effort should be made to achieve a goal blood pressure of below 140/90 mm Hg. In patients with renal insufficiency, recent data suggest that reducing blood pressure to an even lower level may be beneficial (see discussion of renal disease below).

Hypertension in Children and Adolescents

The fifth Korotkoff sound is now used to define DBP for all ages. Definitions of hypertension take into account age and height by sex. Blood pressure at the 95th percentile or greater is considered elevated. Clinicians should be alert to the possibility of identifiable causes of hypertension in younger children. Lifestyle interventions should be recommended, with pharmacological therapy instituted for higher levels of blood pressure or if there is insufficient response to lifestyle modifications. Although the recommendations for choice of drugs are similar in children and adults, dosages of antihypertensive medication should be smaller and adjusted very carefully for children. ACE inhibitors and angiotensin II receptor blockers should not be used in pregnant or sexually active girls.

Uncomplicated elevated blood pressure alone should not be a reason to restrict asymptomatic children from participating in physical activities, particularly because exercise may lower blood pressure and prevent hypertension. Use of anabolic steroid hormones for the purposes of body-building should be strongly discouraged. Efforts should be made to discover other risk factors (e.g., smoking) in children, and interventions should be made if they are present. Detailed recommendations regarding hypertension in children and

---

*Source: Joint National Committee on Detection, Evaluation, and Treatment of High Blood Pressure, "The Sixth Report of the Joint Committee on Detection, Evaluation, and Treatment of High Blood Pressure," National Heart, Lung, and Blood Institute, NIH Publication No. 98-4080, November 1997.

adolescents can be found in the 1996 report by the National Health Blood Pressure Education Program (NHBPEP) Working Group on Hypertension Control in Children and Adolescents.

Hypertension in Women

Large, long-term clinical trials of antihypertensive treatment have included both men and women and have not demonstrated clinically significant sex differences in blood pressure response and outcomes. Recent trials of older persons support a similar approach to hypertension management in men and women.

Hypertension Associated with Oral Contraceptives

Women taking oral contraceptives experience a small but detectable increase in both SBP and DBP, usually within the normal range. Hypertension has been reported to be two to three times more common in women taking oral contraceptives, especially in obese and older women, than in those not taking oral contraceptives. Women age 35 and older who smoke cigarettes should be strongly counseled to quit; if they continue to smoke, they should be discouraged from using oral contraceptives.

If hypertension develops in women taking oral contraceptives, it is advisable to stop their use. Blood pressure will normalize in most cases within a few months. If high blood pressure persists, if the risks for pregnancy are considered to be greater than the risks for hypertension, and if other contraceptive methods are not suitable, then oral contraceptives may have to be continued and therapy for hypertension begun. A prudent approach to the use of oral contraceptives is to prescribe no more than a six-month supply at a time in order to measure blood pressure on a semiannual basis.

Hypertension in Pregnancy

Chronic hypertension is high blood pressure that is present and observable before pregnancy or that is diagnosed before the twentieth week of gestation. The goal of treatment for women with chronic hypertension in pregnancy is to minimize the short-time risks of elevated blood pressure to the mother while avoiding therapy that compromises the well-being of the fetus. If taken before pregnancy, diuretics and most other antihypertensive drugs, except ACE inhibitors and angiotensin II receptor blockers, may be continued. Methyldopa has been evaluated most extensively and is therefore recommended for women whose hypertension is first diagnosed during pregnancy. Beta-blockers compare favorably with methyldopa with respect to efficacy and are considered safe in the latter part of pregnancy; however, their use in early pregnancy may be associated with growth retardation of the fetus (see exhibit "Antihypertensive Drugs Used in Pregnancy." ACE inhibitors and angiotensin II receptor blockers should be avoided because serious neonatal problems, including renal failure and death, have been reported when mothers have taken these agents during the last two trimesters of pregnancy.

Preeclampsia. Preeclampsia, a pregnancy-specific condition, is increased blood pressure accompanied by proteinuria, edema, or both and at times by abnormalities of coagulation and renal and liver function that may progress rapidly to a convulsive phase, eclampsia. Preeclampsia occurs primarily during first pregnancies and after the twentieth week of gestation. It may be superimposed on preexisting chronic hypertension. Large trials have not confirmed the benefit of prophylactic low-dose aspirin or supplemental calcium to prevent preeclampsia. A detailed summary of hypertension in pregnancy was published in a report by the NHBPEP Working Group on High Blood Pressure in Pregnancy. More recent reviews have been published.

Hormone Replacement Therapy and Blood Pressure Response

The presence of hypertension is not a contraindication to postmenopausal estrogen replacement therapy. A recent study indicated that blood pressure does not increase significantly with hormone replacement therapy in most women with and without hypertension and that hormone replacement therapy has a beneficial effect on overall cardiovascular risk factor profiles. However, a few women may experience a rise in blood pressure attributable to estrogen therapy. Therefore, it is recommended that all women treated with hormone replacement therapy have their blood pressure monitored more frequently after such therapy is instituted. The effect of transdermal estrogen and progestogen on blood pressure has not been established.

Hypertension in Older Persons

Hypertension is extremely common in older Americans. Among Americans age 60 and older examined in the third National Health and Nutrition Examination Survey (NHANES III), elevated blood pressure was found in 60 percent of non-Hispanic whites, 71 percent of non-Hispanic African Americans, and 61 percent of Mexican Americans. Especially among older persons, SBP is a better predictor of events (CHD, cardiovascular disease, heart failure, stroke, end-stage renal disease, and all-cause mortality) than is DBP. Recently, it has become clear that an elevated pulse pressure (SBP minus DBP), which indicates reduced vascular compliance in large arteries, may be an even better marker of increased cardiovascular risk than either SBP or DBP alone.

ANTIHYPERTENSIVE DRUGS USED IN PREGNANCY*

The report of the (NHBPEP) Working Group on High Blood Pressure in Pregnancy permits continuation of drug therapy (except ACE inhibitors) in women with chronic hypertension. In addition, angiotensin II receptor blockers should not be used during pregnancy. In women with chronic hypertension with diastolic levels of 100 mm Hg or greater (lower when end organ damage or underlying renal disease is present) and in women with acute hypertension when levels are 105 mm Hg or greater, the following agents are suggested.

Suggested Drug	Comments
Central alpha-agonists	Methyldopa (C) is the drug of choice recommended by the NHBPEP Working Group.
Beta-blockers	Atenolol (C) and metoprolol (C) appear to be safe and effective in late pregnancy. Labetalol (C) also appears to be effective (alpha- and beta-blockers).
Calcium antagonists	Potential synergism with magnesium sulfate may lead to precipitous hypotension. (C)
ACE inhibitors, angiotensin II receptor blockers	Fetal abnormalities, including death, can be caused, and these drugs should not be used in pregnancy. (D)
Diuretics	Diuretics (C) are recommended for chronic hypertension if prescribed before gestation or if patients appear to be salt-sensitive. They are not recommended in preeclampsia.
Direct vasodilators	Hydralazine (C) is the parenteral drug of choice based on its long history of safety and efficacy.

*Adapted from Sibai and Lindheimer. There are several other antihypertensive drugs for which there are very limited data. The U.S. Food and Drug Administration classifies pregnancy risk as follows: C, adverse effects in animals, no controlled trials in humans, use if risk appears justified; D, positive evidence of fetal risk. ACE indicates angiotensin-converting enzyme.

Source: Joint National Committee on Detection, Evaluation, and Treatment of High Blood Pressure, "The Sixth Report of the Joint Committee on Detection, Evaluation, and Treatment of High Blood Pressure," National Heart, Lung, and Blood Institute, NIH Publication No. 98-4080, November 1997.

This is particularly relevant to older individuals who frequently have an isolated elevation of SBP (140 mm Hg or greater with a DBP below 90 mm Hg) (see exhibit "Classification of Blood Pressure"). Those with stage 1 isolated systolic hypertension are at significantly increased cardiovascular risk, but the benefits of treatment in those individuals have not yet been demonstrated in a controlled trial.

Primary hypertension is by far the most common form of hypertension in older persons. However, clinicians must recognize that certain identifiable causes of hypertension (e.g., atherosclerotic renovascular hypertension, primary aldosteronism) may occur more frequently in older persons, especially in those whose hypertension first presented after age 60 or is resistant to treatment.

Blood pressure must be measured in older persons with special care because some older persons have pseudohypertension (falsely high sphygmomanometer readings) due to excessive vascular stiffness. In addition, more older persons with hypertension, especially women, may have "white-coat hypertension" and excessive variability in SBP. In the absence of target organ damage, clinicians should consider pseudohypertension or "white-coat hypertension" and should obtain readings outside the office. In addition, older patients are more likely than younger patients to exhibit an orthostatic fall in blood pressure and hypotension; thus, in older patients, blood pressure should always be measured in the standing as well as seated or supine positions.

Treatment of hypertension in older persons has demonstrated major benefits. Large trials of patients older than age 60 have shown that antihypertensive drug therapy reduces stroke, CHD, cardiovascular disease, heart failure, and mortality.

Hypertension therapy in older persons, as in younger persons, should begin with lifestyle modifications. Older patients will respond to modest salt reduction and weight loss. If goal blood pressure is not achieved, then pharmacological treatment is indicated. The starting dose in older patients should be about half of that used in younger patients. Thiazide diuretics or beta-blockers in combination with thiazide diuretics are recommended because they are effective in reducing mortality and morbidity in older persons with hypertension as shown in multiple randomized controlled trials. When compared to each other, diuretics (hydrochlorothiazide with amiloride hydrochloride) are superior to the beta-blocker atenolol. In older patients with isolated systolic hypertension, diuretics are preferred because they have significantly reduced multiple endpoint events. In addition, an RCT in such patients taking the dihydropyridine nitrendipine showed a 42 percent reduction in fatal and nonfatal stroke over an average two-year interval. The concomitant reductions in coronary events and heart failure did not reach statistical significance, although a favorable trend was reported and all cardiovascular disease mortality was significantly reduced. Because nitrendipine is not available in the United States, other long-acting dihydropyridine calcium antagonists are considered to be appropriate alternatives in these patients.

The goal of treatment in older patients should be the same as in younger patients (to below 140/90 mm Hg if at all possible), although an interim goal of SBP below 160 mm Hg may be necessary in those patients with marked systolic hypertension. Any reduction in blood pressure appears to confer benefit—the closer to normal, the greater the benefit. Drugs that exaggerate postural changes in blood pressure (peripheral adrenergic blockers, alpha-blockers, and high-dose diuretics) or drugs that can cause cognitive dysfunction (central alpha$_2$-agonists) should be used with caution. Additional recommendations about hypertension in older persons can be found in the report by the NHBPEP Working Group on Hypertension in the Elderly.

Patients with Hypertension and Coexisting Cardiovascular Diseases

Patients with Cerebrovascular Disease

Clinically evident cerebrovascular disease is an indication for antihypertensive treatment. However, immediately after the occurrence of an ischemic cerebral infarction, it is appropriate to withhold treatment (unless blood pressure is very high) until the situation has been stabilized. Even when treatment has been withheld temporarily, the eventual goal is to reduce blood pressure gradually while avoiding orthostatic hypotension. Patients with acute ischemic stroke who are treated with fibrinolytic agents require careful blood pressure monitoring, especially over the first 24 hours after starting treatment. SBP of 180 mm Hg or greater or DBP of 105 mm Hg or greater may be controlled with intravenous agents with careful monitoring for worsening of neurological status.

Patients with Coronary Artery Disease

Patients with coronary artery disease and hypertension are at particularly high risk for cardiovascular morbidity and mortality. The benefits and safety of antihypertensive therapy in such patients are well established. Excessively rapid lowering of blood pressure, particularly when it causes reflex tachycardia and sympathetic activation, should be avoided. Blood pressure should be lowered to the usual target range (below 140/90 mm Hg), and even lower blood pressure is desirable if angina persists.

Beta-blockers or calcium antagonists may be specifically useful in patients with hypertension and angina pectoris; however, short-acting calcium antagonists should not be used. After myocardial infarction, beta-blockers without intrinsic sympathomimetic activity should be given because they reduce the risk for subsequent myocardial infarction or sudden cardiac death. ACE inhibitors are also useful after myocardial infarction, especially with left ventricular systolic dysfunction, to prevent subsequent heart failure and mortality.

If beta-blockers are ineffective or contraindicated, verapamil hydrochloride or diltiazem hydrochloride may be used because they have been shown to reduce cardiac events and mortality modestly in two circumstances: (1) following non–Q-wave myocardial infarction, and (2) after myocardial infarction with preserved left ventricular function.

Some patients with hypertension, especially when accompanied by severe left ventricular hypertrophy (LVH), may experience angina without evidence of coronary atherosclerosis. This is thought to reflect an imbalance between myocardial oxygen supply and demand, due in part to changes in the coronary microcirculation. Treatment should be directed at blood pressure control, reversal of LVH, and avoidance of tachycardia, which may exacerbate the supply–demand mismatch.

Patients with Left Ventricular Hypertrophy

Development of LVH permits cardiac adaptation to the increased afterload imposed by elevated arterial pressure. However, LVH is a major independent risk factor for sudden cardiac death, myocardial infarction, stroke, and other cardiovascular morbid and mortal events. Evidence shows that antihypertensive agents (except direct vasodilators such as hydralazine and minoxidil), weight reduction, and decrease of excessive salt intake are capable of reducing increased left ventricular mass and wall thickness. In one study in men with hypertension, treatment with a diuretic and an ACE inhibitor was better than treatment with other drug classes tested for regressing LVH at one year. Observational data indicate that the regression of electrocardiographic evidence of LVH is associated with a reduction in the risk for cardiovascular events. However, no controlled studies demonstrate that such reversal of LVH offers additional benefits beyond that offered by reduction of blood pressure. The electrocardiogram remains valuable not only for detecting left atrial hypertrophy and LVH but also for identifying evidence of myocardial ischemia and arrhythmia. Echocardiography is more sensitive and specific for identifying LVH, but it is too expensive for routine use. Limited echocardiography will identify LVH at a cost that may justify its use in some patients (e.g., those with untreated stage 1 hypertension, no cardiovascular risk factors, no evidence of clinical cardiovascular disease, and no target organ damage).

Patients with Cardiac Failure

In patients with hypertension, structural alterations in the left ventricle (LVH or left ventricular remodeling with dilation) as well as myocardial ischemia from coronary artery atherosclerosis may contribute to the development of heart failure. Some patients with hypertension (current or past) develop heart failure with a normal ejection fraction, implying diastolic dysfunction. Reports from the Framingham Heart Study have demonstrated that hypertension continues to be the major cause of left ventricular failure in the United States. Control of elevated arterial pressure using lifestyle changes and drug therapy improves myocardial function and prevents and reduces heart failure and cardiovascular mortality. After myocardial infarction, therapy with ACE inhibitors prevents subsequent heart failure and reduces morbidity and mortality. In treating heart failure, ACE inhibitors, used alone or in conjunction with digoxin or diuretics, are effective in reducing morbidity and mortality. When ACE inhibitors are contraindicated or not tolerated, the vasodilator combination of hydralazine hydrochloride and isosorbide dinitrate is also effective in these patients. The alpha-beta-blocker carvedilol added to ACE inhibitors has been shown to be beneficial, and, in one trial, the angiotensin II receptor blocker losartan potassium was superior to captopril in reducing mortality. The dihydropyridine calcium antagonists amlodipine besylate and felodipine have been demonstrated to be safe in treating angina and hypertension in patients with advanced left ventricular dysfunction when used in addition to ACE inhibitors, diuretics, or digoxin; other calcium antagonists are not recommended in these patients.

Patients with Peripheral Arterial Disease

Hypertension is one of the major risk factors for the development of carotid atherosclerosis and peripheral arterial disease with intermittent claudication and aneurysms. However, data are not available to determine whether antihypertensive therapy will alter the course of these processes. Early multicenter trials demonstrated a reduction in deaths from dissecting aortic aneurysms.

Patients with Hypertension and Other Coexisting Diseases

Patients with Renal Parenchymal Disease

Pathophysiology. Hypertension may result from any form of renal disease that reduces the number of functioning nephrons, leading to sodium and water retention. Hypertensive nephrosclerosis is among the most common causes of progressive renal disease, particularly in African Americans. Follow-up of large numbers of men screened for the Multiple Risk Factor Intervention Trial and of male veterans has provided the most conclusive and direct evidence of a relationship between blood pressure and end-stage renal disease.

Strategies for slowing progressive renal failure in patients with hypertension. Early detection of hypertensive renal damage is essential. Small elevations of serum creatinine reflect significant losses in glomerular filtration rate. Evaluation should include urinalysis to detect proteinuria or hematuria and possibly renal sonography to exclude lower tract obstruction, to exclude autosomal dominant polycystic kidney disease, and to determine the size of the kidneys. Reversible causes of renal failure should always be sought and treated.

Blood pressure should be controlled to 130/85 mm Hg—or lower (125/75 mm Hg) in patients with proteinuria in excess of one gram per 24 hours—with whatever antihypertensive therapy is necessary. Reducing dietary sodium to a level lower than that recommended for uncomplicated hypertension (less than 100 mmol per day of sodium) helps control high blood pressure in patients with renal insufficiency. If dietary protein restriction is instituted, close attention must be paid to total energy (caloric) intake to prevent malnutrition. Restriction of dietary potassium and phosphorus in patients with creatinine clearances below 30 mL per minute is needed to prevent hyperkalemia and to help prevent secondary hyperparathyroidism.

Antihypertensive drug recommendations for patients with hypertension and renal disease. The most important action to slow progressive renal failure is to lower blood pressure to goal. All classes of antihypertensive drugs are effective, and, in most cases, multiple antihypertensive drugs may be needed. Impressive results have been achieved with ACE inhibitors in patients with Type I diabetic nephropathy, in patients with proteinuria greater than one gram per 24 hours, and in patients with renal insufficiency. Consequently, patients with hypertension who have renal insufficiency should receive, unless contraindicated, an ACE inhibitor (in most cases, along with a diuretic) to control hypertension and to slow progressive renal failure. In patients with a creatinine level of 265.2 mmol/L (3 mg/dL) or greater, ACE inhibitors should be used with caution.

An initial transient decrease in glomerular filtration rate may occur during the first three months of treatment as blood pressure is lowered. If patients are euvolemic and creatinine rises 88.4 mmol/L (1mg/dL) above baseline levels, creatinine and potassium should be remeasured after several days; if they remain persistently elevated, consideration should be given to the diagnosis of renal artery stenosis and ACE inhibitors or angiotensin II receptor blockers should be discontinued because these drugs can markedly reduce renal perfusion in patients with bilateral renal artery stenosis or renal artery stenosis to a solitary kidney.

Thiazide diuretics are not effective with advanced renal insufficiency (serum creatinine level of 221.0 mmol/L [2.5 mg/dL] or greater), and loop diuretics are needed (often at relatively large doses). Combining a loop diuretic with a long-acting thiazide diuretic, such as metolazone, is effective in patients resistant to a loop diuretic alone. Potassium-sparing diuretics should be avoided in patients with renal insufficiency.

Patients with Renovascular Disease

Hemodynamically significant renal artery stenosis may be associated with all stages of hypertension, but it is more commonly found with stage 3 or resistant hypertension and, when bilateral, can lead to reduced kidney function (ischemic nephropathy).

Clinical clues to renovascular disease include (1) onset of hypertension before age 30, especially without a family history, or recent onset of significant hypertension after age 55; (2) an abdominal bruit, particularly if it continues into diastole and is lateralized; (3) accelerated or resistant hypertension; (4) recurrent (flash) pulmonary edema; (5) renal failure of uncertain cause, especially with a normal urinary sediment; (6) coexisting, diffuse atherosclerotic vascular disease, especially in heavy smokers; and (7) acute renal failure precipitated by antihypertensive therapy, particularly ACE inhibitors or angiotensin II receptor blockers.

In patients with indications of renovascular disease, captopril-enhanced radionuclide renal scan, duplex Doppler flow studies, and magnetic resonance angiography may be used as noninvasive screening tests. Three-dimensional images can be obtained by spiral computed tomography, a technique that unfortunately requires intravenous contrast. Definitive diagnosis of renovascular disease requires renal angiography, which carries some risk, particularly radiocontrast–induced acute renal failure or atheroembolism in older patients.

Management. In younger patients with fibromuscular dysplasia, results of percutaneous transluminal renal angioplasty (PTRA) have been excellent and comparable to surgical revascularization. Patients with normal renal function and atherosclerotic renal artery stenosis that is focal, unilateral, and nonostial, without widespread vascular disease, are managed similarly to those with fibromuscular dysplasia. Renal artery stenting has become an important adjunct to PTRA, being used to counteract elastic recoil and to abolish the residual stenosis often observed after PTRA.

Even though many patients with high-grade renal artery stenosis remain stable for prolonged periods, if blood pressure is well controlled, surgical revascularization or PTRA with renal artery stenting may be needed to preserve renal function.

Patients with Diabetes Mellitus

To detect evidence of autonomic dysfunction and orthostatic hypotension, blood pressure should be measured in the supine, sitting, and standing positions in all patients with diabetes mellitus. Automated ambulatory blood pressure monitoring may be especially helpful.

Antihypertensive drug therapy should be initiated along with lifestyle modifications, especially weight loss, to reduce arterial blood pressure to below 130/85 mm Hg. ACE inhibitors, alpha-blockers, calcium antagonists, and diuretics in low doses are preferred because of fewer adverse effects on glucose homeostasis, lipid profiles, and renal function. Although beta-blockers may have adverse effects on peripheral blood flow, prolong hypoglycemia, and mask hypoglycemic symptoms, patients with diabetes who are treated with diuretics and beta-blockers experience a similar or greater reduction of CHD and total cardiovascular events compared with persons without diabetes. In patients with diabetic nephropathy, ACE inhibitors are preferred. If ACE inhibitors are contraindicated or are not well tolerated, angiotensin II receptor blockers may be considered. Renoprotection also has been shown by the use of a calcium antagonist.

Insulin resistance. Obese patients with hypertension have resistance to insulin-mediated glucose uptake by skeletal muscle, which can lead to impaired glucose tolerance and Type II diabetes. Some nonobese persons with normal blood pressure who have first-degree relatives with hypertension also have insulin resistance. It is uncertain whether the higher peripheral insulin levels or the insulin resistance may cause hypertension. These metabolic disturbances as well as the hypertension respond to weight loss, exercise, insulin-sensitizing agents, vasodilating antihypertensive drugs, and certain lipid-lowering drugs.

Patients with Dyslipidemia

The common coexistence and increased risk of dyslipidemia and hypertension mandate aggressive management of both conditions. Because lifestyle modifications are the first approach to the treatment of both conditions, great emphasis must be placed on control of weight; reduced intake of saturated fat, cholesterol, sodium chloride, and alcohol; and increased physical activity in patients with elevated lipids and high blood pressure.

In high doses, thiazide diuretics and loop diuretics can induce at least short-term increases in levels of total plasma cholesterol, triglycerides, and LDL cholesterol. Dietary modifications can reduce or eliminate these effects.

Low-dose thiazide diuretics do not produce these effects. In the Systolic Hypertension in the Elderly Program and the Hypertension Detection and Follow-Up Program, which both used diuretics as initial monotherapy or in combination, the risks for cerebrovascular and coronary events were reduced equally in persons with normal lipid levels and in those with elevated lipid levels.

Beta-blockers may increase levels of plasma triglycerides transiently and reduce levels of HDL cholesterol. Despite this, beta-blockers have been shown to reduce the rate of sudden death, overall mortality, and recurrent myocardial infarction in patients with previous myocardial infarction.

Alpha-blockers may decrease serum cholesterol concentration to a modest degree and increase HDL cholesterol. ACE inhibitors, angiotensin II receptor blockers, calcium antagonists, and central adrenergic agonists have clinically neutral effects on levels of serum lipids and lipoproteins.

Recent trials have shown that aggressive lipid reduction, especially with beta-hydroxy-beta-methylglutaryl coenzyme A (HMG-CoA) reductase inhibitors (statin drugs), provides both primary and secondary protection against CHD. Lifestyle changes and hypolipidemic agents should be used to reach appropriate goals in patients with hypertension and hyperlipidemia. Guidance in the selection of appropriate cholesterol-lowering therapy is available in the guidelines of the National Cholesterol Education Program.

Patients with Sleep Apnea

Obstructive sleep apnea, characterized by loud snoring and disrupted breathing or gasping during sleep, is more common in patients with hypertension and is associated with a number of adverse clinical consequences. Undiagnosed sleep apnea may explain the difficulty in controlling high blood pressure in some patients. Improved hypertension control has been reported in patients after treatment of their sleep apnea.

Patients with Bronchial Asthma or Chronic Airway Disease

Elevated blood pressure is relatively common in acute asthma and may be related to treatment with systemic corticosteroids or beta-agonists.

Beta-blockers and alpha-beta-blockers may exacerbate asthma; therefore, these agents should not be used in patients with asthma except in special circumstances. In addition, the topical ophthalmic application of beta-blockers such as timolol maleate may worsen asthma.

Bronchial reactivity to histamine and kinin remains unchanged with ACE inhibitors, which are safe in most patients with asthma. If a cough related to ACE inhibitor use occurs, angiotensin II receptor blockers are an alternative.

Many over-the-counter medications sold as decongestants and cold and asthma remedies may contain a sympathomimetic agent that can raise blood pressure. Nevertheless, these medications are generally safe when taken in limited doses in patients with hypertension who are receiving adequate antihypertensive therapy. Cromolyn sodium, ipratropium bromide, or corticosteroids by inhalation can be used safely for nasal congestion in persons with hypertension.

Patients with Gout

Hyperuricemia is a frequent finding in patients with untreated hypertension and may reflect a decrease in renal blood flow. In addition, all diuretics can increase serum uric acid levels but rarely induce acute gout. In patients with gout, diuretics should be avoided if possible. Diuretic-induced hyperuricemia does not require treatment in the absence of gout or urate stones.

Patients Undergoing Surgery

Blood pressure of 180/110 mm Hg or greater is associated with a greater risk for perioperative ischemic events. When possible, surgery should be delayed until blood pressure is brought down to lower levels. The perioperative risk for any patient, and especially patients with hypertension, is in part related to the adrenergic arousal before, during, and after surgery. Those without prior antihypertensive therapy may be best treated with cardioselective β-blocker therapy before and after surgery.

Adequate potassium supplementation should be provided to correct hypokalemia well in advance of surgery. Surgical candidates who are controlling their blood pressure adequately with medication should be maintained on their regimen until the time of surgery, and therapy should be reinstated as soon as possible after surgery. If oral intake must be interrupted, parenteral therapy with diuretics, adrenergic inhibitors, vasodilators, ACE inhibitors, or transdermal clonidine hydrochloride may be used to prevent the rebound hypertension that may follow sudden discontinuation of some adrenergic-inhibiting agents. Two studies have indicated a need for caution with calcium antagonists because of an increase in surgical bleeding.

Miscellaneous Causes for Increased Blood Pressure

Cocaine

The majority of cocaine-dependent individuals are normotensive, and no evidence suggests that ongoing cocaine abuse causes chronic hypertension. However, cocaine abuse must now be considered in all patients presenting to an emergency department with hypertension-related problems. Clues include the presence of chest pain, tachycardia, dilated pupils, combativeness, altered mental status, and seizures. Cocaine may induce severe ischemia from coronary and cerebral vasoconstriction as well as acute renal failure due to rhabdomyolysis.

Nitroglycerin is indicated to reverse cocaine-related coronary vasoconstriction, but its antihypertensive efficacy may be inadequate and other parenteral agents may be needed (see the "Parenteral Drugs" exhibit). Nonselective b-blockers such as propranolol should generally be avoided because of the risk of a paradoxical rise in blood pressure as well as coronary vasoconstriction due to the exaggerated effect of catecholamines on unblocked alpha-receptors.

Amphetamines

Acute amphetamine toxicity is similar to that of cocaine but longer in duration, lasting up to several hours. Cerebral and systemic vasculitis and renal failure may occur. Treatment for amphetamine toxicity is similar to that for cocaine toxicity.

Immunosuppressive Agents

Immunosuppressive regimens based on cyclosporine, tacrolimus, and steroids increase blood pressure in 50 percent to 80 percent of recipients of solid organ transplants. When cyclosporine is used alone in nontransplant applications, hypertension develops in 25 percent to 30 percent of patients. The rise in blood pressure reflects widespread vasoconstriction. Renal vasoconstriction leads to reduced glomerular filtration and enhanced sodium reabsorption. Therapy is based on vasodilation, often including dihydropyridine calcium antagonists. Diuretics are effective but may exaggerate prerenal azotemia and may precipitate gout.

Erythropoietin

Recombinant human erythropoietin increases blood pressure in 18 percent to 45 percent of patients when used in the treatment of end-stage renal disease. Hypertension is produced by a rise in systemic vascular resistance, partly related to direct vascular effects of recombinant human erythropoietin, and is not closely related to hematocrit or viscosity. Management includes optimal volume control, antihypertensive agents, and, in some cases, reducing the erythropoietin dose or changing administration from the intravenous to subcutaneous route.

Other Agents

Hypertension may be induced by numerous other chemical agents and toxins, such as mineralocorticoids and derivatives, anabolic steroids, monoamine oxidase inhibitors, lead, cadmium, and bromocriptine.

DEMOGRAPHIC DATA ON HEIGHT/BLOOD PRESSURE
DISTRIBUTION CURVES OF STUDY POPULATION

Source	Age (year)	Boys	Girls	Black	Hispanic	White	Asian	Native American	Other	Missing	Persons[a] (Visits) SBP Available	Persons[b] (Visits) DBP (K5) Available	Total No. of Persons[c] (Visits)
NIH	6-17	1,901	1,751	600	0	2,968	0	0	84	0	3,647 (3,647)	3,614 (3,614)	3,652 (3,652)
Pittsburgh	1-5	150	137	109	0	177	0	0	0	1	287 (899)	0 (0)	287 (899)
Dallas	13-17	5,916	5,649	5,266	1,570	4,729	0	0	0	0	11,565 (21,860)	11,565 (21,852)	11,565 (21,860)
Bogalusa	1-17	3,752	3,611	2,483	0	4,880	0	0	0	0	7,363 (15,922)	0 (0)	7,363 (15,922)
Houston	3-17	1,457	1,378	638	1,341	748	23	0	0	85	2,835 (2,835)	0 (0)	2,835 (2,835)
South Carolina	4-17	3,167	3,264	3,110	0	3,321	0	0	0	0	6,431 (6,431)	6,369 (6,369)	6,431 (6,431)
Iowa	5-17	2,100	1,993	0	0	4,093	0	0	0	0	4,093 (4,093)	0 (0)	4,093 (4,093)
Providence	1-3	231	231	24	4	432	0	0	2	0	462 (906)	371 (566)	462 (906)
Minnesota	9-17	9,995	9,425	3,422	556	11,320	1,678	644	1,800[d]	0	19,420 (19,420)	19,217[e] (19,217)	19,420 (19,420)
NHANES III	5-17	2,489	2,609	1,793	1,851	1,334	64	10	12	34	5,027 (5,027)	4,291[e] (4,291)	5,098 (5,098)
Total	1-17	31,158	30,048	17,445	5,322	34,002	1,765	654	1,898	120	61,130 (81,040)	45,427 (55,909)	61,206 (81,116)
Percent of Total Number of People		(51)	(49)	(29)	(9)	(56)	(3)	(1)	(3)	(0)			

SBP = systolic blood pressure; DBP = diastolic blood pressure; K5 = fifth Korotkoff sound; NIH = National Institutes of Health.
[a]Number of persons (visits) at which SBP was available.
[b]Number of persons (visits) at which DBP (K5) was available.
[c]Number of persons (visits) at which either SBP or DBP (K5) was available.
[d]These children were mostly of mixed ancestry, with the predominant categories white/black or white/Hispanic.
[e]Excludes subjects with a value of 0 for the fifth Korotkoff sound.

Source: *Update on the Task Force Report on High Blood Pressure in Children and Adolescents: A Working Group Report from the National High Blood Pressure Education Program,* NIH Publication No. 96-3790, National Heart, Lung, and Blood Institute, National Institutes of Health, September 1996.

PHARMACOLOGIC THERAPY FOR PREGNANCY-INDUCED HYPERTENSION*

Complications of pregnancy-induced hypertension (PIH) remain a leading cause of maternal mortality in the United States.[1,2] Although theories are abundant, the etiology of the disease has yet to be elucidated. The pathologic effects of PIH on maternal cardiovascular, renal, hepatic, hematologic, neurologic, and uteroplacental systems have been well described.[3] Present strategies for management emphasize prevention and control of eclamptic seizure and hypertensive crisis and correction of fluid imbalance.

Prevention and Control of Seizures

Eclampsia is the occurrence of seizures after gestation week 20 in a woman with PIH that are not caused by any coincidental neurologic disease.[4] The etiology of eclamptic seizures is unclear. Neuropathologic processes, any of which can induce seizure, may include diffuse cerebral edema; subarachnoid, subcortical, and petechial hemorrhages; small infarctions of the cerebral cortex; and hypertensive or metabolic encephalopathy.[5] Seizures arise from damaged excitable neurons whose abnormal discharge spreads to other areas of the brain, leading to secondarily generalized tonic-clonic seizures.[5,6] The electroencephalogram is abnormal in the majority of eclamptic patients, showing focal and diffuse slowing and focal and generalized epileptiform activity.[7] Seizures may appear before, during, or after delivery, but they usually occur within the first 24 postpartum hours.[8]

The three most widely prescribed drugs for the prevention and control of eclamptic seizures are magnesium sulfate, phenytoin, and diazepam.[5,6] Each of these is described in detail. Chlormethiazole, another antiepileptic agent, is popular in other parts of the world but is not available in the United States and will not be described here.[5]

Magnesium Sulfate

Magnesium sulfate has been the mainstay of prevention and treatment of eclamptic seizures in the United States for 80 years. According to Pritchard,[9] one proven therapeutic action of magnesium sulfate parenterally administered in appropriate dosage is the arrest of convulsions in women with eclampsia and the prevention of convulsions in women with severe preeclampsia. Outside the United States, however, it is used infrequently for this purpose.[6,10] Two small,

prospective, controlled trials seem to support the efficacy of magnesium sulfate. One reported that magnesium sulfate offers advantages over diazepam, including fewer recurrent seizures.[11] The second also compared magnesium sulfate with phenytoin and found similar results.[12] Generalizing the results of either of these studies is problematic because of their small sample sizes. After a comprehensive review of the literature, Sibai[13] concluded that magnesium sulfate is the ideal anticonvulsant in preeclampsia and eclampsia.[6] Most recently, a study validated the use of magnesium sulfate for the prevention of eclampsia in a large, prospective, randomized trial.[10] Investigators found that 10 of 1089 women randomly assigned to the phenytoin regimen had seizures, whereas none of the 1049 women assigned to the magnesium sulfate regimen developed them.

Some investigators have cautioned that, from the neurologic point of view, magnesium sulfate is not an effective anticonvulsant and should not be used for management of seizures when anticonvulsants with proven efficacy are available.[6,14] It has also been suggested that eclampsia is the result of hypertensive encephalopathy, and therefore it is argued that magnesium sulfate has limited usefulness because it is not an antihypertensive.[15] Nevertheless, the American College of Obstetricians and Gynecologists recommends the routine use of magnesium sulfate for this purpose.[16] Although the controversy continues, magnesium sulfate endures as the drug of choice for eclamptic seizure prophylaxis and control in the United States.

The mechanism by which magnesium sulfate exerts its action is not understood.[6,17] Magnesium sulfate may act peripherally at the neuromuscular junction, or its action may be predominantly central.[13] An increase in serum magnesium levels does have an effect on cell membranes and blocks neuromuscular and cardiac conduction.[17] The blockade of neuromuscular synapses in hypermagnesemia is due to magnesium's competition with calcium in the presynaptic membrane, inhibiting acetylcholine and calcium ion dependent release.[18] Magnesium may also exert a central effect. Cerebral vasospasm, known to occur with eclampsia, is induced by a high calcium ion concentration and is alleviated by increasing magnesium ion concentration.[19]

Cerebral ischemia causes a high intracellular calcium ion concentration that eventually leads to irreversible cell damage.[16] One route of calcium influx during ischemia is through ion channels linked to the N-methyl-D-aspartate (NMDA) receptor.[16] An increased magnesium ion concentration blocks the NMDA receptor and impedes calcium entry into the cell; in experimental models, this protects the cell from damage.[16] The NMDA receptor has been identified as one of the excitatory amino acid receptors that, when stimulated, can lead to electroencephalographic seizures and tonic-clonic convulsions.[19] Under experimental conditions, magnesium

*Source: Melissa C. Sisson, MN, RN, and Patricia M. Sauer, MSN, RNC, "Pharmacologic Therapy for Pregnancy-Induced Hypertension," *The Journal of Perinatal and Neonatal Nursing,* Vol. 9:4, Aspen Publishers, Inc., © March 1996.

inhibits activation of the NMDA receptors.[19] In theory, this magnesium blockage may prevent neuronal damage that can lead to seizure.[5,19,20]

The two most widely used regimens for the administration of magnesium sulfate are intramuscular injection and continuous intravenous infusion.[13] Based on optimal serum magnesium levels, an intravenous loading dose of 4 to 6 g followed by a maintenance dosage of 2 g/hour is prescribed.[13,17] For recurrent seizures, an intravenous bolus dose of 2 g may be administered.[13] Maternal vital signs and fetal heart rate (FHR) are monitored frequently during bolus dosing in maintenance therapy. When given intravenously, magnesium has an immediate onset of action, and its duration is 30 minutes.[17] It is excreted primarily in urine, and 90% of the dose is excreted the first 24 hours after discontinuation of the drug.[17] Its half-life is 4 hours in patients with normal renal function.[17]

Magnesium sulfate toxicity is rare and most often associated with inadvertent overdose.[17] Magnesium is therapeutic at levels from 4 to 7 mEq/L or 4 to 8 mg/dL. Deep tendon reflexes (DTRs), urine output, and respiratory rate should be assessed often because significant changes in baseline will predict toxicity. The loss of DTRs is a sign that cannot be ignored because of its correlation with a high magnesium level. If toxicity is suspected, the magnesium infusion should be decreased or discontinued until a serum magnesium level can be obtained. Because magnesium is excreted by the kidneys, oliguria can rapidly predispose to toxicity. A urine output exceeding 30 mL/hour is reassuring. Depression of respiratory rate can also occur at high magnesium levels. A rate of less than 16 breath/min may warn of respiratory arrest (see the box titled "Serum Magnesium Levels: Therapeutic Levels and Toxicity"). The antidote for magnesium is calcium gluconate, which should be kept at the bedside. The usual dosage is 1 g of 10% solution administered by intravenous push over 1 to 2 minutes.

Reports on the effects of magnesium sulfate on the fetus and newborn are inconclusive.[13,17] Among the findings in the newborn are increased, decreased, and no effect on FHR variability; low Apgar scores; respiratory depression; hypotonia; and hypocalcemia.[13,17] It is known that magnesium ions cross the placenta and achieve equilibrium between mother and fetus.[4] It is probable that infants of mothers receiving the appropriate dosage according to a defined protocol are not born with clinically significant hypermagnesemia.[4]

Magnesium sulfate is easy to administer and monitor, rapidly effective, and reliable.[17] It has the additional advantage of being universally known to obstetricians and perinatal nurses practicing in the United States.[13] At present, there is little evidence with which to refute magnesium sulfate as the preferred drug for the prevention and treatment of eclamptic seizures.

Phenytoin

In the nonpregnant patient, phenytoin is the preferred drug for seizure prophylaxis.[21] In the United Kingdom, Australia, and Canada, it has been advocated for the prevention and treatment of eclamptic convulsions. Some internists and neurologists in the United States are also recommending phenytoin for this purpose. Recent investigation seems to indicate that further study is warranted, however. An evaluation of a phenytoin regimen based on maternal weight in 26 patients found no seizures or significant maternal or neonatal adverse effects.[22] Another study reported that patients receiving phenytoin tended toward more rapid cervical dilation, smaller decreases in postpartum hematocrit, and fewer side effects than patients in the magnesium sulfate group.[23] Magnesium may actually predispose to these effects because it impairs smooth muscle contraction. After randomization of mild preeclamptics to phenytoin and magnesium sulfate groups, no significant differences in patient tolerance, adverse reaction, or neonatal outcomes were discovered.[24] Another study made a similar comparison and found that phenytoin produced fewer side effects and had better patient acceptance.[6] In contrast, other studies have reported seizures in patients with therapeutic phenytoin levels.[10,12,25,26] It has been hypothesized that phenytoin may be less effective in severe preeclampsia and eclampsia, possibly as a result of decreased cerebral perfusion.[26]

The precise mechanism of action of phenytoin is unknown, but some studies suggest that it modulates sodium and calcium exchange and prostaglandins.[6] It can also inhibit the vasoconstrictive effect of norepinephrine.[6] Phenytoin has a stabilizing effect on all neuronal membranes and suppresses episodes of repetitive firing.[12] It enters the brain rapidly, and anticonvulsant activity is present within minutes.[12]

A variety of treatment regimens have been recommended. Lucas et al[27] administered 1 g of phenytoin intravenously followed by 500 mg orally 10 hours later and concluded that

---

Serum Magnesium Levels: Therapeutic Levels and Toxicity

Therapeutic level	4–8 mg/dL
Loss of patellar reflexes	9–12 mg/dL*
Respiratory arrest	15–17 mg/dL
Cardiac arrest	30–35 mg/dL

*Early signs and symptoms of toxicity include nausea, weakness, warm sensation, flushing, somnolence, double vision, and slurred speech.
Source: Data from Sibai.[13]

a universal dosing regimen comparable to that for magnesium sulfate is feasible. The therapeutic range for anticonvulsant activity is 10 to 20 µg/mL.[17] There is potential for cardiotoxicity with intravenous administration of phenytoin, and therefore continuous electrocardiographic monitoring during infusion may be prudent.[6,17] It is free phenytoin that exerts its therapeutic effects, but 90% is bound to plasma proteins. Plasma proteins are typically low in PIH, and in theory this could produce a high free phenytoin level because there is less protein to bind phenytoin. It has been hypothesized that a low dosage of 12.5 mg/min will reduce the likelihood of a high free phenytoin level.[6] Chronic administration of phenytoin has been associated with alteration in vitamin K-dependent coagulation.[6]

Phenytoin is metabolized by hepatic microsomal enzymes and should be used cautiously when liver function is impaired. For this reason, the administration of phenytoin in the PIH patient with elevated serum oxaloacetic transaminase may be ill advised. Features of phenytoin toxicity are related to disturbances in the cerebellum and vestibular system and include nystagmus, ataxia, and lethargy at levels of 20, 30, and 40 µg/mL, respectively[6] (see the box titled "Serum Phenytoin Levels: Therapeutic Levels and Toxicity").

Phenytoin crosses the placenta and is teratogenic during early pregnancy.[17] When phenytoin is administered during the intrapartum period, however, neonatal side effects are not observed.[6]

The advantages of phenytoin over magnesium sulfate include a long half-life and the availability of an oral preparation.[27] These benefits should be weighed against potential disadvantages as the application of phenytoin therapy in obstetrics continues to be evaluated.

Diazepam

Diazepam has long been recognized as the drug of choice for the management of status epilepticus.[17] In epilepsy models, the benzodiazepines may inhibit the propagation of seizure activity without suppressing the seizure focus.[6] The widespread use of this class of drugs is related to their safety and ease of administration. In Britain, diazepam is routinely used in eclamptic patients to stop seizures and prevent recurrence.[17] The usual dose is 10 mg administered intravenously up to 30 mg. Doses in excess of 30 mg may cause sedation and increase the risk of maternal aspiration.[17] Diazepam has also been reported to result in neonatal hypotonia, hypothermia, lethargy, apnea, and poor sucking effort.[5,17] In the United States, diazepam has been used as an adjunct to magnesium sulfate for the control of seizures.[10,17]

Management of Hypertensive Crisis

Hypertension in PIH is secondary to generalized arterial vasoconstriction.[4,28] Hypertensive crisis that produces vascular damage is defined as a systolic blood pressure exceeding 200 mm Hg or a diastolic blood pressure exceeding 120 mm Hg.[28,29] Severe hypertension can lead to intracerebral hemorrhage, hypertensive encephalopathy, acute renal failure, congestive heart failure, ventricular dysrhythmias, and placental abruption with disseminated intravascular coagulopathy.[28] Intracerebral hemorrhage is the most common cause of maternal death in eclampsia.[3] Autoregulation of cerebral circulation normally protects the brain from fluctuations in systemic blood pressure. Autoregulation fails at a mean arterial pressure (MAP) of 150 to 170 mm Hg, and if pressure continues to rise arterial wall damage ensues.[29] In experimental models, histologic abnormalities are present within 10 minutes of exposure to high pressures, and damage becomes extensive within 1 hour.[30] Most investigators recommend drug therapy for maternal blood pressures of 170/110 or higher.[4,5,13,30]

The goal of antihypertensive therapy is to reduce maternal blood pressure rapidly but not precipitously, with the end point being maintenance of a blood pressure not less than 130/90.[30] Further reduction of blood pressure may not be tolerated by a mother and/or fetus accustomed to the high pressures. A number of effective antihypertensives are available, although new agents are introduced cautiously into obstetric practice because of potential effects on the fetus.[28] The following discussion covers the drugs that are currently used (see the box titled "Nursing Implications in Antihypertensive Therapy").

Hydralazine

Hydralazine is a direct-acting vasodilator that dilates arteries and arterioles and has little impact on venous capacitance vessels.[28] It is the most widely prescribed drug for the rapid control of hypertension in pregnancy in the United States.[4] A reflex tachycardia and renin-mediated fluid retention may increase cardiac output, which may increase uteroplacental

---

Serum Phenytoin Levels: Therapeutic Levels and Toxicity

Therapeutic level	10–20 µg/mL*
Nystagmus	20 µg/mL
Ataxia	>30 µg/mL
Lethargy	>40 µg/mL

*Hypotension, tachycardia, and sedation may occur during loading dose. These signs and symptoms are usually transient with no long-term sequelae.
Source: Data from Repke et al[6] and Naidu et al.[26]

Nursing Implications in Antihypertensive Therapy

Avoid precipitous drops in blood pressure by administering agents slowly

Monitor for drops in blood pressure:
- Monitor blood pressure carefully when administering agent
- Monitor FHR changes that may indicate maternal hypotension and decreased cardiac output:
  - bradycardia
  - tachycardia
  - late decelerations
  - prolonged decelerations
  - loss of short-term variability

If hypotension occurs:
- Use lateral positioning
- Use the modified Trendelenburg position
- Evaluate for hypovolemia
- Monitor for FHR changes
- Ensure adequate intravenous hydration

blood flow.[17,30,31] Excessive reduction of blood pressure can occur when the dose is repeated or when shorter intervals or continuous infusions are used.[17,30]

Hydralazine is metabolized by the liver.[17] Side effects are headache, tremor, tachycardia, flushing, nausea, and vomiting.[17] A reversible lupuslike syndrome occurs only with long-term treatment. Although these effects are uncomfortable for the patient, none is serious.

Hydralazine crosses the placenta, and fetal serum concentration is equal to or greater than that of the mother.[13] Because hydralazine is a potent antihypertensive, an abrupt reduction in blood flow can reduce oxygen delivery to the fetus. A nonreassuring FHR pattern on electronic fetal monitoring (EFM) indicating overshoot hypotension has been reported.[17,32]

Hydralazine is the oldest antihypertensive in clinical practice. Its safety and efficacy in pregnancy have been demonstrated over many years, and consequently it remains the standard antihypertensive agent for blood pressure control in severe preeclampsia.[3,4]

Labetalol Hydrochloride

Labetalol lowers arterial pressure by reducing systemic vascular resistance. It is a combination α- and β-adrenergic blocking agent and may also cause vasodilation via β_{+2}-receptor stimulation.[28,30] The sympathetic nervous system has both α and β receptors that enable it to exert its effect on

target organs and tissues. The α receptors affect vascular smooth muscle and produce vasoconstriction when stimulated. The β receptor types are subdivided, with β_1 affecting the heart and β_2 affecting primarily the lungs. Labetalol exerts its effect on blood pressure by nonselectively blocking α and β receptors.

A comparison of labetalol with hydralazine found that hydralazine lowers MAP more but that labetalol has a more rapid onset; furthermore, duration of action and dosage were variable in the labetalol group.[33] It was also found that labetalol is less likely to produce excessive hypotension and rebound tachycardia, both of which are seen with hydralazine.[33]

Labetalol is metabolized by the liver and excreted in the urine.[17] Maternal side effects include flushing and tremulousness.[17] Labetalol-treated subjects were found to have fewer malignant ventricular dysrhythmias compared with those treated with hydralazine; the investigators in this study concluded that β blockade improves myocardial oxygenation.[32] No deleterious fetal or neonatal effects have been reported.[17] One study did suggest that fetal β blockade may occur after maternal administration of labetalol based on the observation of reduced umbilical artery pulsatility index.[34]

Labetalol is not known to decrease uterine blood flow.[17] It appears to be a safe alternative to hydralazine, but further study of its effect on the fetus and neonate is indicated.[30]

Nifedipine

Nifedipine is an arterial vasodilator that acts by relaxation of smooth muscle through slow calcium channel blockade.[12,28] When calcium entry into smooth muscle or myocardial cells is impeded, excitation and contraction cannot occur. Nifedipine acts directly on vascular smooth muscle to produce vasodilation and has little cardiac effect.

A study was conducted that compared nifedipine with hydralazine in 49 preeclamptic patients.[35] Subjects had blood pressures exceeding 160/110, and all were receiving magnesium sulfate. Patients in both groups experienced minor side effects. Patients in the hydralazine group experienced transient increases in heart rate and dizziness. Hot flashes and headaches occurred in the nifedipine-treated group. A nonreassuring FHR pattern on EFM possibly associated with the administration of hydralazine occurred in 11 of 27 subjects. The investigators concluded that nifedipine is superior to hydralazine because it is more effective at controlling blood pressure, response is more predictable, and administration is more convenient.

Maternal adverse effects include headache, palpitation, and cutaneous flushing.[36] Nifedipine has been used for the inhibition of preterm labor, and its administration for blood pressure control may interfere with labor.[17] It does not appear to reduce uteroplacental blood flow or to cause FHR abnormality.[17,36] There are reports of exaggerated hypotension and muscle weakness when nifedipine and magnesium sulfate are administered concomitantly.[37] Magnesium is known to compete with calcium at the presynaptic membrane and therefore may potentiate the effects of calcium channel blockers.[17]

Nifedipine is increasingly used in PIH, especially when response to other agents is insufficient.[37] Its rapid onset when taken orally is advantageous. Care should be exercised when the patient is also on magnesium sulfate, however, because of a potential synergistic effect. Although nifedipine appears safe for treatment of hypertensive crisis in pregnancy, further controlled clinical trials are necessary before general clinical use can be advocated.[38]

Sodium Nitroprusside

Sodium nitroprusside is a potent direct vasodilator. Its exact mechanism of action is unknown, but it appears to interact with membrane-bound sulfhydryl groups to produce vasodilation.[31] It reduces preload by acting on venous capacitance vessels and reduces afterload by arteriolar dilation.

Sodium nitroprusside's onset of action is immediate and because of its short half-life the duration of effect is 1 to 3 minutes after discontinuation of the drug. It combines with hemoglobin to produce methemoglobin and cyanide.[31] Cyanide is metabolized in the liver to thiocyanate, which is excreted in urine.[17,31] Sodium nitroprusside crosses the placenta, and cyanide can accumulate if it is not converted to thiocyanate by the fetal liver after administration of large doses or prolonged administration or in the presence of altered metabolism.[17] Regarding maternal adverse effects, some investigators have warned that circulatory distress and paradoxic bradycardia can occur, apparently secondary to maternal hypovolemia associated with severe preeclampsia.[39] Correction of maternal hypovolemia before the administration of antihypertensives is essential to avoid profound hypotension.[38] Also, arterial blood gases should be monitored regularly because metabolic acidosis is a sign of cyanide toxicity. An intraarterial line for continuous blood pressure monitoring is indicated.[40]

Concern about fetal cyanide toxicity has limited the use of sodium nitroprusside during pregnancy to patients whose hypertension is refractory to other agents.[3,17] Treatment duration should be short when sodium nitroprusside is used in the antepartum patient.

Prevention and Control of Fluid Imbalance

Recent literature suggests that plasma volume in PIH is contracted in comparison with that in normal pregnancy. Derangements in the forces controlling fluid balance in PIH can lead to complications such as oliguria and pulmonary edema. Judicious fluid therapy is a mainstay of the successful management of PIH.

Regulation of Fluid Balance

Whenever a membrane between two fluid compartments is permeable to water but not to certain particles within the fluid, and the concentration of particles is greater on one side of the membrane than on the other, water will move through the membrane to the compartment with the most particles.[41] Colloids are high-molecular weight proteins that cannot cross uninjured semipermeable membranes. In contrast, crystalloids are low-molecular weight particles that freely cross semipermeable membranes. The plasma colloid proteins are albumin, globulin, and fibrogen, with albumin having the highest concentration. Colloids are also found in the interstitial space. Fluid moves from the space with the highest concentration of colloids to the space with the lowest concentration of colloids when the semipermeable membrane is intact. The pressure gradient that exists across the membrane is directly proportional to the fluid shifts that result from nonmovement of the colloid molecules.[42] This pressure exerted by plasma proteins is referred to as colloid osmotic pressure (COP). The wall of the capillary is the semipermeable membrane across which fluid shifts.

As described, the movement of fluid between the intravascular space and the interstitial space is determined by COP and also by the integrity of the capillary membrane. Another force that affects the movement of fluid is capillary hydrostatic pressure. Hydrostatic pressure represents the pressure exerted by the fluid within the vessels, and it directly opposes COP.[43] COP is the pulling force that holds fluid within the capillary. Hydrostatic pressure is the pushing force that results in the movement of fluid out of the capillary. An increase in capillary hydrostatic pressure, a decrease in COP, and an increase in capillary permeability are all factors that may cause excessive movement of fluid and proteins into the interstitial space.[41] These are also factors that may be altered in PIH.

COP is measurable and is decreased in both the normal pregnancy and the pregnancy complicated by PIH (Table 1). Low COP values in preeclampsia are probably the result of serum protein movement across damaged capillaries into subcutaneous tissues and across damaged glomerular capillaries into the urine.[42] The end result is protein loss from plasma and hypoalbuminemia. Capillary endothelial damage is a hallmark of the disease process.

Fluid Therapy

Intravenous fluids contain colloids or crystalloids. Examples of crystalloid solutions are lactated Ringer's solution and 5% dextrose in water. Blood products, albumin, and

Table 1. COP Values

Period	COP (mm Hg)	
	Normal	Preeclampsia
Pregnancy (term)	22.4±0.54	17.9±0.7
Postpartum (24 hours)	15.4±2.1	13.7±0.5

Source: Adapted from Moise and Cotton.[42]

Plasmanule are examples of colloid solutions. Infusion of crystalloid solutions reduces COP because of a dilutional effect.[42] Infusion of colloid solutions in the absence of damaged capillary membranes draws fluid into the intravascular space.[42]

Use of colloid solutions to expand plasma volume in PIH has generated controversy for years.[41] Maternal hypovolemia can be corrected by adding colloids to the colloid-depleted intravascular space. The danger is that colloids can leak into the interstitial space through the damaged vascular endothelium caused by preeclampsia.[42,43] If colloid concentration in the interstitial space exceeds that in the intravascular space, then fluid can follow the colloids into the interstitial space.[42,43] When an imbalance such as this occurs in the lungs, the result can be pulmonary edema. Many investigators have concluded that the routine use of colloid solutions for correction of low COP in the PIH patient is not justified.[3,42]

The preferred fluid therapy in PIH is crystalloid infusion, usually with lactated Ringer's solution or normal saline.[3] The recommended rate of infusion is 100 to 125 mL/hour. Fluid intake and urinary output should be monitored often because of the potential for imbalance between oncotic and hydrostatic forces. Overhydration can quickly lead to pulmonary edema in the patient with PIH.

Hypovolemia

Severe preeclampsia is often accompanied by relative hypovolemia, and consequently intravascular volume expansion has a role in its acute management.[44] As discussed previously, when vasodilator therapy is introduced in patients with hypertensive crisis who are also volume depleted, the result may be profound hypotension. To obtain a smooth response to antihypertensive therapy, repletion of intravascular volume is recommended.[44]

Epidural anesthesia is associated with maternal hypotension secondary to sympathetic blockade. When it is preceded by volume loading, it is safe and effective in severe preeclampsia and may improve intervillous blood flow.[44] An intravenous bolus of 1000 to 1500 mL of crystalloid solution is recommended.[3]

If urine output falls below 25 to 30 mL/hour over 2 consecutive hours, oliguria is present.[3] Its cause may be considered prerenal or volume related on most occasions, and the treatment is administration of 500 to 1000 mL fluid challenge with normal saline or lactated Ringer's solution over 30 minutes.[45] If urine output does not respond within 1 hour, other causes of oliguria must be suspected. Pulmonary artery catheterization may be indicated to determine the exact nature of oliguria that persists after fluid challenge. Neglect of persistent oliguria can lead to acute renal tubular or cortical necrosis.[45]

Fluid Overload

Inadvertent fluid overload may place the patient with PIH at increased risk for pulmonary edema. The incidence of pulmonary edema associated with PIH is 3%.[3] Reduction of COP, elevated pulmonary capillary wedge pressure, and increased capillary permeability may all promote extravasation of fluid into the interstitial and alveolar spaces with resulting pulmonary edema.[3] Crystalloid infusion is known to reduce COP.[46] Iatrogenic fluid overload may result in hydrostatic pulmonary edema with normal left ventricular function.[3] The most common time for pulmonary edema to occur is 15 hours after delivery, when COP (the pulling force) is low and hydrostatic pressure (the pushing force) is rising as fluid begins to shift from the extravascular to the intravascular space.[47] The combination of a low COP and an increasing hydrostatic pressure due to postpartum fluid shift and intravenous solutions explains pulmonary edema.[48] Colloid solutions should be used selectively, if at all, in patients with severe preeclampsia.

Conclusion

Current pharmacologic management of PIH focuses upon the prevention and control of eclamptic seizures, prevention of hypertensive crisis, and correction of fluid imbalance. Selection of the most appropriate agents for achieving these management priorities can be controversial and is often based on successful past experience with the agents. Additional clinical trials are needed to establish efficacy of both old and new agents. One reason for the slow introduction of new agents for the management of PIH is the need to establish these agents' safety for the fetus and newborn. This requires an unhurried and deliberative process. The arsenal of drugs for management of PIH will expand as research continues.

REFERENCES

1. Atrash HK, Rowley D, Hogne CJ. Maternal and perinatal mortality. *Curr Opin Obstet Gynecol.* 1992;4:61–71.

2. Rochat RW, Koonin LM, Atrash HK, Vewett JJ. Maternal mortality in the United States: Report from the Maternal Mortality Collaborative. *Obstet Gynecol.* 1988;73:91–97.

3. Clark SL, Cotton DB, Hankins GD, Phelan JP. *Critical Care Obstetrics.* 2nd ed. Boston; Mass: Blackwell Scientific; 1991.

4. Pritchard JA, MacDonald PC, Gant NF. *Williams Obstetrics.* 18th ed. Norwalk, Conn: Appleton & Lange; 1993.

5. Kaplan PW, Repke JT. Eclampsia. *Neurol Clin.* 1994;12:565–581.

6. Repke JT, Friedman SA, Kaplan PW. Prophylaxis of eclampic seizures: Current controversies. *Clin Obstet Gynecol.* 1992;35:365–375.

7. Sibai BM, Spinnato JA, Watson DL, et al. Effect of magnesium sulfate in electroencephalographic findings in preeclampsia-eclampsia. *Obstet Gynecol.* 1984;64:261–266.

8. Sibai BM. Eclampsia VI. Maternal-perinatal outcome in 254 consecutive cases. *Am J. Obstet Gynecol.* 1990;163:1049–1053.

9. Pritchard JA. The use of magnesium sulfate in preeclampsia-eclampsia. *J Reprod Med.* 1979;23:107–113.

10. Lucas MJ, Leveno KJ, Cunningham FG. A comparison of magnesium sulfate with phenytoin for the prevention of eclampsia. *N Engl J. Med.* 1995;333:201–205.

11. Crowther C. Magnesium sulphate versus diazepam in the management of eclampsia. *Br J Obstet Gynaecol.* 1990;97:110–117.

12. Dommisse J. Phenytoin sodium and magnesium sulphate in the management of eclampsia. *Br J Obstet Gynaecol.* 1990;97:104–109.

13. Sibai BM. Magnesium sulfate is the ideal anticonvulsant in preeclampsia-eclampsia. *Am J Obstet Gynecol.* 1990;162:1141–1145.

14. Kaplan PW, Lesser RP, Fisher RS, et al. No, magnesium sulfate should not be used in treating eclamptic convulsions. *Arch Neurol.* 1988;45:1361–1364.

15. Donaldson JO. Eclampsia and other causes of peripartum convulsions. In: Donaldson JO, ed. *Neurology of Pregnancy.* Philadelphia, Pa: Saunders; 1978.

16. American College of Obstetricians and Gynecologists (ACOG). *Management of Preeclampsia.* Washington, DC: ACOG; 1986. ACOG technical bulletin 91.

17. McCombs J. Preeclampsia-eclampsia. *Clin Pharm.* 1992;11:236–244.

18. Sadeh M. Action of magnesium sulfate in the treatment of preeclampsia-eclampsia. *Stroke.* 1989;20:1273–1275.

19. Altura BT, Altura BM. The role of magnesium in etiology of strokes and cerebrovasospasm. *Magnesium.* 1982;1:277–291.

20. Cotton DB, Hallak M, Jannez C, Intenkauf SM, Berman RF. Central anticonvulsant effects of magnesium sulfate on *N*-methyl-D-aspartate-induced seizures. *Am J Obstet Gynecol.* 1993;168:974–978.

21. Ryan G, Lange IR, Naugler M. Clinical experience with phenytoin prophylaxis in severe preeclampsia. *Am J Obstet Gynecol.* 1989;161:1297–1304.

22. Slater RM, Wilcox FL, Smith WD, et al. Phenytoin infusion in severe preeclampsia. *Lancet.* 1987;1:1417–1420.

23. Friedman SA, Lim K, Baker CA, Repke JT. Phenytoin versus magnesium sulfate in preeclampsia—A pilot study. *Am J Perinatol.* 1993;10:233–237.

24. Appleton MP, Kuchl TJ, Racbel J, Adams HR, Knight AB, Gold WR. Magnesium sulfate versus phenytoin for seizure prophylaxis in pregnancy-induced hypertension. *Am J Obstet Gynecol.* 1991;165:907–913.

25. Tuffnell D, O'Donovan P, Lilford RJ, Prys-Davies A, Thoraton JG. Phenytoin in preeclampsia. *Lancet.* 1989;2:273–274.

26. Naidu S, Moodley J, Botha J, McFadyen L. The efficacy of phenytoin in relation to serum levels in severe preeclampsia and eclampsia. *Br J Obstet Gynaecol.* 1992;99:881–886.

27. Lucas MJ, Depalma RT, Peters MT, Leveno KJ, Person D, Cunningham FG. A simplified phenytoin regimen. *Am J Perinatol.* 1994;11:153–156.

28. Barton JR, Sibai BM. Acute life-threatening emergencies in preeclampsia-eclampsia. *Clin Obstet Gynecol.* 1992;35:402–413.

29. Sauer PM, Harvey CJ. Pregnancy-induced hypertension. *Crit Care Nurs Clin North Am.* 1992;4:703–710.

30. Naden RP, Redman CW. Antihypertensive drugs in pregnancy. *Clin Perinatol.* 1985;12:521–538.

31. Simon R, Reynolds HN. Afterload reduction. *Crit Care Rep.* 1990;1:415–421.

32. Bhorat IE, Naidoo DE, Rout CE, Moodley J. Malignant ventricular arrhythmias in eclampsia: A comparison of labetalol with hydralazine. *Obstet Gynecol.* 1993;4:1292–1296.

33. Mabie WE, Gonzalez AR, Sibai BM, Amon E. A comparative trial of labetalol and hydralazine in the acute management of severe hypertension complicating pregnancy. *Obstet Gynecol.* 1987;70:328–333.

34. Harper A, Murnaghan GA, Maternal and fetal hemodynamics in hypertensive pregnancies during maternal treatment with intravenous hydralazine or labetalol. *Br J Obstet Gynaecol.* 1991;98:453–459.

35. Fenakel K, Fenakel G, Appelman Z. Nifedipine in the treatment of severe preeclampsia. *Obstet Gynecol.* 1991;77:335–337.

36. Walters BNJ, Redman CWG. Treatment of severe pregnancy-associated hypertension with the calcium antagonist nifedipine. *Br J Obstet Gynaecol.* 1984;91:330–336.

37. Waisman GD, Mayorga LM, Camera MI, Vignolo CA, Martinotti A. Magnesium plus nifedipine: Potentiation of hypotensive effect in preeclampsia? *Obstet Gynecol.* 1988;159:308–309.

38. Dildy GA, Phelan JP, Colton DB. Complications of pregnancy-induced hypertension. In: Clark SK, et al, eds. *Critical Care Obstetrics.* Boston; Mass: Blackwell Scientific; 1991.

39. Wasserstrum N. Nitroprusside in preeclampsia hypertension. 1991;18:79–84.

40. Doary W, Brinkman CR. Antihypertensive drugs in pregnancy. *Clin Perinatol.* 1987;14:783–800.

41. Guyton AC. *Textbook of Medical Physiology.* 8th ed. Philadelphia, Pa: Saunders; 1991.

42. Moise KJ, Cotton DB. The use of colloid osmotic pressure in pregnancy. *Clin Perinatol.* 1986;13:827–841.

43. Stewart LS. Pulmonary edema during pregnancy. *Clin Issues Perinat Women's Health Nurs.* 1992;3:454–460.

44. Wasserstrum N, Cotton DB. Hemodynamic monitoring in severe pregnancy-induced hypertension. *Clin Perinatol.* 1986;13:781–799.

45. Clark SL, Greenspoon JS, Aldahl D, Phelan JP. Severe preeclampsia with persistent oliguria: Management of hemodynamic subsets. *Am J Obstet Gynecol.* 1985;154:490–494.

46. Strauss RG, Kecfen R, Burke T. Hemodynamic monitoring of cardiogenic pulmonary edema complicating toxemia of pregnancy. *Obstet Gynecol.* 1980;55:170–174.

47. Jones MM, Longmire S, Cotton DB, Dorman KF, Skjonsby BS. Influence of crystalloid vs colloid infusion on peripartum colloid osmotic pressure changes. *Obstet Gynecol.* 1986;68:659–661.

48. Benedetti TJ, Kates R, William V. Hemodynamic observations in severe preeclampsia complicated by pulmonary edema. *Am J Obstet Gynecol.* 1985;152:330–334.

TREATMENT OF HYPERTENSION IN PATIENTS WITH DIABETES*

Approximately three million Americans have both hypertension and diabetes.[1,2] For patients with noninsulin dependent diabetes mellitus (NIDDM), the incidence of essential hypertension increases with age and exists in about one out of every two patients.[2,3] In patients with both insulin-dependent diabetes mellitus (IDDM) and NIDDM, diabetic nephropathy is also an important factor for the development of hypertension.[4] Uncontrolled hypertension and diabetes are risk factors for cardiovascular mortality and morbidity, renal dysfunction, and retinopathy.[5,6] In patients with diabetes, the presence of hypertension may lead to premature and more severe cardiovascular events as well as perpetuate renal and retinal dysfunction. The relationship between diabetes and hypertension is not fully understood, but it is clear that these diseases are interrelated.[3] Hyperinsulinemia (insulin resistance) may affect the sympathetic and renin-angiotensin systems' sodium excretion by the kidneys and interfere with peripheral vasodilation.[7-9] These effects may contribute, in part, to elevations in blood pressure. Furthermore, hyperinsulinemia may contribute to or is associated with dyslipidemia and obesity.[10] Although the exact interrelation between hypertension and diabetes is unknown, patients with both conditions are at increased risk for associated morbidity and mortality than with either hypertension or diabetes alone. For these reasons, patients with hypertension and diabetes should be treated early and aggressively.[3] To accomplish this goal, a number of consensus statements on the management and treatment of hypertension and diabetes have been developed and promulgated.[3,11,12,13]

Consensus Statements

A number of expert panels and government agencies have offered consensus statements with respect to the detection, management, and treatment of hypertension and diabetes. To this end, the goal of these efforts, in general, is to increase awareness of the impact of hypertension and diabetes as well as guide health care providers to provide optimal care for patients with diabetes and hypertension. For example, The National High Blood Pressure Education Program Working Group has published and updated its report on diabetes and hypertension.[3,14]

The goal blood pressure to be attained in hypertensive diabetic patients is less than 130/85 mm Hg. To achieve this goal, nondrug therapies and lifestyle modifications should be employed for three months. If an inadequate response or

*Source: Bradley G. Phillips, Pharm D, "Treatment of Hypertension in Patients with Diabetes," *Pharmacy Practice Management Quarterly*, Vol. 17:3, Aspen Publishers, Inc., © October 1997.

considerable progress has not been achieved, drug therapy should be initiated. Drugs from various classes that include angiotensin converting enzyme (ACE) inhibitors, alpha blockers, calcium channel antagonists, and low-dose diuretics may be initially considered while continuing nondrug and lifestyle modification efforts. Due to the compelling and growing evidence for the renal protective effects of ACE inhibitors, they are now considered the drugs of choice in insulin-dependent and noninsulin-dependent diabetic patients who have albuminuria or proteinuria. If initial monotherapy with any of the above agents does not provide an adequate response, the dose may be increased, another agent may be tried, or a second agent may be added to the therapy. Failing this, a second or third antihypertensive agent may be added to attain the desired blood pressure. If not prescribed for initial therapy, low-dose diuretic therapy should be included in subsequent therapy. Beta blockers, although effective in controlling blood pressure, are reserved for those hypertensive diabetic patients who have a clear indication other than hypertension for beta-blocker therapy. This treatment algorithm outlines general treatment strategies that should be considered along with other patient and drug-related issues and considerations before a specific treatment plan is formulated for each diabetic patient.[14]

Therapy Considerations

Selection of the optimal antihypertensive agent in each patient with diabetes should be based on the agent's impact on morbidity and mortality, glucose, electrolytes, insulin resistance, and lipids, as well as the cost of therapy and associated drug-induced adverse effects. Thiazide diuretics and beta blockers have been shown to reduce cardiovascular morbidity and mortality in patients with hypertension.[15-18] For these reasons, they are considered the initial drugs of choice in the treatment of hypertension by the Joint National Committee on the Detection, Evaluation, and Treatment of High Blood Pressure (JNC).[19] However, no study to date has evaluated the impact of these agents, or others, on cardiovascular morbidity and mortality in the diabetic population. It is assumed that diuretics and beta blockers will indeed confer the same beneficial effect on morbidity and mortality in hypertensive diabetic patients as they do in nondiabetic patients. There are several studies to give support to or possibly refute this presumption. The Systolic Hypertension in the Elderly Program (SHEP) evaluated the efficacy of low-dose diuretic, with atenolol and reserpine if needed, with placebo in 4,736 patients with an average baseline systolic blood pressure of 160 mm Hg or greater and a diastolic blood pressure of less than 90 mm Hg.[20] The study found that with an average of four and a half years of active treatment, there was a 36 and 27 percent decrease in fatal and nonfatal strokes and myocardial infarctions, respectively, compared to those patients receiving placebo. A subsequent analysis to compare study outcomes in patients with NIDDM to patients without diabetes enrolled in SHEP revealed that both groups had a 34 percent reduction in cardiovascular disease rate at five years.[21] Further, the absolute risk reduction for treatment compared to placebo in patients with NIDDM was twice as great compared to patients without diabetes.[21] Conversely, Warram and colleagues found an increase in cardiovascular mortality in 759 hypertensive diabetic patients receiving diuretic therapy.[22] This finding is supported by another study, which reported a similar outcome for hypertensive diabetics receiving diuretic therapy.[23]

These conflicting results have fostered, in part, divergent opinions on the role of diuretic and beta-blocker therapies in patients with diabetes. Regardless, many consensus statements support low-dose diuretics for the treatment of hypertension in the diabetic population.[3,13,14] Other antihypertensive therapies (e.g., ACE inhibitors, calcium channel antagonists, and alpha blockers) are currently being evaluated in ongoing trials that are designed to evaluate the impact of treatment on morbidity and mortality in hypertensive patients.

The clinical implications of insulin resistance are a possible effect on blood pressure, lipids, and obesity. Antihypertensive agents have varying effects on insulin sensitivity. In general, ACE inhibitors, alpha blockers, and calcium channel antagonists improve insulin sensitivity and lipidemia, or are lipid neutral.[24–26] Conversely, beta blockers and diuretics may worsen insulin sensitivity and the lipid profile (see Table 1).[27,28] Electrolyte imbalances may be provoked by ACE inhibitors and diuretics. Although it is unclear if these possible drug-induced changes produce clinically relevant changes in the long-term, it would seem prudent to consider these effects in each diabetic patient at the time the decision is made to initiate a specific agent to treat high blood pressure. For example, in a patient with documented hyperinsulinemia or insulin resistance, it may be prudent to select an agent that does not worsen insulin sensitivity.

Pharmacologic selection to treat blood pressure in patients with diabetes should also take into consideration the patient's concomitant disease states, medical history, and ability to pay for medications. In doing so, an antihypertensive that has a proven beneficial impact on other disease states, independent of its effect on blood pressure, may be prescribed. For example, an ACE inhibitor may be considered over other antihypertensive therapies in a patient who has diabetes and also has congestive heart failure or left ventricular hypertrophy.[29–31] Similarly, an alpha blocker may be favored if the patient suffers from benign prostatic hypertrophy. Therefore, the efficacy of the agent to control blood pressure and its effect on body chemistry should be considered in concert with its documented benefit in other disease states (see Table 2). Ultimately, drug therapy will be doomed to failure, regardless of its efficacy and beneficial effects on other disease states, if the patient cannot afford to pay for the medication.

Perhaps the most important consideration is to treat hypertension, diabetes, and dyslipidemia aggressively, as each is associated with significant morbidity and mortality.[3] Therefore, in striving to attain optimal blood pressure control, the same effort should be directed to maintain glycemic control. Intensive insulin therapy in IDDM has been reported to delay the onset and slow the progression of diabetic neuropathy, retinopathy, and nephropathy.[32] It is unknown, however, if intensive insulin therapy in NIDDM would produce similar outcomes. As insulin resistance may play more of a role in the progression and severity of diabetic complications in patients with NIDDM, insulin therapy may be withheld until oral agents have been initiated and optimized. To this end, patients with NIDDM may be prescribed oral sulfonylureas and, now, newer agents like metformin and acarbose in an attempt to control glycemia without aggravating insulin resistance.

Specific treatment measures and unique issues common to each specific class of antihypertensive drugs are delineated below with specific reference to the hypertensive diabetic population.

Table 1. The Impact of Various Classes of Antihypertensive Agents on Body Chemistry

	ACE inhibitors	Alpha blockers	Beta blockers	Calcium channel antagonists	Diuretics
Insulin sensitivity	↑	↑	↓	- ↑	- ↓
Electrolytes	- ↑	-	-	-	↓ ↑
Lipidemia	-	↓	- ↑	-	↑
Glycemia	- ↓	-	↑	-	↑

Notes: ↑ = increase, ↓ = decrease, - = neutral.

Table 2. Treatment Considerations with Various Disease States or Conditions

Coexisting condition	ACE inhibitor	Alpha blocker	Beta blocker	Calcium channel antagonist	Diuretic
DM	++	++	-	+	+/-
Aged	+/-	+	+/-	++	++
CHF	+++	+/-	-	-	++
CAD	+	+	++	+/-	+/-
LVH	+	+/-	+	+	+/-

Notes: DM = diabetes mellitus; CHF = congestive heart failure; CAD = coronary artery disease; LVH = left ventricular hypertrophy; + = treatment benefit; - = treatment detriment; +/- = treatment neutral.

Nondrug Therapy

Nondrug treatment measures should always be employed prior to initiating drug therapy in diabetic patients with mild to moderate hypertension or in concert with drug therapy in diabetic patients with more severe hypertension.[3,14] Nondrug therapy, in general, should focus on the modification of lifestyle to include regular aerobic activity, an attempt to attain and maintain ideal body weight, cessation of smoking, and moderation of alcohol intake.[3,14] Dietary changes and physical activity can lead to improvements in glycemic, lipemic, and blood pressure control. For example, restricting sodium intake to less than 2.3 and or attaining up to a 10 lb. weight loss has been shown to lower blood pressure and improve glycemic control.[3] Daily alcohol intake should be limited to no more than 1 oz. of ethanol (equivalent to 24 oz. of beer, 8 oz. of wine, or 2 oz. of hard liquor). Patients should be encouraged and assisted in smoking cessation. Lifestyle modifications may be tried for three months in order to control and maintain blood pressure before drug therapy is initiated.

Antihypertensive Therapy

ACE Inhibitors

ACE inhibitors decrease the progression of diabetic nephropathy independent of their blood-pressure-lowering properties.[33] In patients with IDDM and renal disease, ACE inhibitor therapy has been shown to reduce the combined endpoint of death, dialysis, or renal transplant by 50 percent.[33] These beneficial effects on the progression of diabetic nephropathy are also apparent in patients with NIDDM. In two recent, randomized, double-blind, placebo-controlled studies, ACE inhibitor therapy was associated with a decline in the loss of glomerular filtration rate (GFR), albuminuria, and maintenance of serum creatinine levels.[34,35] The retarda-

tion of declining GFR was observed for patients with mild (no more than 300 mg/24 hours) and overt (more than 300 mg/24 hours) proteinuria present at the start of the study. These findings are in accordance with a metaanalysis that reported that ACE inhibitors decrease proteinuria independent of the type of diabetes, stage of renal disease, or duration of therapy.[36] Other reasons that may predicate ACE inhibitor therapy in diabetic patients include the improvement in insulin sensitivity and the neutral effect on lipids. For these reasons, ACE inhibitors are the preferred antihypertensive agents in diabetic patients with microalbuminuria or overt diabetic nephropathy.[3,14]

The potential beneficial effects for ACE inhibitor therapy do, however, need to be considered along with several important associated adverse effects. Perhaps most important is that ACE inhibitors may worsen renal insufficiency. This is particularly important in those patients who have preexisting renal dysfunction and in those who are more dependent on the renin-angiotensin system to maintain adequate renal perfusion. For example, patients with severe congestive heart failure or renal artery disease should be monitored more frequently for an increase in serum creatinine. Likewise, ACE inhibitors may cause a dramatic and abrupt decline in renal function in patients with bilateral renal artery stenosis, a condition that is more common in patients with diabetes.[3] Caution should also be exercised when initiating therapy in patients with diabetes who are on diuretic therapy to avoid a more pronounced decline in blood pressure when these agents are prescribed together. As part of patient follow-up, serum electrolytes should be monitored to avoid hyperkalemia, which is associated with ACE inhibitor therapy.

Alpha-1 Blockers

Alpha-1 blockers are attractive antihypertensive medications for diabetic patients as they may produce a beneficial effect on lipids, improve insulin sensitivity, and possess a favorable adverse effect profile.[26,37] In addition, the longer-acting alpha-1 blockers can be administered once daily, which may lead to a better compliance rate. The main drawback associated with this class of agents is that they may provoke orthostatic hypotension. To limit this unwanted side effect, the lowest dose should be initially prescribed and the dose titrated slowly after sitting and standing blood pressures have been measured and evaluated. In addition, the first dose may be given just prior to bedtime. Unlike the central acting alpha agonists, peripheral alpha antagonists are less likely to be associated with a more pronounced or severe orthostatic hypotension in diabetics with known or suspected autonomic dysfunction.

Beta Blockers

Beta blockers should be considered for the treatment of hypertension in patients with diabetes under select conditions where there is a clear benefit (i.e., myocardial infarction or angina).[3] The reasons for limiting beta-blocker therapy to those patients who would obtain a demonstrable benefit from therapy are secondary to drug-related effects on metabolism and on the cardiovascular and nervous systems. Beta blockers without intrinsic sympathomimetic activity (ISA; e.g., atenolol and metoprolol) may aggravate lipids and decrease insulin sensitivity.[28] In addition, by blunting the sympathetic response to a hypoglycemic event, beta blockers can prolong recovery and mask symptoms the patient may rely on to signal an event. Further, beta blockers can increase claudication in patients with diabetes with peripheral vascular disease. However, these potential drug adverse effects may be outweighed in patients with diabetes following myocardial infarction, as acute and long-term beta-blocker therapy (without ISA) can improve morbidity and mortality.[38,39] Although beta blockers with ISA may have fewer of the above-mentioned adverse effects, they offer no clear advantage over other agents. There is also some evidence that when beta-blocker and diuretic therapies are combined in older adult obese patients, the risk of developing NIDDM is increased compared to controls.[40] For these reasons, beta-blocker therapy is usually reserved for those patients with diabetes for whom the benefits of therapy outweigh the risks and in select hypertensive diabetic patients for whom other antihypertensives are contraindicated, ineffective, or not tolerated.

Calcium Channel Antagonists

Calcium channel antagonists (CCAs), alone or in combination with other antihypertensive agents, are viable treatment options to control blood pressure in the diabetic population. In general, these agents are lipid neutral and do not interfere with diabetic control. CCAs, as a class, tend to be more effective with age, which make them an attractive therapy in older patients with NIDDM.[41] In addition, studies have shown that CCAs, with the exception of nifedipine, may improve diabetic nephropathy by decreasing proteinuria and microalbuminuria.[42] However, not all studies are in agreement with this finding, and it is unknown if this beneficial effect is maintained with continued long-term therapy.[42] It has also been proposed that an additive effect may be produced by combining a CCA with an ACE inhibitor in patients with diabetic nephropathy.[43] Clearly, more well-controlled studies are needed to clarify the impact of specific CCAs on diabetic renal disease and to determine if combination therapy with an ACE inhibitor produces a synergistic effect.

Orthostatic hypotension, constipation, and peripheral edema are the main side effects associated with CCAs. Initiating therapy at the lowest possible dose and titrating slowly may be the best means of curtailing these unwanted side effects. Also, extra caution should be exercised to avoid orthostatic hypotension in diabetics with known or suspected neuropathy. As highlighted recently in the literature, short-acting agents (e.g., nifedipine) should be avoided in general for the chronic treatment of hypertension secondary to a possible increase in the risk of myocardial infarction.[44,45]

Diuretics

Thiazide diuretics have been shown to provoke adverse effects on lipid metabolism, blood glucose, and blood chemistry (e.g., potassium, magnesium, and urea).[13] However, when prescribed in low dose (25 mg or less a day of hydrochlorothiazide), these unwanted side effects may not be as pronounced and may be of little clinical importance.[3] Of note, loop diuretics have not been shown to have these effects and are preferred over thiazides when a patient's renal function worsens (serum creatinine greater than 2.5 mg/dL).[19] As patients with diabetes can be described as having an expanded plasma volume, diuretic therapy may be a necessary and effective therapy to control blood pressure in this population.[46] Further, combination therapy with an ACE inhibitor can produce a synergistic effect in lowering blood pressure and therefore can be considered for patients with diabetes who require more than one antihypertensive agent to control blood pressure.[47]

Conclusion

Hypertension in patients with diabetes should be treated early and aggressively. Pharmacologic and nondrug therapies combined with lifestyle modifications are important measures to achieve optimal treatment outcomes. Antihypertensive drugs, including ACE inhibitors, alpha blockers, CCAs, and low-dose diuretics, should be initiated if needed to attain and maintain optimal blood pressure control. Prior to initiating antihypertensive therapy, consideration and careful evaluation of drug-related effects on morbidity and mortality, possible effects on body chemistry, and the impact of therapy on concomitant disease states should be made. As a result, the best antihypertensive agent or combination of agents can be delineated for each patient. These measures to control hypertension should mirror efforts to optimize glycemic and lipemic control in each patient with diabetes.

REFERENCES

1. American Diabetes Association, *Diabetes 1993 Vital Statistics* (Alexandria, VA: 1993).

2. P.M. Dodson, "Epidemiology and Pathogenesis of Hypertension in Diabetes," in *Hypertension and Diabetes*, eds. A.H. Barnett and P.M. Dodson (London: Science Press, 1990).

3. The National High Blood Pressure Education Program Working Group, "National High Blood Pressure Education Program Working Group Report on Hypertension in Diabetes," *Hypertension* 23 (1994): 145–158.

4. M. Epstein, and J.R. Sowers, "Diabetes Mellitus and Hypertension," *Hypertension* 19 (1992): 403–418.

5. J.M. Flack, and J.R. Sowers, "Epidemiologic and Clinical Aspects of Insulin Resistance and Hyperinsulinemia," *American Journal of Medicine* 91, suppl. 1A (1991): 11S–21S.

6. J.S. Skyler et al., "Hypertension in Patients with Diabetes Mellitus," *American Journal of Hypertension* 8 (1995): 100S–105S.

7. A.R. Christlieb et al., "Vascular Reactivity to Angiotensin II and to Noradrenaline in Diabetic Subjects," *Diabetes* 25 (1976): 268–274.

8. R.A. De Fronzo, "The Effect of Insulin on Renal Sodium Metabolism," *Diabetologia* 21 (1981): 165–171.

9. P. Weidmann et al., "Pressor Factors and Responsiveness in Hypertension Accompanying Diabetes Mellitus," *Hypertension* 7, suppl. 2 (1985): 43–48.

10. P.M. Bell, "Clinical Significance of Insulin Resistance," *Diabetic Medicine* 13 (1996): 504–509.

11. R.E. Gilbert et al., "Diabetes and Hypertension. Australian Diabetes Society Position Statement," *The Medical Journal of Australia* 163 (1995): 372–375.

12. K.G. Dawson et al., "Report of the Canadian Hypertension Society Consensus Conference: 5. Hypertension and Diabetes," *Canadian Medical Association Journal* 149 (1993): 821–826.

13. American Diabetes Association, "Treatment of Hypertension in Diabetes," *Diabetes Care* 16 (1993): 1,394–1,401.

14. J.R. Sowers, and M. Epstein, "Diabetes Mellitus and Associated Hypertension, Vascular Disease, and Nephropathy: An Update," *Hypertension* 26, part 1 (1995): 869–879.

15. S. MacMahon et al., "Blood Pressure, Stroke, and Coronary Heart Disease. Part 1: Prolonged Differences in Blood Pressure: Prospective Observational Studies Corrected for the Regression Dilution Bias," *Lancet* 335 (1990): 765–774.

16. Medical Research Council Working Party, "Medical Research Council Trial of Treatment of Hypertension in Older Adults: Principal Results," *British Medical Journal* 304 (1992): 405–412.

17. B. Dahlof et al., "Morbidity and Mortality in the Swedish Trial in Old Patients with Hypertension (STOP-Hypertension)," *Lancet* 338 (1991): 1,281–1,285.

18. R. Collins et al., "Blood Pressure, Stroke, and Coronary Heart Disease. Part 2: Short-term Reductions in Blood Pressure: Overview of Randomized Drug Trials in their Epidemiological Context," *Lancet* 335 (1990): 827–838.

19. Joint National Committee, "The Fifth Report of the Joint National Committee on Detection, Evaluation, and Treatment of High Blood Pressure," *Archives of Internal Medicine* 153 (1993): 154–183.

20. SHEP Cooperative Research Group, "Prevention of Stroke by Antihypertensive Drug Treatment in Older Persons with Isolated Systolic Hypertension: Final Results of the Systolic Hypertension in the Elderly Program (SHEP)," *JAMA* 265 (1991): 3,255–3,264.

21. J.D. Curb et al., "Effect of Diuretic-based Antihypertensive Treatment on Cardiovascular Disease in Older Diabetic Patients with Isolated Systolic Hypertension," *JAMA* 276 (1996): 1,886–1,892.

22. J.H. Warram et al., "Excess Mortality Associated with Diuretic Therapy in Diabetes Mellitus," *Archives of Internal Medicine* 151 (1991): 1,350–1,356.

23. R. Klein et al., "Relation of Ocular and Systemic Factors to Survival in Diabetes," *Archives of Internal Medicine* 149 (1989): 266–272.

24. T. Pollare et al., "A Comparison of the Effects of Hydrochlorothiazide and Captopril on Glucose and Lipid Metabolism in Patients with Hypertension," *New England Journal of Medicine* 321 (1989): 868–873.

25. W.H.H. Sheu et al., "Comparison of the Effects of Atenolol and Nifedipine on Glucose, Insulin, and Lipid Metabolism in Patients with Hypertension," *American Journal of Hypertension* 4 (1991): 199–205.

26. A. Lehtonen, "Doxazosin Effects on Insulin and Glucose in Hypertensive Patients. The Finnish Multicenter Study Group," *American Heart Journal* 121 (1991): 1,307–1,311.

27. H.O. Lithell, "Effect of Antihypertensive Drugs on Insulin, Glucose, and Lipid Metabolism," *Diabetes Care* 14 (1991): 203–209.

28. T. Pollare et al., "Sensitivity to Insulin During Treatment with Atenolol and Metoprolol: A Randomized, Double Blind Study of Effects on Carbohydrate and Lipoprotein Metabolism in Hypertensive Patients," *British Medical Journal* 298 (1989): 1,152–1,157.

29. SOLVD Investigators, "Effect of Enalapril on Survival in Patients with Reduced Left Ventricular Ejection Fractions and Congestive Heart Failure," *New England Journal of Medicine* 325 (1991): 293–302.

30. SOLVD Investigators, "Effect of Enalapril on Mortality and the Development of Heart Failure in Asymptomatic Patients with Reduced Left-ventricular Ejection Fractions," *New England Journal of Medicine* 327 (1992): 685–691.

31. F.G. Dunn et al., "Enalapril Improves Systemic and Renal Hemodynamics and Allows Regression of Left Ventricular Mass in Essential Hypertension," *American Journal of Cardiology* 53 (1984): 105–108.

32. The Diabetes Control and Complications Trial Research Group, "The Effect of Intensive Treatment of Diabetes on the Development and Progression of Long Term Complications in Insulin Dependent Diabetes Mellitus," *New England Journal of Medicine* 329 (1993): 977–986.

33. E.J. Lewis et al. for the Collaborative Study Group, "The Effect of Angiotensin-converting Enzyme Inhibition on Diabetic Nephropathy," *New England Journal of Medicine* 329 (1993): 1,456–1,462.

34. H.E. Lebovitz et al., "Renal Protective Effects of Enalapril in Hypertensive NIDDM: Role of Baseline Albuminuria," *Kidney International* 45 (1994): S150–S155.

35. M. Ravid et al., "Long-term Stabilizing Effect of Angiotensin-converting Enzyme Inhibition on Plasma Creatinine and on Proteinuria in Normotensive Type II Diabetic Patients," *Annals of Internal Medicine* 118 (1993): 577–581.

36. B.L. Kasiske et al., "Effect of Antihypertensive Therapy on the Kidney in Patients with Diabetes: A Meta-regression Analysis," *Annals of Internal Medicine* 118 (1993): 129–138.

37. R.R. Luther et al., "The Effects of Terazosin and Methylchlorothiazide on Blood Pressure and Serum Lipids," *American Heart Journal* 117 (1989): 842–847.

38. ISIS-1 (First International Study of Infarct Survival) Collaborative Group, "Randomized Trial of Intravenous Atenolol Among 16,027 Cases of Suspected Acute Myocardial Infarction: ISIS-1," *Lancet* 12 (1986): 57–66.

39. G. Olsson et al., "Long-term Treatment with Metoprolol after Acute MI: Effect on 3 Year Mortality and Morbidity," *Journal of the American College of Cardiology* 5 (1985): 1,428–1,437.

40. L. Mykkanen et al., "Increased Risk of Non-insulin Dependent Diabetes in Elderly Hypertensive Subjects," *Journal of Hypertension* 12 (1994): 1,425–1,432.

41. W. Zing et al., "Calcium Antagonists in Elderly and Black Hypertensive Patients," *Archives of Internal Medicine* 151 (1991): 2,154–2,162.

42. D.D. Hoelscher et al., "Hypertension in Diabetic Patients: An Update of Interventional Studies to Preserve Renal Function," *Journal of Clinical Pharmacology* 35 (1995):73–80.

43. G.L. Bakris et al., "Treatment of Arterial Hypertension in Diabetic Humans: Importance of Therapeutic Selection," *Kidney International* 41 (1992): 912–919.

44. B.M. Psaty et al., "The Risk of Myocardial Infarction Associated with Antihypertensive Drug Therapies," *JAMA* 274 (1995): 620–625.

45. B.G. Phillips et al., "Calcium-channel Blockers and Risk of Myocardial Infarction: More Hype Than Harm," *American Journal of Health System Pharmacy* 52 (1995):1,460–1,462.

46. G.W. Edelson, and J.R. Sowers, "Treatment of Hypertension in Selected Patient Groups: An Emphasis on Diabetes Mellitus and Hypertension," *The Endocrinologist* 4 (1995):205–210.

47. B. Dahlof et al., "Controlled Trial or Enalapril and Hydrochlorothiazide in 200 Hypertensive Patients," *American Journal of Hypertension* 1 (1988):38–41.

HYPERTENSION IN AN INNER-CITY MINORITY POPULATION*

Managing the cardiovascular problems of vulnerable populations presents unique challenges to nurses. The sequelae of cardiovascular disease (CVD) have been especially devastating to the minority populations who may lack funds and/or access to adequately resolve their problems. The term *minority* refers to those at a societal disadvantage because of such factors as race, ethnicity, or age.[1] Relatively little research on the impact of health promotion on older people has been done.[2] In the small body of literature on older people, low-income and minority older people have been underrepre-sented.[3] The sample described herein is part of a larger community sample secured by random digit telephone

dialing for the purposes of describing hypertension awareness in an inner-city minority population. Intervention strategies focused on attempts by health care providers to be responsive and resourceful in assessing and implementing a community awareness strategy. The sample in this article consists of adult African Americans (n = 965) described in relation to awareness of hypertension and health perception.

Hypertension is a major risk factor for cardiovascular disease. African Americans have been shown to be disproportionately affected by hypertension.[4] National prevalence estimates indicate that 30% of African American adults aged 18 to 74 years have hypertension compared with 19% of white Americans.[5] The sequelae of uncontrolled hypertension are well documented and include stroke, renal failure, and heart disease. Controlling hypertension has been shown to reduce mortality rates for some of these conditions.[6] Consistent with the increased prevalence of hypertension, African Americans have an approximately 50% greater risk of heart disease mortality and 100% greater risk of stroke mortality compared with that of white Americans.[7] Reduction of blood pressure with drugs clearly decreases cardiovascular mortality and morbidity in patients with diastolic blood pressure greater than 90 mm Hg and in those with isolated systolic hypertension (systolic > 160 mm Hg and diastolic > 90 mm Hg).[8] Increased patient knowledge has a significant impact on compliance with hypertension drug regimens in minority older people.[9]

Minority populations face many barriers to health improvement. Frequently, these populations lack knowledge of, and belief in, the value of health promotion and disease prevention; they experience frustration at the lack of appropriate, relevant, and usable health information.[10] Among people who are aware of their hypertension and who remain under treatment, lack of adequate blood pressure control may be partially related to noncompliance with treatment protocols or may simply be a factor of tolerance by health care providers of moderately elevated blood pressure status. Finding a means to increase knowledge and confidence of minority populations in an adequate hypertension control regimen is a paramount step in increasing treatment adherence.

Conceptual Framework

The conceptual orientation of this descriptive analysis is the Health Belief Model, which proposes that people fail to engage in health-promoting activities because they do not believe such actions will improve their conditions or they do not perceive their conditions to be dangerous or life-threatening.[11] The Diffusion Model was also used because it advocates a saturation methodology for bringing new ideas into an ethnic community by using culturally homogeneous providers and existing systems.[12] Health belief is important because

*Source: K. Lynn Wieck, PhD, RN, "Hypertension in an Inner-City Minority Population," *The Journal of Cardiovascular Nursing*, Vol. 11:4, Aspen Publishers, Inc., © July 1997.

the condition of hypertension is largely asymptomatic. Furthermore, in an effort to empower people to be responsible for their own health, they must first believe that they can influence the condition for which they are at risk. A key part of the study strategy was to communicate to the community that they could control their blood pressure and to remind them to do so. Diffusion provides a guide for communicating an innovation into a society for the purpose of changing behavior, in contrast to the purpose of changing knowledge or attitude. Assuming that health belief is affected by communication, information of a culturally complementary nature was diffused into the target community. Rogers[12] asserts that the most effective communication occurs when the source of information and receiver are similar; therefore, when possible, an effort was made to provide services and messages featuring African Americans. Community leaders were involved in the awareness effort from the inception of the study.

Review of the Literature

High blood pressure is much more common among African Americans of both genders than it is among the total population.[13] More patients visit physicians and receive prescriptions for the treatment of hypertension than for any other medical disorder.[14] Additionally, a number of large epidemiologic studies have demonstrated increased prevalence of hypertension in minorities, along with increased morbidity and mortality.[15-17] These findings present a strong case for the management of minority hypertension in a proactive way. The ability to influence lifestyle choices and medication adherence in hypertensive African American populations is a key to the successful management of hypertension.

Minority Issues

The accelerating demographic shift in this country toward an older America is underway, and the fastest growth in that direction is among minorities.[18] Health care issues of an aging population must begin with the most vulnerable populations that include minorities.

Although stroke and cardiovascular mortality have declined, and progress has been made in controlling hypertension among African Americans, a gap still exists among hypertension prevalence, heart disease, and stroke mortality between African Americans and both Hispanics and non-Hispanic whites. In 1989, African Americans were 1.4 times as likely as white Americans to develop heart disease and 1.9 times more likely than white Americans to develop cerebrovascular disease.[19] Death and disability from cerebrovascular disease is greater in African Americans than it is in whites. African Americans experience stroke three to six times more frequently than do whites.[20] It seems reasonable that individual awareness of risk factors plays a role in the effectiveness of prevention strategies.

Knowledge of the symptoms of CVD differs significantly between whites and African Americans. In a community-based study, Folsom et al[21] found African Americans were more likely to mention hypertension and overexertion as causes of CVD ($P<.05$, n = 1,252). Although a large proportion of this sample (32% of African Americans and 54% of whites) were aware that smoking was a major risk factor for CVD, African Americans were less likely than whites to identify high cholesterol (25% of African Americans and 39% of whites) as a risk factor.

The natural history of hypertension in African Americans is characterized by early onset, increased severity, markedly greater end-organ damage, and a lower degree of control.[14] These factors suggest physiologic as well as sociologic differences between the majority of white hypertensive clients and most, if not all, African American hypertensive clients. Because African American patients often present with advanced disease, cardiac diagnostic testing may need to be modified, including close assessment of atypical chest pain, comprehensive risk factor assessment with lipid analysis, and echocardiography to detect left ventricular hypertrophy.[14] Treatment differences based on race, such as delay of treatment and altered reactions to specific medications, have been documented.[22]

Many myths surround the treatment of hypertension in African Americans. It is *not* true that African Americans are unresponsive to drug therapy. In hypertensive African Americans, diuretics are more effective than in white Americans, while angiotensin-converting enzyme (ACE) inhibitors and beta blockers are not as effective. Diuretics as a monotherapy are efficacious in treating African Americans, and compliance may be higher because such treatments are low-cost, have fewer side effects, and can be given once a day.[23] Compliance with drug therapy will be improved if the health care provider chooses a simplified drug regimen and avoids drugs that produce intolerable side effects. Multiple drug therapy and multiple daily doses should be avoided whenever possible.[4] User-friendly prescriptive practices and increased awareness may lead to increased control of hypertension in the inner-city, low-income, minority community.

Correlates and Sequelae of CVD in Minority Populations

The risk of CVD increases with age. The Cardiovascular Health Study (CHS) was a community-based cohort study of people (n = 5,201 men) 65 years of age and older (*m* = 73 years) that described factors which correlated with blood pressure. Major correlates were heart rate, aortic root dimension, creatinine, hematocrit, alcohol use, ethnicity, internal carotid artery wall thickness, mitral early/late peak flow velocity, white blood cell count, cigarette smoking, and age. African Americans had significantly higher blood pressure than did non-African Americans (P<.001). Older age and being of the African American race were independent predictors of diastolic blood pressure increases. Systolic blood pressure seemed to climb throughout life; however, diastolic blood pressure decreased slightly after age 50 or 60 years, even through the age of 90 years.[24]

Hypertension has been reported to be responsible for up to 33% of renal failure in some African American populations. The incidence of end-stage renal disease (ESRD) continues to increase among minorities. The relative risk estimates of hypertensive ESRD in African Americans have ranged from 4.4 to 18.1 times higher than white Americans. Although the excessive ESRD risk in African Americans is not explained by hypertension alone, the classic risk factors of hypertension, Type II diabetes mellitus, and possibly Type I diabetes mellitus pose an increased risk for ESRD.[25]

Noncompliance with drug therapy and high therapy dropout rates are common among hypertensive populations. One of the many reasons for this phenomenon may be the absence of significant clinical symptoms. This problem is exacerbated in low-income populations where poor health may be caused by environmental exposures, material deficiencies, and lack of access to health care.[13] Access to primary care providers is also limited in inner-city areas, where African Americans do not receive enough early, routine, and preventive health care.[13] Seeking food and shelter may take precedence over seeking to improve health. The long waiting lines often associated with public clinics, as well as crowded clinic conditions, are barriers to receiving care for many low-income individuals. Moreover, the cost of an antihypertensive regimen may not seem worthwhile when the condition is asymptomatic. Even when public services are used, the client must get to the clinic, arrange child care or bring the children to the clinic, and obtain meals during the clinic visit. Furthermore, if the client is a member of the working poor, wages will be lost when a day of work is given up to go to a clinic.[4]

In a summary of health priorities for the next century, the US Department of Health and Human Services points out in the epic *Healthy People 2000*[13] that high blood pressure is much more common among African Americans of both genders than it is among the total population. Furthermore, obesity, a common comorbid condition to hypertension, is a problem for 44% of African American women over age 20, as compared with 37% of low-income women in general and 27% of all women. The goal for the year 2000 is to increase to 90% the proportion of hypertensive people who are taking positive health actions to control their condition. The barriers to positive health care behaviors present challenges to the health care industry, which seeks to improve quality of life while decreasing the needless pain, suffering, and expense associated with the negative sequelae of CVD. The following analysis sought to identify the state of hypertension awareness and health perception in a large inner-city minority population based on the identified needs.

Methodology

The hypothesis guiding this study was that most African Americans were not aware of their hypertension. Furthermore, the researcher wished to determine whether there was a difference between older African Americans and their younger counterparts in awareness and health perception. Because the focus was on awareness, a random digit dialing (RDD) phone survey was instituted to determine prevalence of self-reported hypertension and current treatment patterns in a geographically defined area with a predominantly minority population. The RDD methodology is reported elsewhere (Unpublished Observations: Hyman et al. Blood pressure measurement and antihypertensive treatment in a low-income African American population.).

A subsample (n = 965) of the randomly dialed respondents who agreed to participate in a personal interview and screening were asked to come to a central location in the community. It is recognized that this sample is biased because they agreed to come for the interview for compensation. All people had their blood pressure measured and were asked to complete health-related questionnaires. People 65 years of age and older (n = 148) were compared with people under 65 years of age (n = 817) to identify hypertensive status, awareness of hypertension, and perception of health.

Findings

The older people who came in for a personal interview (n = 148) had a mean age of 71.57 years (SD = 6.06). Those under 65 years of age (n = 817) had a mean age of 42.89 years (SD = 13.11). The older sample was 44% male and 56% female, while the younger sample was 41% male and 59% female. The older sample was significantly more likely to have been told that they were hypertensive (x^2 = 28.75, df = 2, P = .00). Sixty-four percent of older people (n = 94) were self-reported hypertensives, while only 40% (n = 326) of the younger subjects had been told that they had hypertension. When asked about the use of antihypertensive medications, older individuals were significantly more likely to be taking antihypertensives than were individuals in the younger group (x^2 = 31.00, df = 2, P = .00). Of the older, self-proclaimed hypertensive subjects, 75% (n = 71) stated they were on antihypertensive medications. A smaller percentage of the younger group was on medications for their hypertension (63.5%, n = 207). The mean systolic blood pressure of the older hypertensive sub-sample was 142.75 mm Hg

(SD = 20.66), and mean diastolic blood pressure was 75.93 mm Hg (SD = 10.59). The maximum systolic pressure was 204 mm Hg, and the maximum diastolic pressure was 106 mm Hg. The younger group had a mean systolic pressure of 128.88 mm Hg (SD = 20.23) and a mean diastolic pressure of 78.24 mm Hg (SD = 12.10).

Information was gathered about the health perception of these two sample groups. Overall, health perception for both groups was positive with 64% (n = 614) reporting excellent, very good, or good health; 32% (n = 307) reporting fair health; and only 4% (n = 39) reporting poor health (see "Self-rated Health of African American Community Sample"). No attempt was made to control for comorbidity. Chi-square analysis demonstrated no difference between the older and younger sample subjects regarding how they perceived their health. When asked to compare their health with how they felt 1 year ago, half of the respondents stated that their health was the same (50.9%, n = 491) while 36% (n = 348) reported that it was better (see "Health Compared to a Year Ago by African American Community Sample"). Again, there was no difference between the younger and older sample subjects. Comparing themselves with other people, 71% (n = 689) did not think they became sick more easily than did other people and 55% (n = 527) believed they were as healthy as anybody they knew. While there was no difference between the two groups relating to their perception of getting sick more easily than other people, x^2 analysis did demonstrate a difference in the belief that they were as healthy as anybody they knew (x^2 = 12.43, *df* = 5, *P* = .03), with older people having a slightly better view of their stamina than did their younger counterparts (see "Comparative Health Perception of Older and Younger African American Community Sample"). Consistent with this somewhat optimistic outlook, 72% (n = 694) reported that they did not expect their health to get worse.

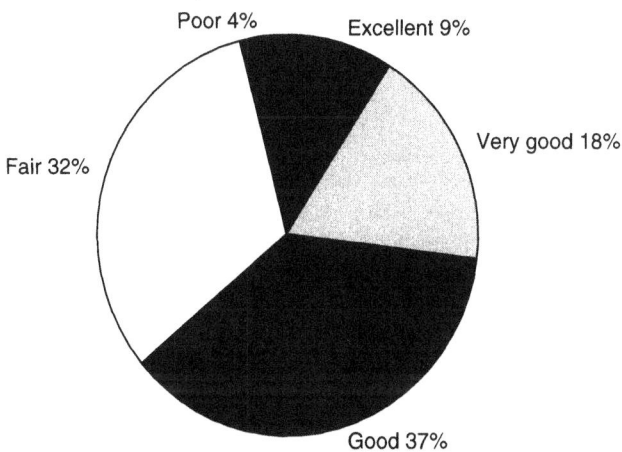

Health compared to a year ago by African American community sample. n = 965.

Discussion of Findings

While there appeared to be a high rate of blood pressure measurement and hypertension awareness in this low-income, minority population, the presence of higher systolic levels, particularly among the older subjects, remains disconcerting. Health promotion efforts in the past have been aimed at locating "hard-to-reach" populations, identifying potential health problems, and getting patients into treatment; it appears that the awareness aspect of this strategy is working. The problem of keeping the population engaged in an adequate treatment regimen seems to be the key to future health promotion efforts. Because the person does not feel sick, treatment compliance does not assume a top priority among sustenance and daily living needs. Although there is a heightened awareness of the presence of hypertension, there is also, unfortunately, a heightened tolerance for higher levels of systolic and diastolic blood pressure levels by both the health care providers and the patients themselves. Increasingly, the importance of elevation in systolic blood pressure is being recognized and emphasized.[26] The reasons for the tolerance of sustained systolic elevation may be outdated practice methods, a reluctance to change the client's medication regimen, a desire to keep medication regimen simple and easy to follow, or a fluctuation in the health care provider sites used by the minority person attempting to navigate the changing health care delivery system. Most of the study participants had a private physician whom they consulted for care. However, the number of minority older people using the emergency center for primary care (18%) is problematic. Factors that influence providers' treatment styles as well as health services used by hypertensive minorities need to be studied.

A positive finding of this study was the general level of optimism demonstrated by this group of hypertensive Afri-

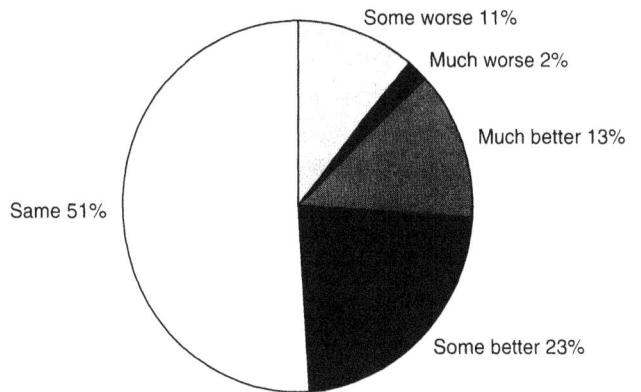

Self-rated health of African American community sample. n = 965.

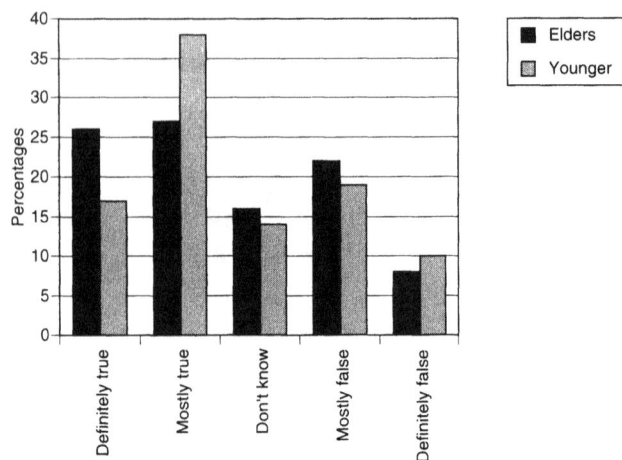

Comparative health perception of older (n = 148) and younger (n = 817) African American community sample to the statement "I am as healthy as anyone I know."

can Americans regarding their health outlook. They generally perceived themselves to be in good health and did not expect that their health would get worse in the future. This optimistic view of health may contribute to African Americans' disbelief that an asymptomatic condition like hypertension could actually be life-threatening. Nevertheless, the finding that the participants had a positive outlook regarding their health is important to nurses as they try to capitalize on that health optimism by contributing to the education and support of this vulnerable group.

Nursing Implications

Efforts to prevent, treat, and control hypertension will require more intensive interventions that focus on raising awareness and supporting ongoing lifestyle behavior changes. Because no differences were found in the level of health optimism demonstrated by this inner-city older and younger African American population, health intervention efforts that focused on positive health behaviors seem efficacious for both groups. Efforts to prevent hypertension in normotensive minority groups need to focus on limiting salt and fat intake along with weight reduction efforts. Treatment of hypertensive people who are on medication should be focused on reinforcing positive behaviors and continued adherence to their medication regimen.

Lifestyle intervention to complement drug therapy remains an essential component of hypertension management.[27] Because older people were more likely to be hypertensive and more likely to be on medication, intervention strategies should be aimed at community centers and nutrition assistance centers where older people are more likely to congre-

gate. For the younger African American population, interventions must continue to focus on knowledge of the sequelae of hypertension and debunking the myths regarding hypertension, such as "all blood pressure medicine causes impotency," "I control my stress so I will never get high blood pressure," or "I know I don't have high blood pressure because I don't feel sick." Current screening methods seem to be succeeding in raising awareness of hypertension in all ages. These efforts at churches, grocery stores, schools, and other areas where people congregate should be continued.

REFERENCES

1. Holzberg C. Ethnicity and aging: anthropological perspectives on more than just the minority elderly. *Gerontologist.* 1982;22: 249–257.

2. US Department of Health and Human Services. *Healthy Older People: The Report of a National Health Promotion Program.* Washington, DC: Office of Disease Prevention and Health Promotion; September, 1990.

3. Haber D. Health promotion to reduce blood pressure level among older blacks. *Gerontologist.* 1986;26:119–121.

4. Francis CK. Hypertension, cardiac disease, and compliance in minority populations. *Am J Med.* 1991;91(suppl 1A):29S–36S.

5. Burt VL, Cutler JA, Higgins M, et al. Trends in the prevalence, awareness, treatment and control of hypertension in the adult US population. *Hypertension.* 1995;26:60–69.

6. Rocella E, Horan M. The national high blood pressure education program: measuring progress and assessing its impact.*Health Psychol.* 1988;7(Suppl):297–303.

7. National Center for Health Statistics. *Health, United States, 1992.* Hyattsville, Md: Public Health Service; 1993.

8 SHEP Cooperative Research Group. Prevention of stroke by antihypertensive drug treatment in older persons with isolated systolic hypertension. Final results of the Systolic Hypertension in the Elderly Program (SHEP). *JAMA.* 1991;265:3,255–3,264.

9. Wieck KL. Education needs of low-income elderly women in a large metropolitan city in the USA. *Int Nurs Rev.* 1992;Fall:4.

10. US Department of Health and Human Services. *Executive Summary: Strategies for Diffusing Health Information to Minority Populations: A Profile of a Community-based Model.* Washington, DC: National Heart, Lung and Blood Institute; September 1987.

11. Becker M. The health belief model and sick role behavior. *Health Educ Monogr.* 1978;2:409–419.

12. Rogers EM. *Communication of Innovations: A Cross-cultural Approach,* 2nd ed. New York, NY: The Free Press; 1971.

13. US Department of Health and Human Services.*Healthy People 2000.* Washington, DC: Public Health Service; 1990.

14. Francis CK. Hypertension and cardiac disease in minorities. *Am J Med.* 1990;88(suppl 3B):3S–8S.

15. National Blood Pressure Education Program Working Group on Risk and High Blood Pressure. An epidemiological approach to describing risk associated with blood pressure levels. *Hypertension.* 1985;7:641.

16. National Center for Health Statistics. *Blood Pressure Levels in Persons 18–74 Years of Age in 1976–1980, and Trends in Blood Pressure from 1960–1980 in the United States.* Vital Health Statistics, Series 11, No. 234, publication # (PHS) 86-1684. Washington, DC: US Department of Health and Human Services; 1986.

17. Sempos D, Cooper R, Kovar M, McMillen M. Divergence of the recent trends in coronary mortality for the four major race-sex groups in the United States. *Am J Public Health.* 1988;78:1,422–1,427.

18. American Association for Retired People. *Health Promotion for Older Minority Adults.* The National Resource Center on Health Promotion and Aging; 1991.

19. Division of Vital Statistics. *Current Estimates from the National Health Interview Survey.* Washington, DC: National Center for Health Statistics; 1994. Series 10, No. 189, DHHS Publication no. (PHS) 94-1517, Appendix II.

20. Gillum RF. Stroke in blacks. *Stroke.* 1988;19:1–9.

21. Folsom A, Sprafka JM, Luepker R, Jacobs D. Beliefs among black and white adults about causes and prevention of cardiovascular disease: The Minnesota heart survey. *Am J Prev Med.* 1988;4: 121–127.

22. Naumberg EH, Franks P, Bell B, Gold M, Engerman J. Racial differences in the identification of hypercholesterolemia. *J Fam Pract.* 1993;36:425–430.

23. Saunders E. Tailoring treatment to minority patients. *Am J Med.* 1990;88(suppl 3B):21S–23S.

24. Tell GS, Rutan GH, Kronmal RA, et al. Correlates of blood pressure in community-dwelling older adults: the cardiovascular health study. *Hypertension.* 1994;23:59–67.

25. Ferguson R, Morrissey E. Risk factors for end-stage renal disease among minorities. *Transplant Proc.* 1993;25:2,415–2,420.

26. National High Blood Pressure Education Program. *Working Group Report on Primary Prevention of Hypertension.* Washington, DC: US Dept. of Health and Human Services; 1993. NIH Publication #93-2669.

27. Nothwehr F, Elmer P, Hannan P. Prevalence of health behaviors related to hypertension in three blood pressure treatment groups: The Minnesota heart health program. *Prev Med.* 1994;23:362–368.

PREDICTORS OF AMBULATORY BLOOD PRESSURE: IDENTIFICATION OF HIGH-RISK ADOLESCENTS*

Hypertension affects 50 million Americans ages 6 and older, but it is not equally distributed among subgroups of the population. In 1992, the death rate from high blood pressure was approximately five times higher among Black Americans than among White Americans.[1] Less is known about blood pressure levels among Hispanic Americans, but in general, the data point toward slightly lower blood pressure levels among Mexican American adults compared with those for non-Hispanic Black and White adults in the United States.[2] Since the precursors of cardiovascular disease become evident during childhood and adolescence,[3] it is important to study factors affecting high blood pressure as they emerge early in life.

*Source: Janet C. Meininger, RN, FAAN, et al., "Predictors of Ambulatory Blood Pressure: Identification of High-Risk Adolescents," *Advances in Nursing Science,* Vol. 20:3, Aspen Publishers, Inc., © March 1988.

This study focused on adolescence, a critical period in biologic, social, and psychologic development. This stage is not only a transitional phase during which adult patterns of health behavior are established,[4] but also a pivotal transition in the evolution of risk for hypertension and other cardiovascular morbidity. Epidemiologic studies of adolescent blood pressure as a predictor of risk for adult hypertension in the same individuals have used resting blood pressure levels of mature adolescents as the predictor.[5] In the present research, measures that go beyond resting blood pressure were incorporated; specifically, blood pressure reactivity in the laboratory and 24-hour ambulatory blood pressure were investigated. With these multiple methods it may be possible to develop protocols for identifying high-risk individuals at earlier stages of development.

The purpose of this study was to examine the extent to which ambulatory blood pressure could be predicted by blood pressure levels exhibited during talking segments of a laboratory protocol and by resting blood pressure in 15- and 16-year-old male and female adolescents from three ethnic groups: African, European, and Mexican Americans. The investigators hypothesized that blood pressure levels during laboratory reactivity testing would be better predictors of ambulatory blood pressure levels than levels of blood pressure measured at rest using a standard protocol. If laboratory blood pressure patterns could be used to predict which individuals have high levels of blood pressure during the course of daily activities, the laboratory protocol may be a useful screening tool, identifying high-risk individuals. A secondary purpose was to test for ethnic group differences in adolescent ambulatory blood pressure.

Conceptual Framework

The model that served as the framework for this study (see "Emergence of Risk for Cardiovascular Mobidity and Mortality: A Life Span Perpective on Prevention and Research") was developed to analyze the methods currently available to prevent the occurrence of cardiovascular diseases and to identify gaps in our knowledge base that need to be substantiated with further research.[6] This framework is based on the classic work of Leavell and Clark,[7] who proposed that any effort directed toward health promotion and disease prevention must be based on a clear understanding of the natural history of the processes responsible for the etiology of the disease.

The etiology of coronary artery disease involves a web of factors, each of which has a modest impact on the risk of disease. The relative risk associated with a single risk indicator is not large; nevertheless, reduction or elimination of major factors such as high blood pressure, hyperlipidemia, and obesity could have a very substantial impact on public health because these risk factors are so prevalent in our population. Therefore, preventive efforts should focus on those risk factors that are associated with an increase in risk of disease, are prevalent in the population, and have the potential to respond positively to changes in environment and lifestyle. Cardiovascular diseases account for a large proportion of disease, disability, and death in the United States. Incidence, that is, the number of new cases over a period of time, is one measure of morbidity. There are about 1.5 million heart attacks a year and 0.5 million strokes. Approximately 42% of mortality in the United States is attributable to cardiovascular causes. Of the total yearly deaths, 513,200 are attributed to heart attack, 149,200 to stroke, and 30,900 to hypertension.[1]

In this framework, prevention is viewed from a life span perspective, encompassing a whole spectrum of activities from tertiary prevention, otherwise known as rehabilitation, to primary prevention, which is directed toward averting initiation of the disease process itself. Primary prevention can begin very early in life and continue throughout the life span. It is achieved by health promotion and by specific protection against environmental factors. In the case of cardiovascular diseases, this level of prevention would need to begin early in life in order to precede the onset of pathological atherosclerotic or hypertensive processes. Prevention can target the lifestyles of individuals within the population or can target environmental factors directly. Secondary prevention is relevant after the emergence of a high-risk profile or in the very early phases of clinically apparent disease, such as stage 1 hypertension.[8] This can begin as early as adolescence and young adulthood and extend throughout the remainder of the life span. In the absence of diagnostic tools to detect very early stages of atherosclerosis, we presume that individuals with high-risk cardiovascular profiles are at least in the beginning stages of pathogenesis. Thus, intervention with individuals with risk factors such as high blood pressure, adverse lipid and lipoprotein profiles, and obesity is at the level of secondary prevention. Tertiary prevention is directed toward individuals with clinically diagnosed disease and is aimed toward restoration of functional capabilities, prevention of disability, and prevention of death from cardiovascular diseases. These activities are conducted with clinical populations, usually those in middle to late adulthood.

EMERGENCE OF RISK FOR CARDIOVASCULAR MORBIDITY AND MORTALITY: A LIFE SPAN PERSPECTIVE ON PREVENTION AND RESEARCH

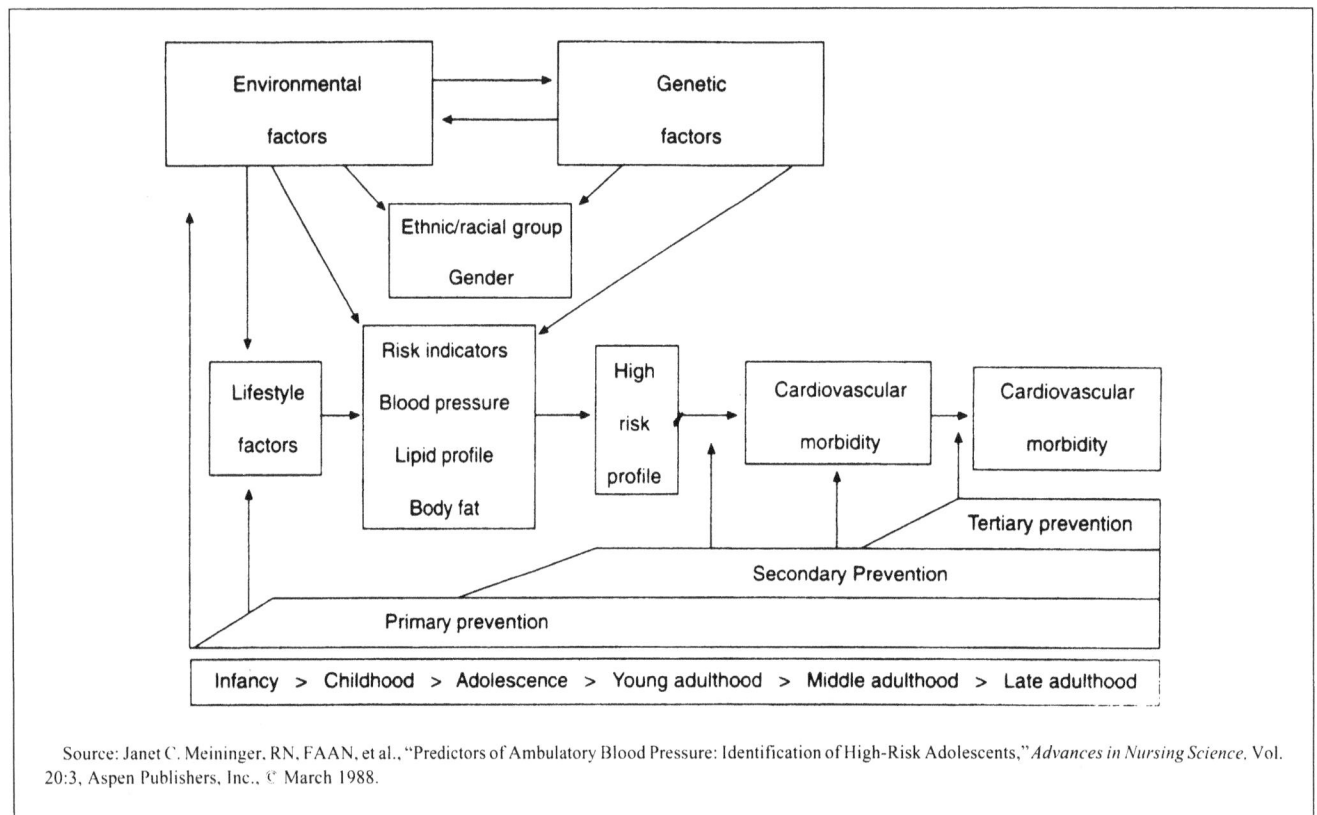

Source: Janet C. Meininger, RN, FAAN, et al., "Predictors of Ambulatory Blood Pressure: Identification of High-Risk Adolescents," *Advances in Nursing Science*, Vol. 20:3, Aspen Publishers, Inc., © March 1988.

Background

Epidemiologic data that compare ethnic groups within the same study are rare. Available studies are inconsistent in the age at which higher levels of blood pressure are observed for African Americans compared with European Americans, but the general trend is that differences between ethnic groups emerge in adolescence and increase with age. A recent review indicates that resting blood pressures are not substantially different between Black and White children in the United States under the age of 12.[9] In young adults in the Coronary Artery Risk Development in Young Adults Study (CARDIA),[10] ethnic differences in blood pressure for both men and women were greater for the age group 25 to 30 years than for the group 18 to 24 years old. At ages 25 to 30 years, Black male participants had systolic blood pressure (SBP) 1.5 mmHg ($p < .05$) and Black female participants had SBP 1.8 mmHg ($p < .01$) higher than White participants after controlling for body mass index, physical fitness, cigarette smoking, and alcohol intake. With similar adjustments there were no significant ethnic group differences in either age group for diastolic blood pressure (DBP). It is possible that ambulatory measurements will allow for the detection of group differences at younger ages. For instance, in a study of adolescents between the ages of 10 and 18 years,[11] Black subjects had higher SBP (108 ± 10 mmHg) compared with White subjects (106 ± 10 mmHg) at night. Similarly, nocturnal DBP was higher ($p = .003$) for Blacks (63 ± 8 mmHg) compared with Whites (60 ± 7 mmHg).

Cardiovascular reactivity refers to the magnitude, patterns, and mechanisms of cardiovascular response associated with exposure to stress.[12] Blood pressure reactivity has been studied with the rationale that it could be an earlier precursor of hypertension than elevated resting blood pressure levels. Several types of psychological stressors have been employed in laboratory protocols including video games and serial subtraction. Talking has been established as a stressor accompanied by blood pressure reactivity in subjects of varying age and health status.[13–16] Blood pressure increased regardless of speech content, but talking about anger and other personally relevant content was associated with the greatest increases.[17,18] With relatively few exceptions, the research studies on cardiovascular reactivity have been conducted in the laboratory. There is a need for further research on the extent to which blood pressure responses to standardized laboratory protocols predict levels of blood pressure sustained during the course of daily activities. The availability of lightweight ambulatory monitors allows for measurement of blood pressure in an unobtrusive manner over 24-hour intervals.

Although laboratory studies of adolescents' blood pressure responses to mental stressors are not uncommon, few of these studies have examined blood pressure responses during talking. Those that have[19,20] were limited by small sample sizes or lack of ethnic group representation. A pertinent exception to this is a program of research by Ewart and Kolodner,[21] who examined blood pressure response during a self-disclosure speaking task with several other mental stressor tasks (video game, mirror drawing, mental arithmetic) in 14- to 15-year-old Black (n = 153) and White (n = 107) adolescents. The sample was restricted to those students who had systolic or diastolic blood pressure above the 66th percentile of the distribution of ninth graders of the same race and gender in two Baltimore public high schools. SBP and DBP increased approximately 13 mmHg above baseline during speaking as compared with increases of 8 mmHg for the other tasks ($p < .01$). Blood pressure responses to speaking were not significantly different by ethnic group.

A subsequent study of this sample by Ewart and Kolodner[22] linked blood pressure response to the laboratory interview with 24-hour ambulatory blood pressures. Blood pressure response to the laboratory interview predicted ambulatory blood pressure in the total sample and in Blacks, Whites, females, and males. In a similar study of undergraduate students by Linden and Con,[23] cardiovascular reactivity in response to a 5-minute discussion of a recent interpersonal conflict situation predicted ambulatory systolic and diastolic blood pressure. These two studies provide support for examining cardiovascular response to talking as the laboratory stimulus and testing the extent to which laboratory blood pressure response predicts 24-hour blood pressure levels in adolescents.

There is a growing consensus that ambulatory blood pressure monitoring is considered more representative of the individual's true pressure than individual readings or averages of measurements taken in resting subjects. Its reproducibility, however, is hindered by variability in posture and physical and mental activity.[24] Self-reported ratings of these factors in diaries at each measurement of ambulatory blood pressure have been incorporated in many studies, but this method is limited because the accuracy and completeness of diary entries varies from subject to subject and compliance and accuracy may be lacking except from the most highly motivated subjects. To overcome this problem, simultaneous mechanical or electronic monitoring of physical activity has been incorporated in some studies of ambulatory blood pressure. Stewart and associates[25] in a study of an adult clinical sample, found that, on average, physical activity accounted for 20% of SBP and 26% of DBP variation. The present study incorporated electronic monitoring of physical activity (actigraphy) with ambulatory monitoring of blood pressure over 24 hours.

Methods

Sample

This was a study of 60 adolescents that was conducted to pilot test methods of data collection and analysis in preparation for a larger project. A quota sampling method was used to yield equal numbers of males and females (30 in each group) and equal numbers of African-, European-, and Mexican Americans (20 in each group). The age range in the pilot study was restricted to 15 and 16 years to control for variability introduced by the heterogeneity of subject maturity among younger adolescents. This heterogeneity could obscure the ability to make valid comparisons among male and female subjects but could not be controlled statistically because of the small sample size. The sample was accessed through a public high school in Houston. Students were recruited through health and physical education classes because they are required courses; thus, students would not be excluded on the basis of the particular courses in which they were enrolled. The sample for this report was restricted to 41 subjects who had complete data on all aspects of the protocol pertinent to this analysis: ambulatory blood pressure and activity monitoring, resting blood pressure, and the laboratory protocol. The sample was 51.2% female (n = 21) and 48.8% male (n = 20), 34.1% African American (n = 14), 24.4% European American (n = 10), and 41.5 % Mexican American (n = 17). The mean age of this group was 15.4 years, SD, 1.7. There were no differences in age by gender or ethnic group. Approximately half of the students lived with both of their biological parents (47.5%); the remainder lived with one biological parent, primarily the mother. Most of the parents had graduated from high school; 20% of the fathers and mothers had less than a high school education. Occupations of parents spanned the middle categories of Hollingshead's[26] rankings: 30% were semiskilled workers; 34% were skilled craftsmen, clerical, or sales workers; and 32% were classified in medium business, minor professional, and technical level occupations.

Instruments

Blood pressure. Three instruments were used to measure blood pressure: a mercury sphygmomanometer (Baumanometer) and stethoscope, and two automatic devices that use an oscillometric technique (Dinamap and Spacelabs monitors). With all three of these instruments, an appropriately sized cuff was selected so that the bladder width of the cuff was 40% to 50% of the upper-arm circumference. For auscultatory measurement of blood pressure with the Sphygmomanometer (Baumanometer-300, WA Baum, Inc, Copiague, NY) and stethoscope, procedures outlined by the American Heart Association[27] were followed to measure resting blood pressure. Three measurements were taken after the subject had been sitting quietly for 5 minutes. The second and third measurements were averaged for this analysis. The Dinamap (Model 825XT, Critikon, Tampa, FL) was used to record blood pressure during the laboratory protocol. The cuff automatically inflates and deflates at programmable inter-

vals. The validity of the Dinamap has been documented by comparison of its readings with those obtained simultaneously from direct intraarterial monitoring.[28,29] The ambulatory blood pressure recorder (Spacelabs, model 90207; Spacelabs, Inc; Redlands, WA), was selected because of its reported reliability,[30] predictive validity,[31] and size (12.2 oz with batteries). Concurrent validity with intraarterial readings has been reported.[32] It discriminates between pressure signals, subject movement, and respiratory artifact and is automatically zeroed before each reading. Time of the measurements is programmed. Data are stored within the monitor's memory until they are downloaded to a computer for editing and analysis. The protocols for both oscillometric devices (Dinamap and Spacelabs monitors) included procedures for calibration with a mercury sphygmomanometer.

Physical activity and diary recordings during ambulatory monitoring. Since the conditions under which blood pressure was measured during ambulatory monitoring were not controlled or observed, physical activity of the subject was measured with a Motionlogger actigraph (Ambulatory Monitoring, Inc., Ardsley, NY). This instrument, which is the size of a large wristwatch, collects and stores data on subject activity as a continuous time series.[33] There is strong evidence of reliability and validity of this instrument.[34] The ambulatory blood pressure monitor and the Motionlogger were synchronized so that specific intervals of Motionlogger readings were linked with ambulatory blood pressure readings for analysis. In this study, five readings at 1-minute intervals immediately before the blood pressure reading were used to control for subject activity level at each blood pressure measurement.

In addition, activities and feelings were recorded by the subject each time blood pressure was measured during waking hours. A standard diary format was used to note time of day, position, location, activity, and mood. Ambulatory blood pressure readings outside a specified range for this age group were examined in the context of the subject diary data (eg, activity, position, mood) at the time of blood pressure measurement and through reports of the activity monitor which indicated whether or not the subject was awake or asleep. (See "Editing of Ambulatory Blood Pressure Data" below.)

Height. Stature was measured during a physical examination with an Accustat (Ross Laboratories) wall-mounted anthropometer. Subjects removed their shoes before this measurement. This variable was used in the analysis to control for the effect of body size on blood pressure.[35]

Procedures for Data Collection

Recruitment. The research protocol was approved by the Committee for the Protection of Human Subjects. Students in the age range of interest who were enrolled in health and physical education classes were given information about the study. For those who volunteered to participate, parental consent was obtained. A Spanish translation of the consent form was available for parents who did not speak or understand English. To encourage completion of the study by those who agreed to participate, each adolescent participant who completed all segments of the protocol was reimbursed $30.00. In addition, subjects who were recruited from the same classroom proceeded through the data collection procedures together so that participation in the study became a peer group experience. Subjects were assured that parents and school personnel would not have access to the data obtained from the physical examination or any other information collected for the study. They were informed that an exception to this would be persistently high blood pressures that needed medical assessment.[3]

Laboratory testing. A private, quiet room within the school was used for the laboratory protocol, which was conducted by a trained data collector. The subject was seated in a comfortable chair and a blood pressure cuff of the appropriate size was attached to the subject's left arm and connected to the Dinamap. The 26-minute protocol consisted of 6 minutes of resting followed by two counterbalanced series of 4 minutes of quiet, 2 minutes of talking, and 4 minutes of quiet. During one series the adolescent talked about a usual day (neutral talking); in the other series the subject talked about an anger-provoking situation (angry talking). Blood pressure was taken every 2 minutes throughout the 26-minute protocol except during talking when it was taken every minute. Talking segments were conducted in English and audiotaped. This laboratory protocol was a repeated measures cross-over design. The within-subjects factors were series (angry and neutral talking); period (quiet-talk-quiet in each series); and measurement (measurement one and two in each period). Series was randomly ordered and crossed over for each subject.

Ambulatory monitoring. Blood pressure was monitored for 24 hours using the Spacelabs ambulatory equipment. Activity was simultaneously monitored with the Motionlogger actigraph. Following each ambulatory blood pressure measurement, the subject reported position, location, posture, number of people present and feelings in a diary. At the beginning of the school day, the participant was fitted with the appropriately sized cuff and Motionlogger on the nondominant arm and wrist. The monitors were programmed and synchronized. Blood pressure was recorded every 30 minutes during the day and every hour at night. Entries in the diaries were made immediately following each blood pressure measurement except during the night. Participants were instructed to wear the monitor throughout the 24-hour period except during bathing and to keep their arms still when

the blood pressure cuff automatically inflated. Instructions about the use of the diary were provided and subjects were given an opportunity to practice diary recordings in conjunction with manual triggering of the monitor during a practice session.

Data Editing and Statistical Analysis

Reactor status. Each subject was classified into one of three categories of blood pressure reactor status on the basis of blood pressure recordings during the talking segments of the laboratory session. Blood pressure levels rather than blood pressure change scores were used to create this variable because of greater temporal stability over 6 months for blood pressure levels observed during talking segments of laboratory protocols.[21] Separate classifications were made for systolic and diastolic blood pressures and for male and female subjects. Subjects were classified as "consistently high reactors" if they were in the highest quartile of the distribution of blood pressure for their same-sex counterparts during angry and neutral talking. "Consistently low reactors" were those in the lowest quartile of the distribution of blood pressure during angry and neutral talking. All other subjects were classified as "mixed reactors."

Editing of ambulatory blood pressure data. First, some readings were removed from consideration because they produced a Spacelabs error code. These errors were most likely caused by subject movement during a blood pressure reading. Second, readings outside a specified range for this age group[22] were examined in the context of the subject diary data (activity, position, mood) at the time of blood pressure measurement and through reports of the activity monitor, which indicated whether or not the subject was awake or asleep. The following criteria were used to identify potentially out-of-range readings: (1) pulse pressure less than 20 mmHg; (2) systolic blood pressure above 225 mmHg or less than 50 mmHg; (3) diastolic blood pressure above 110 mmHg or less than 30 mmHg; or (4) the reading was 50 mmHg or more from the previous reading.[22] For example, if a high value occurred at a time when the subject had recorded that the measurement took place during an argument, it was retained. Extremely low values that coincided with activity readings consistent with sleep were retained. Each out-of-range value was evaluated independently by two investigators and disagreements were further evaluated by a third investigator. Fewer than 10 subjects had out-of-range values and usually there was only one of these per subject.

Statistical analysis. A mixed-effects model for repeated measures data proposed by Laird and Ware[36] was used for testing relationships between ambulatory blood pressure, and several independent variables including gender, ethnic group, resting blood pressure, blood pressure reactor status during the laboratory protocol, height, and level of activity in the 5-minute interval before each blood pressure measurement. The use of a two-stage model with each participant as the unit of analysis and each repeated measurement of ambulatory blood pressure as the subunit provided a means to effectively deal with the unbalanced dataset and to avoid the variability problem inherent in analysis using individual summary statistics.

Results

Means and standard deviations for blood pressure measured at rest using a standard protocol, during the laboratory protocol and during ambulatory monitoring, are presented by ethnic group and gender (see "Descriptive Statistics for Blood Pressure Measurements by Gender and Ethnic Group"). For females, systolic and diastolic blood pressures were higher for African-Americans compared with the other two groups. For males, the pattern was not as consistent, possibly due to the extremely small sample sizes in some subgroups. The gender and ethnic group differences also varied by the method and circumstances of measurement. During ambulatory blood pressure monitoring, African American males had the highest SBP. European American males had the highest SBP measured at rest using a standard protocol, and Mexican American males had the highest laboratory baseline SBP. Males in the three ethnic groups had similar DBP levels. In all subgroups, laboratory baseline systolic and diastolic blood pressure (oscillometric) were lower than blood pressures measured with the ambulatory monitors (oscillometric).

Descriptive statistics for laboratory blood pressure during talking by reactivity status (high, mixed, and low reactors) are presented by gender (see "Descriptive Statistics for Laboratory Blood Pressure during Talking by Reactivity Status and Gender). Gender differences observed during laboratory reactivity status are much more pronounced for systolic compared with diastolic blood pressure. Males had higher SBP during talking than females.

The mixed effects analysis was applied with ambulatory

DESCRIPTIVE STATISTICS FOR BLOOD PRESSURE MEASUREMENTS BY GENDER AND ETHNIC GROUP (N=41), 15 TO 16-YEAR-OLD ADOLESCENTS, HOUSTON, TX

	Resting BP (Physical Exam)		Laboratory BP (Baseline)		Ambulatory BP (Day)		Ambulatory BP (Night)	
	Mean	SD	Mean	SD	Mean	SD	Mean	SD
Males								
Systolic								
African (5)*	117.60	8.65	110.80	5.47	134.80	11.84	125.40	9.63
European (5)	124.10	9.65	109.10	12.39	122.60	10.60	113.00	2.35
Mexican (10)	113.70	8.53	112.55	8.80	123.40	6.77	115.80	6.44
Diastolic								
African	68.10	8.20	56.20	4.71	72.20	4.66	63.20	2.17
European	63.50	5.18	55.30	1.20	68.20	5.17	57.60	6.02
Mexican	63.00	7.35	57.30	6.74	71.30	4.83	63.30	4.47
Females								
Systolic								
African (9)	106.28	9.56	103.17	8.81	121.44	5.66	114.11	4.70
European (5)	103.20	3.13	96.70	5.06	118.80	2.95	112.40	4.22
Mexican (7)	102.57	7.71	96.00	9.10	114.00	2.16	110.43	4.72
Diastolic								
African	65.72	5.82	60.00	7.00	75.00	7.07	66.44	6.97
European	59.50	5.83	55.10	3.52	71.40	4.93	62.60	5.22
Mexican	63.07	8.33	54.79	8.99	68.86	3.98	64.57	3.26

*Numbers in parentheses are subgroup sample size.

Source: Janet C. Meininger, RN, FAAN, et al., "Predictors of Ambulatory Blood Pressure: Identification of High-Risk Adolescents," *Advances in Nursing Science*, Vol. 20:3, Aspen Publishers, Inc., © March 1998.

DESCRIPTIVE STATISTICS FOR LABORATORY BLOOD PRESSURE DURING TALKING BY REACTIVITY STATUS AND GENDER, 15 TO 16-YEAR-OLD ADOLESCENTS, HOUSTON, TX

	High Reactor			Mixed Reactor			Low Reactor		
	n	Mean	SD	n	Mean	SD	n	Mean	SD
Males									
Systolic	5	144.30	14.81	12	122.73	7.14	3	109.08	3.22
Diastolic	7	77.21	6.01	8	66.66	2.54	5	58.85	1.49
Females									
Systolic	4	112.38	1.83	13	107.00	4.68	4	101.69	3.60
Diastolic	5	74.80	4.21	12	65.13	2.42	4	59.94	2.47

Source: Janet C. Meininger, RN, FAAN, et al., "Predictors of Ambulatory Blood Pressure: Identification of High-Risk Adolescents," *Advances in Nursing Science*, Vol. 20:3, Aspen Publishers, Inc., © March 1998.

systolic and diastolic blood pressure (analyzed separately) as the dependent variables (n = 1,537). The independent variables of interest were gender, ethnic group, blood pressure measured at rest using a standard protocol, and blood pressure reactor status during laboratory testing (high, low, mixed). To control for anthropometric differences that are related to blood pressure, the subject's height was included in each analysis. Five activity measurements recorded every minute for 5 minutes before each measurement of ambulatory blood pressure were used for this analysis to control for level of subject activity.

Results for SBP are presented (see "Mixed Effects Model for 24-Hour Ambulatory SBP"). Activity, height, ethnic group, gender, and SBP reactor status during laboratory testing were significant predictors of ambulatory systolic blood pressure. Males had higher SBP than females (+4.08 mmHg, p = .0001). African American adolescents had ambulatory SBP 3.72 mmHg higher (p = .03) than Mexican American adolescents after taking into account other variables in the model. European American adolescents were not significantly different from those of Mexican American background. Activity level was a statistically significant predictor variable (p = .0001) as was height (p = .03), but resting SBP was not. Those who were classified as high SBP reactors on the basis of blood pressures observed during the talking segments of the laboratory protocol had significantly higher 24-hour ambulatory SBP (+8.09 mmHg, p = .0001) than those classified as low reactors; mixed reactors were not significantly different from low reactors.

For 24-hour DBP (see "Mixed Effects Model for 24-Hour Ambulatory DBP"), activity, ethnic group and DBP reactor status during laboratory testing were significant predictors. African Americans had higher DBP (+3.41 mmHg, p = .01) than Mexican Americans. European American subjects were not significantly different from Mexican American subjects

in DBP. Resting DBP was not predictive of 24-hour DBP, but reactor status of DBP during the laboratory protocol was statistically significant. For those classified as high DBP reactors during laboratory testing, DBP was 6.58 mmHg higher than those classified as low DBP reactors (p = .0001). Mixed reactors also had higher ambulatory DBP than low reactors (+5.06 mmHg, p =.0001).

Discussion

In this study, blood pressure measured while talking during laboratory reactivity testing was a better predictor of ambulatory blood pressure levels measured over 24 hours than levels of blood pressure as it was measured at rest using a standard protocol. In multivariable analysis, laboratory indicators of elevated blood pressure induced by talking were significant predictors of 24-hour ambulatory blood pressure in models which controlled for resting blood pressure, activity, height, gender, and ethnic group. For DBP, both high and mixed DBP reactors during the laboratory testing were significantly different from low reactors in 24-hour ambulatory DBP. In contrast, for SBP, only those who were high SBP reactors were significantly different from low reactors in 24-hour ambulatory SBP. This may be due to the higher variability in SBP among mixed reactors during the talking segment of the laboratory protocol compared with the variability of mixed DBP reactors.

These results are consistent with those Ewart and Kolodner[21,22] who studied Black and White adolescents in the same age group who were in the upper tertiles of blood pressure. They are also similar to findings of Linden and Con[23] who studied European and Asian-American male and female undergraduate students. Very few previous studies have used regression methods to control for multiple sources of variation while investigating the strength of the associa-

MIXED EFFECTS MODEL FOR 24-HOUR AMBULATORY SBP (mmHG, N = 1,537), 15 TO 16-YEAR-OLD ADOLESCENTS, HOUSTON, TX

Parameter	Estimate	t	p
Intercept	66.89	4.51	.0001
Height (meters)	18.78	2.30	.03
Activity	0.04	13.88	.0001
Gender (male)*	4.08	2.30	.0001
Ethnic group (European)[†]	-0.08	-0.06	.95
Ethnic group (African)[†]	3.72	2.32	.03
SBP during physical examination	0.08	1.27	.21
High SBP reactor[‡]	8.09	5.01	.0001
Mixed SBP reactor[‡]	0.87	0.70	.49

*Rerence group = female
[†]Reference group = Hispanic
[‡]Reference group = low SBP reactor

Source: Janet C. Meininger, RN, FAAN, et al., "Predictors of Ambulatory Blood Pressure: Identification of High-Risk Adolescents," *Advances in Nursing Science,* Vol. 20:3, Aspen Publishers, Inc., © March 1998.

MIXED EFFECTS MODEL FOR 24-HOUR AMBULATORY DBP (mmHG, N = 1,537), 15 TO 16-YEAR-OLD ADOLESCENTS, HOUSTON, TX

Parameter	Estimate	t	p
Intercept	65.01	6.22	.0001
Height (meters)	-3.85	-0.57	.57
Activity	0.05	16.89	.0001
Gender (male)*	-.42	-0.35	.73
Ethnic group (European)[†]	-1.69	-1.56	.13
Ethnic group (African)[†]	3.41	2.65	.01
DBP during physical examination	-0.04	-0.68	.50
High DBP reactor[‡]	6.58	5.92	.0001
Mixed DBP reactor[‡]	5.06	5.14	.0001

*Reference group = female
[†]Reference group = Hispanic
[‡]Reference group = low DBP reactor

Source: Janet C. Meininger, RN, FAAN, et al., "Predictors of Ambulatory Blood Pressure: Identification of High-Risk Adolescents," *Advances in Nursing Science,* Vol. 20:3, Aspen Publishers, Inc., © March 1998.

tion between laboratory cardiovascular reactivity indicators and levels of blood pressure during ambulatory monitoring.[37] The findings of the present study, when considered in conjunction with previous studies, provide further evidence that blood pressure measured during laboratory tasks that require talking may be a useful predictor of blood pressure levels measured over a period of 24 hours. It appears that blood pressure responses of adolescents induced while talking during laboratory protocols may be more representative of blood pressure over 24 hours than blood pressure measured at rest using a standard protocol. Although these findings are in the direction hypothesized by the investigators, they were based on an extremely small sample of 41 adolescents and should be confirmed in larger samples before generalizing.

It was noted that resting systolic and diastolic blood pressures measured with the auscultatory method were, on average, higher than those measured with the Dinamap, an oscillometric device during the laboratory protocol. It is difficult to discern to what extent this pattern was due to the differences in the circumstances of measurement as opposed to differences in instrumentation. In a previous study that included adolescents,[38] oscillometric systolic blood pressure readings were higher than auscultatory systolic readings, but oscillometric diastolic blood pressure readings were lower than auscultatory diastolic readings.

Gender differences in resting blood pressure, reactive blood pressures during talking, and those observed during ambulatory monitoring are consistent with previous studies.[20-22] Males had higher systolic blood pressure than females. Blood pressure differences by ethnic group reflected rankings similar to those of large population-based samples.[2] Although rankings varied depending on the method of measurement and setting, in general, African-American adolescents had the highest levels of blood pressure compared with European and Mexican Americans. The ethnic subgroups in the present study were extremely small and may not have been representative of the target population. The small sample size also precluded inclusion of multiple anthropometric measurements on subjects that may partially explain large gender and ethnic differences in blood pressure. A strength of the mixed effects model was that it effectively dealt with the multiple but unbalanced number of observations of ambulatory blood pressure on each subject. This study is among the few that have incorporated the mixed levels of the data in the statistical analysis and is the only one of this group that has focused on adolescent subjects.

REFERENCES

1. American Heart Association. *1997 Heart and Stroke Statistical Update*. Dallas, Tex: AHA, 1996.

2. Sorel JE, Ragland DR, Syme, SL, Davis WB. Educational status and blood pressure: the Second National Health and Nutrition Examination Survey 1976–1980 and the Hispanic Health and Nutrition Examination Survey 1982–1984. *Am J Epidemiol*. 1992;135: 1,339–1,348.

3. Task Force on Blood Pressure Control in Children. Report of the Second Task Force on Blood Pressure Control in Children. *Pediatrics*. 1987;9:1–25.

4. Langer LM, Warheit GJ. The Pre-Adult Health Decision-Making Model: linking decision-making directedness/orientation to adolescent health-related attitudes and behaviors. *Adolescence*. 1992;27: 919–994.

5. Lauer RM, Clarke WR. Childhood risk factors for high adult blood pressure: the Muscatine Study. *Pediatrics*. 1989;84:633–641.

6. Meininger JC, Hayman LL. The emergence of cardiovascular risk: opportunities for nursing intervention and research. Symposium presented at the meeting of American Nurse Association Council of Nurse Researchers; September 1989; Chicago, Illinois.

7. Leavell HR, Clark EG. *Preventive Medicine for the Doctor in His Community, an Epidemiologic Approach*. New York: McGraw Hill, 1965.

8. Joint National Committee on Detection, Evaluation and Treatment of High Blood Pressure (1993). Fifth report. *Arch Intern Med*. 153, 154–183.

9. Prineas RJ, Elkwiry ZM. Epidemiology and measurement of high blood pressure in children and adolescents. In: Loggie JMH, ed. *Pediatric and Adolescent Hypertension*. Boston: Blackwell; 199 2:92–103.

10. Liu K, Ballew C, Jacobs DR Jr, et al. Ethnic differences in blood pressure, pulse rate, and related characteristics in young adults: the CARDIA study. *Hypertension*. 1989;14:218–226.

11. Harshfield GA, Pulliam DA, Somes GW, Alpert BS. Ambulatory blood pressure patterns in youth. *Am J Hypertens*. 1993;6:968–973.

12. Sherwood A, Turner JR. Individual differences in cardiovascular response to stress. In: Turner JR, Sherwood A, Light KC, ed. *A Conceptual and Methodological Overview of Cardiovascular Reactivity Research*. New York: Plenum; 1992.

13. Krantz DS, Helmers KF, Bairey CN, Nebel LE, Hedges SM, Rozanski A. Cardiovascular reactivity and mental stress-induced myocardial ischemia in patients with coronary artery disease. *Psychosom Med*. 1991;53:1–12.

14. Matthews KA, Stoney CM. Influence of sex and age on cardiovascular responses during stress. *Psychosom Med*. 1988;50:46–56.

15. Lynch JJ. *The Language of the Heart: The Body's Response to Human Dialogue*. New York: Basic Books; 1985.

16. Liehr P. Uncovering a hidden language: the effects of listening and talking on blood pressure and heart rate. *Arch Psychiatr Nurs*. 1992;6:306–311.

17. Siegman AW. Cardiovascular consequences of expressing, experiencing, and repressing anger. *J Behav Med.* 1993;16:539–569.

18. Thomas SA, Liehr P, DeKeyser F, Friedmann G. Nursing blood pressure research, 1980-1990: a bio-psycho-social perspective. *Image J Nurs Sch.* 1993;25:157–164.

19. Thomas SA, Lynch JJ, Friedmann E, Suginohara M, Hall PS, Peterson C. Blood pressure and heart rate changes in children when they read aloud in school. *Public Health Rep.* 1984;99:77–84.

20. Matthews KA, Manuck SB, Saab PG. Cardiovascular responses of adolescents during a naturally occurring stressor and their behavioral and psychophysiological predictors. *Psychophysiology.* 1986;23: 198–209.

21. Ewart CK, Kolodner KB. Social competence interview for assessing physiological reactivity in adolescents. *Psychosom Med.* 1991;53: 289–304.

22. Ewart CK, Kolodner KB. Predicting ambulatory blood pressure during school: effectiveness of social and nonsocial reactivity tasks in black and white adolescents. *Psychophysiology.* 1993;30:30–38.

23. Linden W, Con A. Laboratory reactivity models as predictors of ambulatory blood pressure and heart rate. *J Psychosom Res.* 1994;38:217–228.

24. Ward MM, Turner JR, Johnston DW. Temporal stability of ambulatory cardiovascular monitoring. *Ann Behav Med.* 1994;16:3–11.

25. Stewart MJ, Brown H, Padfield PL. Can simultaneous ambulatory blood pressure and activity monitoring improve the definition of blood pressure? *Am J Hypertens.* 1993;6:174S–178S.

26. Hollingshead AB. Four Factor Index of Social Status (unpublished working paper). New Haven, Conn: Yale University, 1975.

27. American Heart Association. *Recommendations for Human Blood Pressure Determination by Sphygmomanometers.* Dallas, Tex: AHA; 1987.

28. Ramsey M. Noninvasive automatic determination of arterial pressure. *Med Biol Eng Comput.* 1979;17:11–18.

29. Yelderman M, Ream AK. Indirect measurement of mean blood pressure in the anesthetized patient. *Anesthesiology.* 1979;50: 253-256.

30. James GD, Pickering TG, Yee LS, Harshfield GA, Riva S, Laragh JH. The reproducibility of average ambulatory, home, and clinic pressures. *Hypertension.* 1988; 11:545–549.

31. Parati G, Pomidossi G, Albini F, Malaspina D, Mancia G. Relationship of 24-hour blood pressure mean and variability to severity of target-organ damage in hypertension. *J Hypertens.* 1987;5:93–98.

32. Graettenger WF, Lipson JL, Cheney DG, Wober MA. Validation of portable non-invasive blood pressure monitoring devices: comparisons with intra-arterial and sphygmomanometer measurements. *Am Heart J.* 1988; 116:1,155–1,160.

33. Mason DJ, Redeker N. Measurement of activity. *Nurs Res.* 1993;42: 87–92.

34. Tryon W. *Activity Measurement in Psychology and Medicine.* New York: Plenum; 1991.

35. Rosner B, Prineas RJ, Loggie, JMH, Daniels SR. Blood pressure nomograms for children and adolescents, by height, sex, and age, in the United States. *J Pediatr.* 1993;123:871–886.

36. Laird NM, Ware JH. Random effects models for longitudinal data. *Biometrics.* 1982;34:963–974.

37. Turner JR, Ward MM, Gillman MD, Johnston DW, Light KC, Van Doornen LJP. The relationship between laboratory and ambulatory cardiovascular activity: current evidence and future directions. *Ann Behav Med.* 1994;16:12–23.

38. Abcejo SN, Cardenas MF, Leal MA. The Relationship Between Physical Activity and Blood Pressure Measured by Two Indirect Methods in Adolescents and Their Parents. Master's research project. Houston, Tex: The University of Texas-Houston Health Science Center; 1993.

BLOOD PRESSURE TABLES ADJUSTED FOR HEIGHT*

Body size is the most important determinant of BP in childhood and adolescence. The concept that the differential growth rates present in children would require some adjustments in interpretation of the BP percentile for individual children was suggested in the second task force report. That report included tables from the 90th percentile of height and weight with the sex and age BP distribution curves and indicated that tall children with pressures that seem to be elevated may actually be normotensive if their height for a given age is beyond the 90th height percentile. In a recent report that reanalyzed the national childhood BP data, the BP percentiles were refined and based not only on sex and age but also on height to determine age-, sex-, and height-specific systolic and diastolic BP percentiles. This approach provides information that allows for consideration of different levels of growth in evaluating BP and demonstrates that BP standards that are based on sex, age, and height permit a more precise classification of BP according to body size. More importantly, this approach avoids misclassifying children at the extremes of normal growth. For example, very tall children will not be misclassified as hypertensive, and very short children with high normal BP or even hypertension will not be missed. Although BP clearly is also associated with obesity, this association is believed to be a causal one, wherein the obesity contributes to higher BP and to increased risk for cardiovascular disease.

The BP data in this report on children and adolescents have been updated and reanalyzed to include height percentiles. The report now includes the data presented in the second task force report, the data added in the report by Rosner et al., (Rosner B, Prineas RJ, Loggie JMH, Daniels SR. Blood pressure nomograms for children and adolescents, by height, sex, and age, in the U.S. *J Pediatr.* 1993;123:871–886.) and newly obtained data from the 1988–91 National Health and Nutrition Examination Survey (NHANES III). (Centers for Disease Control and Prevention, National Center for Health Statistics. National Health and Nutrition Examination Survey (NHANES III) 1988–1991, data computed for The Na-

*Source: Update on the Task Force Report on High Blood Pressure in Children and Adolescents: A Working Group Report from the National High Blood Pressure Education Program, NIH Publication No. 96-3790, National Heart, Lung, and Blood Institute, National Institutes of Health, September 1996.

BLOOD PRESSURE LEVELS FOR THE 90TH AND 95TH PERCENTILES OF BLOOD PRESSURE FOR BOYS AGE 1 TO 17 YEARS BY PERCENTILES OF HEIGHT (TABLE 1)

Age	Height Percentiles* → BP† ↓	Systolic BP (mm Hg)							Diastolic BP (mm Hg)						
		5%	10%	25%	50%	75%	90%	95%	5%	10%	25%	50%	75%	90%	95%
1	90th	94	95	97	98	100	102	102	50	51	52	53	54	54	55
	95th	98	99	101	102	104	106	106	55	55	56	57	58	59	59
2	90th	98	99	100	102	104	105	106	55	55	56	57	58	59	59
	95th	101	102	104	106	108	109	110	59	59	60	61	62	63	63
3	90th	100	101	103	105	107	108	109	59	59	60	61	62	63	63
	95th	104	105	107	109	111	112	113	63	63	64	65	66	67	67
4	90th	102	103	105	107	109	110	111	62	62	63	64	65	66	66
	95th	106	107	109	111	113	114	115	66	67	67	68	69	70	71
5	90th	104	105	106	108	110	112	112	65	65	66	67	68	69	69
	95th	108	109	110	112	114	115	116	69	70	70	71	72	73	74
6	90th	105	106	108	110	111	113	114	67	68	69	70	70	71	72
	95th	109	110	112	114	115	117	117	72	72	73	74	75	76	76
7	90th	106	107	109	111	113	114	115	69	70	71	72	72	73	74
	95th	110	111	113	115	116	118	119	74	74	75	76	77	78	78
8	90th	107	108	110	112	114	115	116	71	71	72	73	74	75	75
	95th	111	112	114	116	118	119	120	75	76	76	77	78	79	80
9	90th	109	110	112	113	115	117	117	72	73	73	74	75	76	77
	95th	113	114	116	117	119	121	121	76	77	78	79	80	80	81
10	90th	110	112	113	115	117	118	119	73	74	74	75	76	77	78
	95th	114	115	117	119	121	122	123	77	78	79	80	80	81	82
11	90th	112	113	115	117	119	120	121	74	74	75	76	77	78	78
	95th	116	117	119	121	123	124	125	78	79	79	80	81	82	83
12	90th	115	116	117	119	121	123	123	75	75	76	77	78	78	79
	95th	119	120	121	123	125	126	127	79	79	80	81	82	83	83
13	90th	117	118	120	122	124	125	126	75	76	76	77	78	79	80
	95th	121	122	124	126	128	129	130	79	80	81	82	83	83	84
14	90th	120	121	123	125	126	128	128	76	76	77	78	79	80	80
	95th	124	125	127	128	130	132	132	80	81	81	82	83	84	85
15	90th	123	124	125	127	129	131	131	77	77	78	79	80	81	81
	95th	127	128	129	131	133	134	135	81	82	83	83	84	85	86
16	90th	125	126	128	130	132	133	134	79	79	80	81	82	82	83
	95th	129	130	132	134	136	137	138	83	83	84	85	86	87	87
17	90th	128	129	131	133	134	136	136	81	81	82	83	84	85	85
	95th	132	133	135	136	138	140	140	85	85	86	87	88	89	89

*Height percentile determined by standard growth curves.
†Blood pressure percentile determined by a single measurement.

Source: Update on the Task Force Report on High Blood Pressure in Children and Adolescents: A Working Group Report from the National High Blood Pressure Education Program, NIH Publication No. 96-3790, National Heart, Lung, and Blood Institute, National Institutes of Health, September 1996.

BLOOD PRESSURE LEVELS FOR THE 90TH AND 95TH PERCENTILES OF BLOOD PRESSURE FOR GIRLS AGE 1 TO 17 YEARS BY PERCENTILES OF HEIGHT (TABLE 2)

Age	Height Percentiles* → BP† ↓	Systolic BP (mm Hg)							Diastolic BP (mm Hg)						
		5%	10%	25%	50%	75%	90%	95%	5%	10%	25%	50%	75%	90%	95%
1	90th	97	98	99	100	102	103	104	53	53	53	54	55	56	56
	95th	101	102	103	104	105	107	107	57	57	57	58	59	60	60
2	90th	99	99	100	102	103	104	105	57	57	58	58	59	60	61
	95th	102	103	104	105	107	108	109	61	61	62	62	63	64	65
3	90th	100	100	102	103	104	105	106	61	61	61	62	63	63	64
	95th	104	104	105	107	108	109	110	65	65	65	66	67	67	68
4	90th	101	102	103	104	106	107	108	63	63	64	65	65	66	67
	95th	105	106	107	108	109	111	111	67	67	68	69	69	70	71
5	90th	103	103	104	106	107	108	109	65	66	66	67	68	68	69
	95th	107	107	108	110	111	112	113	69	70	70	71	72	72	73
6	90th	104	105	106	107	109	110	111	67	67	68	69	69	70	71
	95th	108	109	110	111	112	114	114	71	71	72	73	73	74	75
7	90th	106	107	108	109	110	112	112	69	69	69	70	71	72	72
	95th	110	110	112	113	114	115	116	73	73	73	74	75	76	76
8	90th	108	109	110	111	112	113	114	70	70	71	71	72	73	74
	95th	112	112	113	115	116	117	118	74	74	75	75	76	77	78
9	90th	110	110	112	113	114	115	116	71	72	72	73	74	74	75
	95th	114	114	115	117	118	119	120	75	76	76	77	78	78	79
10	90th	112	112	114	115	116	117	118	73	73	73	74	75	76	76
	95th	116	116	117	119	120	121	122	77	77	77	78	79	80	80
11	90th	114	114	116	117	118	119	120	74	74	75	75	76	77	77
	95th	118	118	119	121	122	123	124	78	78	79	79	80	81	81
12	90th	116	116	118	119	120	121	122	75	75	76	76	77	78	78
	95th	120	120	121	123	124	125	126	79	79	80	80	81	82	82
13	90th	118	118	119	121	122	123	124	76	76	77	78	78	79	80
	95th	121	122	123	125	126	127	128	80	80	81	82	82	83	84
14	90th	119	120	121	122	124	125	126	77	77	78	79	79	80	81
	95th	123	124	125	126	128	129	130	81	81	82	83	83	84	85
15	90th	121	121	122	124	125	126	127	78	78	79	79	80	81	82
	95th	124	125	126	128	129	130	131	82	82	83	83	84	85	86
16	90th	122	122	123	125	126	127	128	79	79	79	80	81	82	82
	95th	125	126	127	128	130	131	132	83	83	83	84	85	86	86
17	90th	122	123	124	125	126	128	128	79	79	79	80	81	82	82
	95th	126	126	127	129	130	131	132	83	83	83	84	85	86	86

*Height percentile determined by standard growth curves.
†Blood pressure percentile determined by a single measurement.

Source: Update on the Task Force Report on High Blood Pressure in Children and Adolescents: A Working Group Report from the National High Blood Pressure Education Program, NIH Publication No. 96-3790, National Heart, Lung, and Blood Institute, National Institutes of Health, September 1996.

tional Heart, Lung, and Blood Institute. Atlanta, GA: Centers for Disease Control and Prevention.) These normative tables are based on the first BP measured during screening on 61,206 children, including 31,158 boys and 30,048 girls.

The 90th and 95th percentiles of systolic and diastolic BP (using the fifth Korotkoff phase) for the 5th through 95th percentiles for height by sex and age are given for children in Tables 1 and 2, respectively. The difference in the 90th and 95th percentiles for BP for children of the same age and sex but of different height is apparent in these tables.

The BP tables adjusted for height and age in this report, as compared with the tables using only age, alter the BP percentile estimates of boys and girls at all ages and particularly for very young children. In general, BPs in the 90th and 95th percentiles for sex, height, and age are lower for shorter children than BPs in the 90th and 95th percentiles given for children by age alone. Conversely, tall children are allowed higher normal BPs when their height is taken into consideration than when age alone is used.

To use the tables in a clinical setting, the height percentile is determined from the standard growth charts. The child's measured systolic and diastolic BP is compared with the numbers provided in the table (boys or girls) for age and height percentile. The child is normotensive if BP is below the 90th percentile. If the child's BP (systolic or diastolic) is at or above the 95th percentile, the child may be hypertensive and repeated measurements are indicated. BP measurements between the 90th and 95th percentiles are high-normal and warrant further observation and consideration of other risk factors.

Standards for systolic and diastolic BP for infants younger than 1 year are available in the second task force report. Additional data recently have been published. (Hulman S, Edwards R, Chen YQ, Polansky M, Falkner B. Blood pressure patterns in the first three days of life. *J Perinatol*. 1991;11:231–234; and Zubrow A, Hulman S, Kushner H, Falkner B. Determinants of blood pressure in infants admitted to neonatal intensive care units: a prospective, multicenter study. *J Perinatol*. 1995;15:470–479.)

QUICK-REFERENCE DIAGNOSTIC CHARTS

QUICK-REFERENCE DIAGNOSTIC CHARTS

The quick-reference diagnostic charts are for use in the clinical setting. By following the steps listed below, clinicians can make a quick assessment for classification of blood pressure.

CLASSIFICATION OF BLOOD PRESSURE IN CHILDREN AND ADOLESCENTS*

SBP and DBP < 90th percentile	Normal
SBP or DBP ≥ 90th percentile and < 95th percentile	High-Normal**
SBP or DBP ≥ 95th percentile	Hypertension**

* for age and sex

** for age and sex measured on at least three separate occasions

SBP = systolic blood pressure
DBP = diastolic blood pressure

USING THE CHARTS

1. Use the standard height charts to determine the height percentile.
2. Measure the child's blood pressure. Record SBP and DBP.
3. Use the correct gender chart for 90th percentile of DBP.
4. Find the child's age on the right side of the chart. Follow the age line horizontally across the chart to the intersection of the line for the height percentile (vertical line).
5. Move UP or DOWN the height percentile line to the intersection of measured blood pressure.
   Result on 90th Percentile Chart:

- If you move DOWN on the height percentile line, blood pressure is **NORMAL**. Repeat steps 3 through 5 on the chart for 90th percentile SBP.
- If you move UP on the height percentile line, you must repeat steps 3 through 5 on the chart for 95th percentile DBP.
   Result on 95th Percentile Chart:
- If you move DOWN on the height percentile line, blood pressure is **HIGH-NORMAL.** Repeat steps 3 through 5 on the chart for 95th percentile SBP.
- If you move UP on the height percentile line, **HYPERTENSION*** is indicated. Repeat steps 3 through 5 on the chart for 95th percentile SBP.

Data points for the Quick-Reference Diagnostic Charts are found in Tables 1 and 2.
*Note that hypertension is diagnosed after three consecutive BP readings above the 95th percentile on three separate occasions.

Source: Update on the Task Force Report on High Blood Pressure in Children and Adolescents: A Working Group Report from the National High Blood Pressure Education Program, NIH Publication No. 96-3790, National Heart, Lung, and Blood Institute, National Institutes of Health, September 1996.

TREATMENT OF HYPERTENSION IN CHILDREN AND ADOLESCENTS*

Nonpharmacologic Therapy

Nonpharmacologic therapy comprises weight reduction, exercise, and dietary intervention. Nonpharmacologic therapy should be introduced not only in the care of patients with hypertension but also in children with high-normal BP (90th to 95th percentile BP distribution) and to complement drug therapy for patients with severe hypertension.

Body size is the major determinant for BP among children. In obese children, both systolic and diastolic BP may decrease in response to weight loss. In addition, weight loss offers other benefits. The adverse effect of obesity on cardiovascular function is compounded in the presence of hypertension, and overweight adolescents are at increased risk for cardiovascular disease as adults. Weight loss also has a positive effect on serum lipid profiles, and, in obese children, weight loss diminishes the effect of dietary salt on BP. The prevention of obesity in childhood would convey significant benefits in reducing risks for cardiovascular disease as well as other benefits. When elevated BP is associated with obesity, efforts should be directed at reducing obesity with strategies to lower excessive calorie intake and to increase physical exercise. Correction of obesity is difficult to achieve in children as well as adults. Because of the known benefits of weight control, efforts both to prevent and to control childhood obesity should be pursued. More effective weight loss strategies for children are developing, which should facilitate more effective treatment.

BP also is directly related to degree of physical fitness. The benefit of the increased physical activity occurs gradually over months. When increases in physical activity are combined with weight loss, the reduction in BP is superior to the effect resulting from weight reduction alone. Hypertension usually is not a contraindication to participation in sports and strenuous activity, particularly because exercise has a beneficial effect on BP and other risk factors. Sudden death during sporting events has not been reported in athletes with hypertension as it has in athletes with hypertrophic cardiomyopathy or cardiac arrhythmias.

Although dietary interventions to control or reduce obesity in childhood have demonstrated benefit to BP, limited data support the benefit to BP of other dietary interventions in the young. The preponderance of evidence from published clinical trials suggests that dietary sodium restriction reduces

BP in adults with hypertension. Most studies to determine whether sodium reduction lowers BP in children have been very short term. As yet, no clear evidence supports sodium reduction as beneficial in children or adolescents with mild hypertension. However, because sodium intake is generally well in excess of needs and mild BP elevation often is associated with obesity, a moderate reduction in dietary sodium can be beneficial. Sodium restriction is also of benefit in some types of secondary hypertension such as chronic glomerulonephritis. Practical dietary considerations include an increase in fresh fruits and vegetables, elimination of added salt to home-cooked foods in preparation and at the table, and a reduction in foods with high sodium content.

These strategies for nonpharmacologic therapy should be employed as initial treatment maneuvers for children with BP above the 90th percentile for age, gender, and height. Similarly, these nonpharmacologic methods are appropriate for children and adolescents with other risk factors for hypertension, particularly a strong family history of hypertension. Some childhood data sets indicate that African American children have BP levels that are somewhat higher than those of white children, suggesting that the prevalence of high BP may be greater in African American children than white children. Recent data from California regarding Asian American children show that they also tend to have higher BP than white children. With the known excess prevalence, morbidity, and mortality of essential hypertension among adult African Americans in the United States, it is advisable to be vigilant in monitoring BP and to encourage healthy diet, exercise, and weight control behaviors in African American children, especially in the presence of a family history of hypertension. This approach seems to be prudent for other groups with a higher prevalence of hypertension or individuals with a family history of high BP.

Pharmacologic Therapy

When drug therapy is used, the goal is to reduce BP to below the 95th percentile. The second task force report provided guidelines for the use of antihypertensive drugs in childhood, which continue to be endorsed. These drugs and their dosing recommendations are provided in "Antihypertensive Drug Therapy for Hypertensive Emergencies in Children," which contains the drugs recommended for acute antihypertensive therapy, and in "Antihypertensive Drug Therapy for Chronic Hypertension in Children," which lists the drugs used for chronic antihypertensive therapy. Antihypertensive drug therapy should be individualized, depending on the level of BP, the degree of response, the occurrence of side effects, and the patient's medical history. Diuretics and beta-blockers have been used in treating hypertension in children and adolescents, and these medications continue to be useful. Since publication of the second task force report,

---

*Source: Update on the Task Force Report on High Blood Pressure in Children and Adolescents: A Working Group Report from the National High Blood Pressure Education Program, NIH Publication No. 96-3790, National Heart, Lung, and Blood Institute, National Institutes of Health, September 1996.

ANTIHYPERTENSIVE DRUG THERAPY FOR HYPERTENSIVE EMERGENCIES IN CHILDREN

Drug	Dose
Nifedipine	0.25-0.5 mg/kg oral prn. May be repeated two times, if no response.
Sodium Nitroprusside	0.5-1 mcg/kg/min IV initially. May be increased stepwise to 8 mcg/kg/min maximum.
Labetalol	0.2-1 mg/kg/dose IV. May be increased incrementally to 1 mg/kg/dose until response achieved. 0.25-2 mg/kg/hr maintenance, either bolus or IV infusion.
Esmolol	500-600 mcg/kg IV load dose over 1-2 min then 200 mcg/kg/min. May be increased by 50-100 mcg/kg q 5-10 min to max of 1,000 mcg/kg.
Diazoxide	1-5 mg/kg/dose IV bolus up to max of 150 mg/dose.
Hydralazine	0.2-0.4 mg/kg IV prn. May be repeated two times if no response.
Minoxidil	0.1-0.2 mg/kg oral.

Source: Update on the Task Force Report on High Blood Pressure in Children and Adolescents: A Working Group Report from the National High Blood Pressure Education Program, NIH Publication No. 96-3790, National Heart, Lung, and Blood Institute, National Institutes of Health, September 1996.

a number of newer antihypertensive agents have become available and are described below.

Angiotensin-converting enzyme (ACE) inhibitors have become one of the primary agents for antihypertensive therapy not only because of their effectiveness in reducing BP but also because of their positive benefits on cardiac function, peripheral vasculature, and renal function. ACE inhibitors are effective in children and can be useful in young infants and newborns. Both the potency and the duration of action seem greater in this age group than in older children.

A significant adverse effect of ACE inhibitors on the kidneys is severe reduction in glomerular filtration in patients with bilateral renal artery stenosis or renal artery stenosis in a solitary or transplanted kidney. A more recent observation is the adverse effect of ACE inhibitors on the developing fetus. The use of ACE inhibitors during the second and third trimesters of pregnancy is associated with oligohydramnios and fetal effects of pulmonary hypoplasia, renal tubular dysplasia, and hypocalvaria as well as with hypotension and anuria after birth. Because of the teratogenic risk with fetal exposure, ACE inhibitors should be used with extreme caution in adolescent girls who may be sexually active.

Calcium channel blockers constitute a class of compounds that inhibit intracellular flux of calcium. At the present time, nifedipine is the calcium channel blocker used most often for treatment of childhood hypertension. The usefulness of nifedipine in treating chronic hypertension is limited by a short duration of action. Long-acting preparations have improved the effectiveness of nifedipine, but the tablet strength makes it impractical for use in small children. Because of recent concerns about possible adverse effects of short-term calcium channel blockers used in adults, it has been recommended that physicians exercise caution in their use. Presently there are no long-term data available on children using calcium channel blockers or any classes of antihypertensive agents. Most adverse effects are limited to a brief period of time after initial drug administration. The heart rate and cardiac output increase but usually return to pretreatment levels within a few weeks. Newer calcium channel blocking agents seem to have fewer side effects, although their use in children has been limited.

Benefit may be achieved with pharmacologic intervention at less severe levels of hypertension in some clinical situations. Children with confirmed chronic renal disease such as chronic glomerulonephritis should have therapy to reduce

ANTIHYPERTENSIVE DRUG THERAPY FOR CHRONIC HYPERTENSION IN CHILDREN

Listed in alphabetical order by drug class*

Drug	Dose (mg/kg/day) Initial	Maximum	Dosing Interval
Adrenergic-Blocking Agents			
Alpha-/Beta-Blocker			
Labetalol	1	3	q 6-12 hr
Alpha-Blocker			
Prazosin	0.05-0.1	0.5	q 6-8 hr
Beta-Adrenergic Blockers			
Atenolol	1	8	q 12-24 hr
Propranolol	1	8	q 6-12 hr
Alpha-Agonist			
Clonidine	0.05-0.1**	0.5-.6†	q 6 hr
Calcium Antagonists			
Nifedipine	**0.25**	3	q 4-6 hr
Nifedipine XL	0.25	3	q 12-24 hr
Converting Enzyme Inhibitors			
Captopril			
Children	1.5	6	q 8 hr
Neonates	0.03-0.15	2	q 8-24 hr
Enalapril	0.15	not established	q 12-24 hr
Diuretics			
Bumetanide	0.02-0.05	0.3	q 4-12 hr
Furosemide	1	12	q 4-12 hr
Hydrochlorothiazide	1	2-3	q 12 hr
Metolazone	0.1	3	q 12-24 hr
Spironolactone	1	3	q 6-12 hr
Triamterene	2	3	q 6-12 hr
Vasodilators			
Hydralazine	0.75	7.5	q 6 hr
Minoxidil	0.1-0.2	1	q 12 hr

*Other drugs are available in some classes, but data on dosage in children have not been published.
**Total initial dose in mg.
†Total daily dose in mg.

Source: Update on the Task Force Report on High Blood Pressure in Children and Adolescents: A Working Group Report from the National High Blood Pressure Education Program, NIH Publication No. 96-3790, National Heart, Lung, and Blood Institute, National Institutes of Health, September 1996.

BP to below the 95th percentile to preserve renal function. Children with diabetes constitute another group of patients warranting very careful BP surveillance. There is evidence that some children with diabetes, especially those who have a strong family history of hypertension, are at greater risk for development of diabetic nephropathy. Children, as well as adults, with diabetes are likely to achieve renal protective benefits from therapy to maintain BP below the 90th percentile.

Extensive clinical trials have not been conducted to examine the benefits and risks of antihypertensive therapy in children and adolescents. Because of the limited data available on therapy outcomes, the guidelines for treatment of children with hypertension are conservative. Treatment of children with mild hypertension should focus on lifestyle- or health-related behavioral changes including weight reduction and increased physical activity. Children with secondary hypertension, which may or may not be curable, should have therapy directed at the underlying cause of the hypertension.

Public Health Considerations

In the general population, it is estimated that more than 70 percent of premature morbidity can be attributed to tobacco use, undertreatment of hypertension, and obesity. From a public health perspective, health-related behaviors that reduce the risk of cardiovascular disease should be encouraged for all children and their families. In addition to monitoring BP, appropriate nutrition and exercise should be encouraged and smoking should be strongly discouraged during childhood.

NUTRITION COUNSELING IN TREATMENT OF HYPERTENSION*

Theories and Facts about Nutrition and Hypertension

The *Fifth Report of the Joint National Committee on Detection, Evaluation, and Treatment of High Blood Pressure* states that the goal of treating patients with hypertension is to prevent morbidity and mortality associated with high blood pressure and to control blood pressure by the least intrusive means possible. The committee states that lifestyle

modifications including weight reduction, increased physical activity, and moderation of dietary sodium and alcohol intake are definitive or adjunctive therapy for hypertension. These lifestyle factors form the basis for intervention strategies that have shown promise in the prevention of high blood pressure. However, their capacity to reduce morbidity or mortality in those with elevated blood pressure is not conclusively documented. In spite of this lack of conclusive evidence, lifestyle modifications offer multiple benefits at little cost and with minimal risk. Even when lifestyle modifications are not adequate in themselves to control hypertension, they may reduce the number and doses of antihypertensive medications needed to manage the condition. Researchers have found that lifestyle modifications are helpful in the large proportion of hypertensive patients who have additional risk factors for premature cardiovascular disease, especially dyslipidemias or diabetes. The Joint National Committee states that clinicians should vigorously encourage their patients to adopt these lifestyle modifications. The Joint National Committee also recommends the classification scheme in Table 1 for blood pressure levels.

Research on Weight Control and Hypertension

A compelling body of evidence relates obesity to hypertension. Many studies in epidemiology have shown the relationship of body weight and arterial pressure in both hypertensive and normotensive persons. In smaller studies, body weight and blood pressure have also been correlated in children and adolescents. In adults, relative body weight, body weight change over time, and skin-fold thickness have been directly related to blood pressure levels and to subsequent rate of development of hypertension. In addition, the risk of normotensive persons later becoming hypertensive is related to the degree of obesity. Several additional studies have documented the importance of weight gain in subsequent development of hypertension.

Additional evidence indicates that truncal or abdominal fat deposition may be important to hypertension. The deposition of excess fat in this upper body region correlates with hypertension, dyslipidemia, diabetes, and increased coronary heart disease mortality.

Researchers have provided a variety of evidence that weight reduction induced by calorie restriction lowers blood pressure. Experimental starvation studies have shown falls in systolic pressure from 104 mm Hg (millimeters of mercury) to 93 mm Hg and diastolic pressures from 70 mm Hg to 63 mm Hg. All subjects were normotensive. With refeeding, blood pressure values returned to prestarvation levels.

---

*Source: Linda G. Snetselaar, *Nutrition Counseling Skills for Medical Nutrition Therapy*, Aspen Publishers, Inc., © 1997.

Table 1. Classification of Blood Pressure for Adults Age 18 Years and Older*

Category	Systolic (mm Hg)	Diastolic (mm Hg)
Normal[†]	<130	<85
High normal	130–139	85–89
Hypertension**		
STAGE 1 (Mild)	140–159	90–99
STAGE 2 (Moderate)	160–179	100–109
STAGE 3 (Severe)	180–209	110–119
STAGE 4 (Very Severe)	≥210	≥120

*Not taking antihypertensive drugs and not acutely ill. When systolic and diastolic pressures fall into different categories, the higher category should be selected to classify the individual's blood pressure status. For instance, 160/92 mm Hg should be classified as Stage 2, and 180/120 mm Hg should be classified as Stage 4. Isolated systolic hypertension (ISH) is defined as SBP ≥ 140 mm Hg and DBP <90 mm Hg and staged appropriately (e.g., 170/85 mm Hg is defined as Stage 2 ISH).

[†]Optimal blood pressure with respect to cardiovascular risk is SBP <120 mm Hg and DBP <80 mm Hg. However, unusually low readings should be evaluated for clinical significance.

**Based on the average of two or more readings taken at each of two or more visits following an initial screening.

Note: In addition to classifying stages of hypertension based on average blood pressure levels, the clinician should specify presence or absence of target-organ disease and additional risk factors. For example, a patient with diabetes and a blood pressure of 142/94 mm Hg plus left ventricular hypertrophy should be classified as "Stage 1 hypertension with target-organ disease (left ventricular hypertrophy) and with another major risk factor (diabetes)." This specificity is important for risk classification and management.

Source: Reprinted from the National High Blood Pressure Education Program; National Institutes of Health; National Heart, Lung, and Blood Institute, *The Fifth Report of the Joint National Committee on Detection, Evaluation, and Treatment of High Blood Pressure,* 1994.

Research correlating changes in blood pressure in hypertensive persons with changes in weight began in the 1920s. A study found that weight reduction resulted in lower pressures, and later many researchers reported reduced blood pressure with weight loss.

In the Chicago Coronary Prevention Evaluation Program, a considerable decrease in body weight was associated with decreases in pressure, heart rate, and serum cholesterol. A later Israeli study indicated that most obese hypertensive persons achieved normal pressure when they lost only half of their excess weight, even though they remained very obese. Achieving ideal body weight was not crucial to reducing blood pressure, and the pressure fall persisted as long as the decreased body weight was maintained. Researchers in the Dusseldorf Obesity study found that, for hypertensive persons not receiving antihypertensive medication over four and one-half years, the pressure fall was greatest in those who lost 12 kilograms. In another study, the decrease in blood pressure in subjects who lost weight was associated with contraction of plasma volume and a decline in cardiac output, which in turn was related to slower heart rate and decreases in plasma cholesterol, uric acid, and blood glucose.

Weight reduction reduces blood pressure in a large proportion of hypertensive individuals who are more than 10 percent above ideal weight. A reduction in blood pressure usually occurs early during a weight-loss program, often with weight loss as small as 10 pounds.

Basic conclusions from these studies follow:

- Elevated blood pressure correlates with increased body mass.
- Decreases in blood pressure result when weight is reduced.
- With weight loss, cardiovascular morbidity and mortality will decrease even if pressure does not. For persons on antihypertensive drugs the number and/or dosage of these agents may be reduced with decreases in blood pressure following weight loss.

The 1994 Joint National Committee on Detection, Evaluation, and Treatment of High Blood Pressure issued the following recommendations about weight control and hypertension:

- All hypertensive patients who are above their ideal weight should initially be placed on an individualized, monitored weight-reduction program involving caloric restriction and increased caloric expenditure by regular physical activity.
- In overweight patients with stage 1 hypertension, an attempt to control blood pressure with weight loss and other lifestyle modifications should be tried for at least three to six months prior to initiating pharmacologic therapy. If pharmacologic therapy is needed, patients should continue to pursue vigorously the weight-loss program.

Research on Dietary Sodium Restriction and Hypertension

A second nonpharmacological method for controlling high blood pressure is restricting dietary sodium. Epidemiologic observations and clinical trials support an association between dietary sodium intake and blood pressure. Based on linear regression analysis within populations, a 100 mmol (millimole) per day lower average sodium intake was associated with a 2.2 mm Hg lower systolic blood pressure (SBP) in 10,000 people, and a 5 to 10 mm Hg lower SBP in multiple other studies involving 47,000 participants. Furthermore, a 100 mmol per day lower sodium intake was associated with a 9 mm Hg decrease in the rise of SBP in persons between the ages of 25 and 55 years.

Multiple therapeutic trials document a reduction of blood pressure in response to reduced sodium intake. In short-term trials, moderate sodium restriction in hypertensive individuals on average reduces SBP by 4.9 mm Hg and diastolic blood pressure (DBP) by 2.6 mm Hg. In trials involving people aged 50 to 59 and lasting five weeks or longer, a 50 mmol per day reduction of sodium intake was associated with an average of 7 mm Hg reduction in SBP in hypertensive persons and a 5 mm Hg reduction in normotensive people.

Individuals vary in their blood pressure response to changes in dietary sodium. African Americans, older people, and patients with hypertension are more sensitive to changes in dietary sodium.

The 1994 Joint National Committee on Detection, Evaluation, and Treatment of High Blood Pressure issued the following recommendations about sodium restriction and hypertension.

- Because the average American consumes more than 150 mmol of sodium per day, moderate dietary sodium reduction to a level of less than 100 mmol per day (less than 6 grams of table salt or less than 2.3 grams of sodium per day) is recommended.
- For patients with stage 1 hypertension, the above degree of restriction may result in controlled blood pressure.
- For patients needing drug therapy, dietary sodium restriction may decrease the medication requirements.

Research on Alcohol and Hypertension

A third important nonpharmacological method of helping to lower blood pressure is reduction in alcohol consumption. Epidemiological surveys have shown that consuming more than 60 to 80 grams (1½ to 2 ounces) of alcohol per day is associated with a significantly higher prevalence of hypertension. In one study, 51.5 percent of clients who consumed more than 80 grams of alcohol per day had hypertension (blood pressure greater than 140/90 mm Hg) on admission to a hospital. Following elimination of alcohol, systolic and diastolic pressures decreased; only 9 percent remained hypertensive. Those who abstained from alcohol over time remained normotensive; most of those who reverted back to drinking also reverted to previous elevated levels of blood pressure.

Although these studies point to the importance of abstinence from the standpoint of hypertension, almost all epidemiological evidence has shown lower morbidity and mortality from coronary heart disease in people who consume one to two ounces of ethanol per day compared with those who do not drink.

The 1994 Joint National Committee on Detection, Evaluation, and Treatment of High Blood Pressure issued the following recommendations about alcohol and hypertension:

- Persons with hypertension who drink alcohol-containing beverages should be counseled to limit their daily intake to 1 ounce of ethanol (2 ounces of 100-proof whiskey, 8 ounces of wine, or 24 ounces of beer).
- Significant hypertension may develop during withdrawal from heavy alcohol consumption, but the pressor effect of alcohol withdrawal reverses a few days after alcohol consumption is reduced.

Research on Potassium and Hypertension

A high dietary potassium intake may protect against developing hypertension, and potassium deficiency may increase blood pressure and induce ventricular ectopy. The Joint National Committee on Detection, Evaluation, and Treatment of High Blood Pressure recommends the following:

- Normal plasma concentrations of potassium should be maintained, preferably from food sources.
- If hypokalemia occurs during diuretic therapy, additional potassium may be needed either from potassium-containing salt substitutes, potassium supplements, or use of a potassium-sparing diuretic. Potassium chloride supplements and potassium-sparing diuretics must be used with caution in patients susceptible to hyperkalemia.

Research on Calcium and Hypertension

In many but not all epidemiologic studies, there is an inverse association between dietary calcium and blood pressure. Calcium deficiency is associated with an increased prevalence of hypertension, and a low calcium intake may amplify the effects of a high sodium intake on blood pressure. An increased calcium intake may lower blood pressure in some patients with hypertension. However, the overall effect is minimal, and there is no way to predict which patients will benefit. Based on this evidence, there is currently no rationale for recommending calcium intakes in excess of the recommended daily allowance of 20 to 30 mmol (800 to 1200 mg) in an attempt to lower blood pressure.

Research on Magnesium and Hypertension

Suggestive evidence of an association between lower dietary magnesium intake and higher blood pressures exists. However, the Joint National Committee on Detection, Evaluation, and Treatment of High Blood Pressure states that, given no convincing data, they do not recommend an increased magnesium intake in an effort to lower blood pressure.

Summary of Research Findings

In conclusion, three methods of dietary treatment, weight control, sodium restriction, and alcohol restriction, are recommended for management of hypertension. Evidence is too meager to justify recommendations about other nutrients in relation to hypertension. The research behind recommendations for low-calorie, low-sodium diets adds strength to the overall objective of reducing high blood pressure. The following sections provide research on adherence to changes in eating patterns; examples of inappropriate eating behaviors; methods of assessing those behaviors; and strategies for dealing with lack of knowledge, forgetfulness, and lack of commitment to low-sodium methods of altering high blood pressure. Indeed, persons who are hypertensive at ideal body weight may require only the low-sodium diet to normalize blood pressure.

Research on Adherence to Eating Patterns in Treatment of Hypertension

Contingency contracting was found to be effective in reducing weight in a hypertensive client population. Further, a feasibility test for the Dietary Intervention Study of Hypertension showed that interventions for weight reduction and sodium-potassium modification among hypertensives can be relatively independent, implying that a hypertension education program could be divided into these components or that these interventions could be used separately.

Monitoring of and feedback on urinary sodium levels resulted in successful sodium reductions in recent studies. The simplification of urine sodium estimation procedures through use of overnight instead of 24-hour urine samples and immediate feedback by analysis using chloride titrator strips are important advances in the practicality of these monitoring techniques. It is important to regularly monitor both behavioral (pill counts) and physiological outcome (blood pressure) data to avoid accidentally blaming clients for inadequate therapeutic response. Indeed, a client may be an excellent adherer but show little physiological response if treatment is inappropriate or inadequate. It has been suggested that the primary cause of dietary noncompliance may be inadequate dietary counseling. Nurses trained by the

medical director, a physician, counseled 489 subjects, who received information on the causes and results of hypertension and the elimination of salt at the table and in cooking, and discussed lists of high-sodium foods and substitutes. The 12 subjects in the control group were treated by family physicians in their usual manner, which generally included advice to restrict salt usage but no intensive dietary counseling or extra assistance. The failure to note differences in the two groups in this study was attributed to a lack of nutrition counseling. The counseling sessions involved only the client; yet family support has been found to be important in successful adherence to dietary regimens.

A study in Finland showed favorable results when cooperation between physician and client improved. Physicians began providing oral and written information on hypertension that emphasized the importance of adherence to treatment. Clients also received a blood pressure follow-up card on which the blood pressure reading and the precise time of the next appointment were recorded. Clients who missed their appointments were sent a new invitation.

Many clients believe that taking medicine should make them feel better. Since hypertension is an asymptomatic illness, the client does not obtain symptom relief from the medication or diet.

In chronic health care situations such as hypertension, a belief in shared control or cooperation between clients and health care providers lays the groundwork for optimum treatment outcomes. This finding suggests that other, internal and powerful characteristics may interact in the best interest of the client. Shared responsibility in control of hypertension may be critical to increasing adherence in the client with uncontrolled hypertension.

Components of a structured behavior modification program are described as: (1) self-monitoring of sodium and/or calorie intake, (2) nutrient and behavior goal setting, (3) structured problem solving, and (4) skill training. Prevention of relapse should be addressed in the context of emotional, social, and environmental forces that impinge upon the individual's behavior. Elements in the relapse prevention program include (1) introducing the client to the concept of high-risk situations and assessing previous coping strategies; (2) including skill training and behavior rehearsal to increase the client's coping skills in response to negative emotions, interpersonal conflict, and social pressure; (3) enhancing motivation through an emphasis on the long-term consequences of engaging in prohibited behaviors; (4) teaching clients how to cope cognitively and behaviorally with slips; (5) tailoring the rules of a low-sodium, weight-loss eating pattern to the individual's unique situation; (6) teaching strategies for minimizing high-risk situations; and (7) teaching clients to seek and enhance the social support available for following an antihypertensive eating pattern. Some researchers also emphasized the importance of follow-up contact after completion of the initial program and recommended individual counseling, group meetings, telephone contact, and regular mail contact for at least the first three to six months—the time the majority of relapses occur.

Inappropriate Eating Behaviors

Diets modified in sodium content may be extremely difficult for most clients with whom nutrition counselors must deal. Salt is used as a flavoring agent in nearly every food. Altering such dietary habits means drastic changes for most clients.

Nutrition counselors frequently hear the complaint, "I really miss familiar flavors," or "Everything I eat tastes like sawdust." For unconscious salters (those who salt without tasting), the true flavors of foods may never have come through. They can gradually discover the natural flavors in foods.

The new eating pattern limits clients' food options because most commercial products are very high in sodium. With the trend toward prepackaged commercial meals and other products, clients on a low-sodium regimen are left with fewer choices. This limitation has led to many alterations in old eating habits. Clients not only must change what they usually eat but also must become accustomed to a new and foreign range of food flavors.

The food industry, in an effort to assist these persons, has developed a variety of low-salt products. However, these generate comments such as, "Do you expect me to eat this low-sodium soup? It's terrible." Another complaint is that some salt substitutes leave a bitter aftertaste. Objections to commercial low-sodium products constitute a recurring problem for nutrition counselors.

Assessment of Eating Behaviors

For clients who must follow a low-sodium diet, a baseline assessment is crucial. Such regimens require changes in many foods that individuals routinely and even unconsciously consume. Identifying when, where, with whom, and how much sodium is consumed can be of great benefit in helping to reduce salt intake patterns.

In collecting this information, the clients self-monitor their sodium intake. Before using the form, clients might be asked simply to observe their general behaviors involving sodium consumption (for example, salting before tasting). They might be given ideas on which basic foods are high in sodium.

During the baseline data collection, clients begin counting sodium intake occurrences, along with collecting related information indicated in the form. The following guidelines can be of help:

- The form must be portable and readily available for recording.
- Clients must be familiar enough with high-sodium foods to record all occurrences of the target behavior (sodium intake).
- Clients should record the data as the behaviors occur.
- Clients always should keep written records—memory is not adequate for baseline data collection.

ALGORITHM FOR NUTRITION SCREENING AND INTERVENTION IN HYPERTENSION

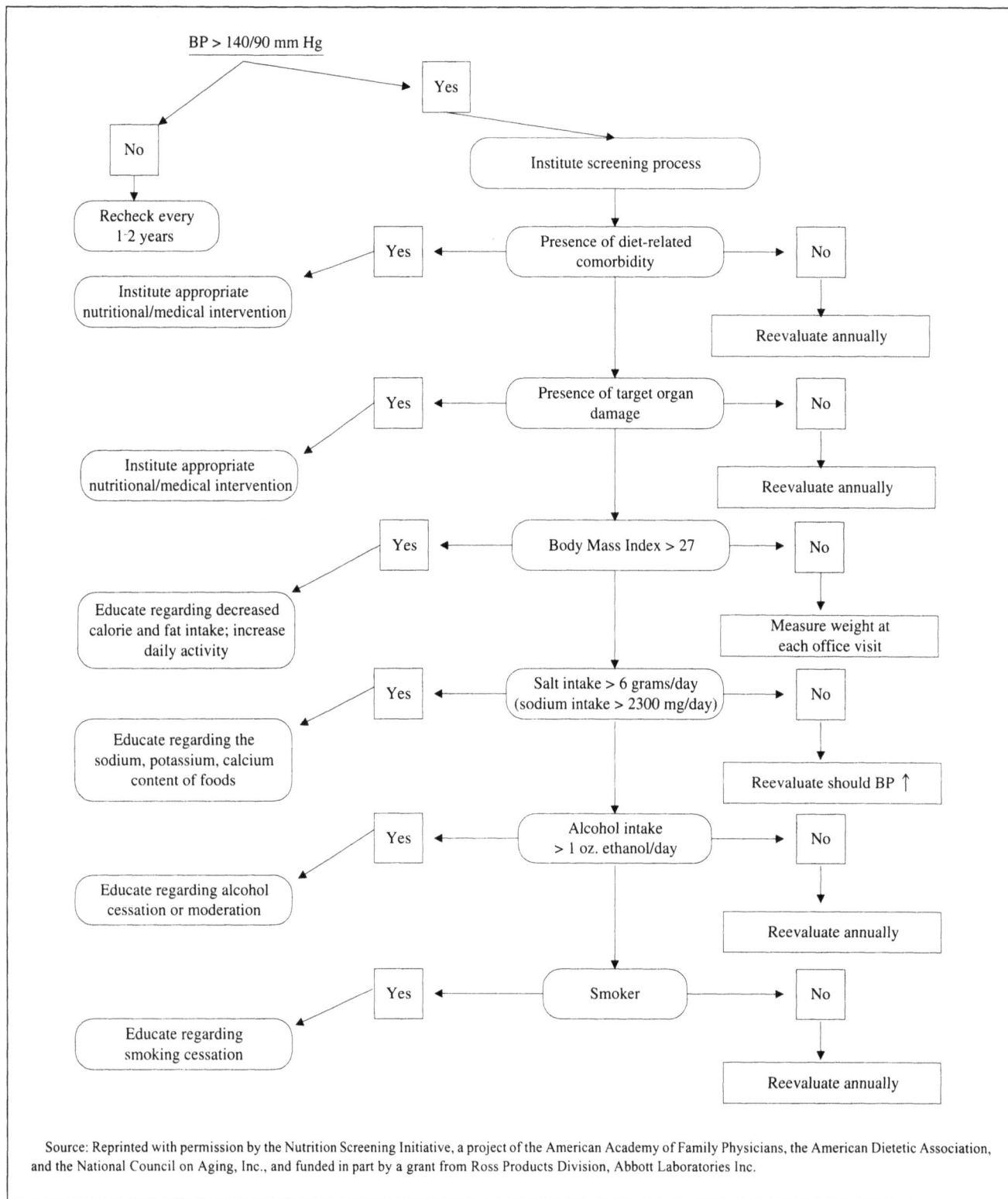

BP > 140/90 mm Hg

```
                          Yes
No

Recheck every                    Institute screening process
1-2 years

                    Yes ←  Presence of diet-related  → No
                           comorbidity

Institute appropriate                              Reevaluate annually
nutritional/medical intervention

                    Yes ←  Presence of target organ  → No
                           damage

Institute appropriate                              Reevaluate annually
nutritional/medical intervention

                    Yes ←  Body Mass Index > 27  → No

Educate regarding decreased                        Measure weight at
calorie and fat intake; increase                   each office visit
daily activity

                    Yes ←  Salt intake > 6 grams/day  → No
                           (sodium intake > 2300 mg/day)

Educate regarding the                              Reevaluate should BP ↑
sodium, potassium, calcium
content of foods

                    Yes ←  Alcohol intake  → No
                           > 1 oz. ethanol/day

Educate regarding alcohol                          Reevaluate annually
cessation or moderation

                    Yes ←  Smoker  → No

Educate regarding                                  Reevaluate annually
smoking cessation
```

Source: Reprinted with permission by the Nutrition Screening Initiative, a project of the American Academy of Family Physicians, the American Dietetic Association, and the National Council on Aging, Inc., and funded in part by a grant from Ross Products Division, Abbott Laboratories Inc.

THE ROLE OF CARDIOVASCULAR REACTIVITY TO STRESSFUL CHALLENGES IN THE ETIOLOGY OF HYPERTENSION*

There is significant variability among individuals in the cardiovascular responses to both physical and psychologic stimuli, a phenomenon called cardiovascular reactivity.[1,2] The magnitude of cardiovascular reactivity may distinguish those prone to develop cardiovascular disease or differentiate pathophysiologic states among individuals who have existing pathologies such as hypertension.[3]

This article presents theoretic and empiric information about the reactivity of the cardiovascular system to stressful challenges and explains what differences in the magnitude of reactivity indicate about the pathophysiologic state of patients. Furthermore, proposed mechanisms underlying the pathophysiology of hyperreactivity are discussed as they relate to the development or maintenance of hypertension.

Cardiovascular Reactivity and Stress

The linear relationship of heart rate, oxygen consumption, and cardiac output to exercise workload serves as the foundation for defining cardiovascular reserve capacity for exercise.[4] The magnitude and linearity of these responses are theoretically related to the metabolic demands of working skeletal muscle and the necessary peripheral blood flow adaptations to meet metabolic demand.[5] Thus, in healthy subjects, dynamic exercise evokes an assumed metabolically proportional stimulus–response relationship. However, the cardiovascular response to psychologic stimuli may be exaggerated relative to the metabolic demand of the stressor.[6] A proportionately greater oxygen consumption for behavioral versus physical stimuli has been reported.[7,8] Studies of reactivity to physical versus psychologic stressors have suggested that the mechanisms underlying the responses to each type of stimulus are different. Psychologic stressors, such as shock avoidance tasks, have been associated with slight reductions in cardiac output and increases in peripheral resistance from baseline levels, whereas exercise tasks are associated with increased cardiac output and decreased peripheral resistance.[9] Psychologic stressors may stimulate an anticipatory reaction to ready the subject for the motor

activity of "fight or flight."[10] However, without the enactment of the anticipated motor activity, the physiologic augmentation of cardiac output is inappropriate to the real needs of muscle tissue and may result in a compensatory autoregulatory vasoconstriction.[11,12]

Obrist[6] proposed that different stress challenges provoke different patterns of autonomic responses. Tasks that require active coping, or sustained mental strategy, to control outcome of their performance, produce responses more influenced by β-adrenergic stimulation than α-adrenergic stimulation. Passive tasks, or those whose outcome cannot be altered by the action of the performer, are proposed as more influenced by α-adrenergic stimulation and have greater vascular responses.[6] However, in a review of 22 studies comparing cardiovascular responses to active versus passive coping, Pickering and Gerin[13] found no evidence for heart rate (β adrenergic) hyperreactivity in borderline or established hypertensive versus control subjects exposed to active coping tasks. The authors of this review concluded that there is evidence for increased systolic blood pressure reactivity in borderline and established hypertensive versus control subjects for behavioral (active and passive coping tasks) as well as for physical challenges (exercise and cold pressor task) although behavioral stimuli tend to produce relatively greater reactivity responses. The results of these studies cannot be interpreted as support for hyperreactivity as a cause of hypertension.[13] Rather, hyperreactivity may be a consequence of hypertension. Support for this latter conclusion comes from studies of physical challenges, where either no differences in reactivity using the cold pressor test[14] or relatively small differences in reactivity using dynamic exercise[15,16] were observed between borderline hypertensives and control subjects but substantial differences in reactivity to both challenges existed between established hypertensives and normotensive controls.

Variability in Cardiovascular Reactivity Responses

Individual differences in cardiovascular reactivity to psychologic stress have been demonstrated in humans exposed to a variety of stressors including aversive reaction time tasks, mental arithmetic tests, video games, and interpersonal challenges such as public speaking as well as to physical challenges including dynamic exercise, isometric exercise, and the cold pressor test.[1] Studies[17–19] in animal models have found that spontaneously hypertensive rats (SHR) are hyperreactive to behavioral stressors and renal nerve stimulation and have greater sodium retention with these stressors when compared to responses observed in control rats.

*Source: Kathleen Potempa, DNSc, "An Overview of the Role of Cardiovascular Reactivity to Stressful Challenges in the Etiology of Hypertension," *The Journal of Cardiovascular Nursing*, Vol. 8:4, Aspen Publishers, Inc., © July 1994.

Matthews and Rakaczky[20] reviewed 27 studies of reactivity in subjects with a family history of hypertension. The most commonly employed test in these studies was the cold pressor test (11 of 19 studies), which can be viewed as primarily a physical challenge. All 19 reports concluded that exaggerated heart rate or blood pressure response to stress (or both) was associated with a positive family history of hypertension. Lawler and associates[21] observed the development of established hypertension in a rat model genetically predisposed to hypertension when exposed to shock-avoidance conflicts, whereas control rats of the same strain did not develop hypertension. Thus, there is evidence that hyperreactivity is a genetically linked trait marker for hypertension. Given this evidence, the question then becomes, Is cardiovascular reactivity a cause of hypertension development?

The Cardiovascular Reactivity Hypothesis

The magnitude of cardiovascular reactivity is an attribute of an individual, most likely having genetic origins, that is distributed along a continuum ranging from high reactivity to low reactivity. The cardiovascular reactivity hypothesis states that individuals who are "hyperreactors" respond to behavioral stress with exaggerated and metabolically inappropriate cardiovascular responses that set in motion pathophysiologic events that eventually lead to sustained hypertension.[3] This hypothesis assumes that the initiating stress is behavioral or emotional and under the influence of cerebral-limbic modulation. It also assumes that the physiologic responses to stress represent anticipatory arousal to support the muscle activity of the classic defense fight or flight response.[6]

Two pathophysiologic scenarios have been constructed from this hypothesis.[22] In the first scenario, the "hyperreactor's" response to the environmental stress initiates abnormal signals from the cerebral-limbic circuits that drive the lower cardiovascular control system, which responds normally, albeit to an abnormal signal.[22] In the second scenario, the behaviorally initiated signals are normal, but the target organ systems respond to the signals abnormally.[22] Much of the current work on the pathophysiologic mechanisms of cardiovascular reactivity is related to these two scenarios. The central nervous system (CNS) mechanisms studied include the sympathetic outflow mechanisms and the opiate system as they relate to the cerebrallimbic signaling system. Additionally, a defect in the baroreflex has also been hypothesized.[13] Peripheral mechanisms studied thus far in relationship to this hypothesis include the peripheral vascular response to sympathetic nervous system activity, the influence of sodium on vascular reactivity, and the role of insulin resistance and compensatory hyperinsulinemia on several mechanisms that foster and maintain hypertension.

Possible Mechanisms Influencing Cardiovascular Reactivity

Central Nervous System Mechanisms

The notion that behavioral stress and hypertension are causally linked suggests a role for the CNS in the determination of the individual differences in responsivity to stressful stimuli.[23] Several nuclei in the brain stem and medulla are related to the maintenance of cardiovascular homeostasis. The medulla also functions to integrate autonomic responses, receiving input from the limbic, cortical, cerebellar, reticular, and other areas of the brain.[24] This centrally mediated integration regulates the final alterations in cardiovascular responses that lead to changes in heart rate, cardiac contractility, peripheral resistance, and the adrenal medullary outflow.[24]

Although the potential influence of the CNS on cardiovascular responses is not clearly elucidated, the sympathetic nervous system (SNS) and the endogenous opiate system have been studied as they relate to cardiovascular reactivity. The assumed interaction of these two systems is through the cortical-limbic modulation of emotional responses as messages; these messages are transacted to lower adrenergic outflow pathways.[25] The baroreflex response has been implicated in the expression of cardiovascular reactivity.

Sympathetic nervous system alterations in cardiovascular reactivity. Several investigators[26–28] have reported elevated resting norepinephrine levels (indicating enhanced SNS activity) in human hypertensives and in animal models of hypertension using a variety of methods. Enhanced sympathetic drive is a well-documented event in normotensive individuals with a family history of hypertension.[29] Patients with borderline hypertension show both an increased sympathetic tone and a decreased parasympathetic tone.[29] Julius[23] suggests that this finding is the strongest argument for the role of the CNS in the pathophysiology of hypertension because the CNS regulates sympathetic drive in an integrated manner.

Manuck and Krantz[30] propose two models to explain the relationship of centrally mediated stress response and elevated blood pressure. In the recurrent activation model, the reactivity observed with behavioral stress in the laboratory should correspond to the magnitude of blood pressure spikes occurring in response to the stresses of everyday life. These blood pressure spikes are characterized by peaks and valleys that return to a baseline blood pressure. In this model, the frequency of blood pressure spikes is theoretically related to the exposure rate to environmental stressors or CNS responsivity to behavioral stimuli (or both). In the second model, the prevailing state model, the reactivity relationship to stressors in the laboratory is indicative of the magnitude of the sympathetically driven constant elevation of blood pressure occurring during waking hours. This continuous outflow may reflect a greater cardiovascular response to the anticipated stresses of the day, a concept consistent with studies of passive coping styles.[3]

Both models are simplistic, and the actual relationship of reactivity to hypertensive state is better represented by a model that combines aspects of the recurrent activation and prevailing state models.[3] This combined model suggests that both high and low reactors begin the day at parallel levels, but high reactors have both greater anticipatory sympathetic outflow and exaggerated responses to some, but not all, stressors.[3] This model is more consistent with current data that show inconsistent relationships between heart rate or blood pressure reactivity measured in the laboratory and casual resting blood pressure and average blood pressure measured during ambulatory monitoring.

Baroreflex mechanism. Pickering and Gerin[13] suggest that the baroreflex response may play a role in the regulation of the blood pressure reactivity responses. Hyperreactivity to external stimuli has been documented as the result of impairment of the baroreflex response through the denervation of the sino-aortic afferent nerve pathway.[31] The baroreflex sensitivity is also reduced during tasks where the blood pressure is normally elevated, such as dynamic exercise,[32] isometric exercise,[33] and mental arithmetic.[34] Also, normotensive subjects with a family history of hypertension show decreased baroreflex sensitivity,[35] and subjects with reduced sensitivity have enhanced blood pressure variability.[36]

Endogenous opioids and cardiovascular reactivity. The enhancement of autonomic tone associated with borderline and early essential hypertension has been related to centrally mediated autonomic outflow.[23] Endogenous opioids, notably endorphins and enkephalins, have been proposed as the likely modulators of central sympathetic outflow.[25] These peptides are released during intense autonomic stimulation and may account for the link between hyperreactivity and the development of essential hypertension.[25]

Opioids are linked functionally to blood pressure control by the observation that they have hypotensive action during systemic shock[26,37] and alter the baroreflex response.[38] The primary role of opioids thus appears to be inhibition or blunting of sympathetically mediated stress responses. A deficiency in the opioid system may result in disinhibition reflected in exaggerated fluctuations in catecholaminergic neurotransmission as well as the resulting cardiovascular responsivity to the initiating stressor.[25] This hypothesis is in line with the first pathophysiologic scenario of cardiovascu-lar reactivity described earlier. In this case, a deficiency in opioid peptide or reduced opioid receptor sensitivity may permit an undampened pathway from stressor to enhanced sympathetic outflow stimulation characteristic of borderline and early hypertension.

Vascular Mechanisms

SNS activity, vascular tone, and vascular reactivity. Authors[39-41] of several studies have reported increased α-adrenergic vascular tone and increased vascular reactivity in association with increased peripheral vascular resistance. An enhanced peripheral resistance is the principal hemodynamic alteration in established hypertension and is inappropriately, but not absolutely, elevated in many borderline hypertensives.[23] Enhanced vascular reactivity to all vasoconstrictors regardless of their receptor type is a consistent finding in established hypertension.[42] This increased vascular reactivity is an example of a positive feedback system where vessels have higher resistance to flow that leads to higher pressure, which then favors an increase in wall thickness and remodeling.[42] Thus, the role of vascular reactivity and vascular tone in the etiology and maintenance of hypertension has been hypothesized.[42] Proposed mechanisms for enhanced vascular tone and reactivity include an increased sympathetic drive, enhanced α receptor sensitivity, derangement of membrane co-transport systems, and vascular remodeling.[42]

The influence of physical and psychologic stress on vascular reactivity is hypothetical. It is proposed that the centrally mediated SNS activity stimulated by stressors will have an eventual influence on a sustained increase in vascular tone, peripheral resistance, and vascular reactivity. However, this chain of events is not straightforward, and it may be a consequence—and not a cause—of hypertension. Enhanced vascular reactivity may contribute to the enhanced cardiovascular responsiveness to stressful challenges observed in some early and well-established hypertensives.

Salt sensitivity in the evolution of hyperreactivity. Excessive dietary intake of salt has been consistently associated with the development of hypertension.[43,44] The blood-pressure-lowering effects of low-sodium diets in humans have been well established.[43] Animal models have revealed a consistent, progressive pathology associated with high salt intake in salt-sensitive rats versus salt-resistant rat strains leading to hypertension development and cardiovascular morbidity.[43,45]

Exploration of the vascular effects of salt sensitivity has revealed a reduced vasodilator response to ischemic forearm exercise in salt-sensitive normotensive and hypertensive subjects given a high-sodium diet.[46,47] These findings suggest an interactive role of salt sensitivity, dietary sodium intake, and vascular tone on the vasodilatory reserve. It has also been shown that vasoconstriction to norepinephrine and serotonin, modulated by endothelium-dependent constricting factor (EDCF), is potentiated in salt-sensitive Dahl rats given a high-salt diet.[48]

Exposure to acute stressors produces short-term slowing of sodium excretion in the hypertensive dog,[49] spontaneously hypertensive rat,[19] and in the Dahl rat model of borderline hypertension.[50] Human investigations have yielded similar results.[43] Although Lawler and colleagues[51] showed the development of hypertension in back-crossed rats with chronic stress exposure without dietary manipulation, others[52] have observed that stress-induced hypertension occurs only in the presence of a high-salt diet in borderline hypertensive Dahl rats. However, high-salt diet alone, in the absence of stress manipulation, produced hypertension in the borderline hypertensive rat if the salt exposure was prolonged.[43,52]

There is a paucity of direct studies of the effect of salt intake on cardiovascular reactivity. The results have been mixed, with more studies showing lower reactivity with high-salt diet, especially in African-American subjects.[53] This contradictory finding is rather difficult to explain. Dimsdale and colleagues[54] concluded that high salt intake does not generally alter blood pressure reactivity, although reactivity may be influenced in some susceptible individuals.

The evidence suggests that there is a role for sodium in the etiology of hypertension. However, the role of sodium and the pathogenesis of hypertension cannot be explicated at this time.

Insulin and blood pressure reactivity development. The often-occurring triad of hypertension, diabetes, and coronary artery disease has introduced the plausibility of a common pathophysiologic defect. Insulin-resistance syndrome is a constellation of symptoms that includes insulin resistance, compensatory hyperinsulinemia, high triglyceride levels, low levels of high-density lipoproteins (HDL), and glucose intolerance.[55] It has been hypothesized that insulin resistance, and compensatory hyperinsulinemia, may be the primary metabolic defect that initiates a pathophysiologic cascade leading to the development of hypertension.[56] Development of type II diabetes and onset of coronary artery disease are included in the sequelae of pathophysiologic events.[57]

The consequence of insulin resistance is augmentation of pancreatic β-cell insulin secretion. Hyperinsulinemia has been observed in animal and human manifestations of hypertension.[56] Insulin may contribute to high blood pressure and the development of hypertension through several possible pathways. Insulin acts at several effector sites, resulting in increased sympathetic activity—particularly increased norepinephrine levels, enhanced sodium retention by the kidney,

and enhanced sodium and calcium influx into vascular smooth muscle cells. Insulin fosters the proliferation of arteriolar smooth muscle cells.[57] Insulin, in the presence or absence of hypoglycemia, produces increased heart rate, increased cardiac output, and enhanced myocardial contractility. The mechanism of these effects has been related to enhanced sympathetic activity.[58]

There are no published studies reporting a direct association between reactivity level and hyperinsulinemia. However, proponents of the reactivity hypothesis suggest that the enhanced sympathetic tone is the theoretic link between behaviorally evoked stress, hyperinsulinemia, and eventual hypertension development.[58] For this proposition to be true, enhanced sympathetic tone must precede or coincide with hyperinsulinemia in genetically insulin-resistant individuals. Although most favor the hypothesis that insulin resistance is the primary defect in the pathophysiologic cascade,[56-58] the possibility that central sympathetic drive is the initiating problem cannot be ruled out at this time.[57]

Perspectives on the Reactivity Hypothesis

It is clear from the discussion so far that there are several possible genetic defects that may foster hypertension. These defects include (1) defects in the manner in which the CNS processes signals from stressors such as the opioid signaling system, (2) derangement in the blood-pressure-sensing mechanism or in the baroreflex mechanism, and (3) derangements in insulin-mediated glucose uptake causing insulin-resistance syndrome and hyperinsulinemia. There is some evidence[59] that the magnitude of cardiovascular reactivity to stressors is genetically determined. However, the question remains whether reactivity is a behaviorally driven trait that plays a key role in hypertension development.

Pickering and Gerin[13] evaluated the reactivity hypothesis on the basis of four criteria: (1) the reliability of the reactivity response over time, (2) the consistency of the reactivity response across behavioral stimuli, (3) the presence of a strong relationship between reactivity and the blood pressure elevation during normal life stresses, and (4) the prospective evidence that hyperreactivity is an independent predictor of hypertension. They concluded that the test-retest reliability of reactivity is only modest (coefficients ranging from .4 to .7) and that generalizability of reactivity response across tasks is most valid for similar task groups such as behavioral and physical stimulus groups. They conceded that reliability improves with the use of continuous rather than intermittent measures of blood pressure. Furthermore, they concluded that hypertensives do tend to show greater reactivity to all stressors than do normotensives, especially to behavioral stress. This reactivity may be a consequence and not a cause of hypertension.

In a meta-analysis of reactivity literature, Frederickson and Matthews[1] concluded that borderline hypertensives exhibit higher blood pressure and heart rate reactivity predominantly to stressors that elicit active coping skills. They also found that normotensive offspring of hypertensive parents showed elevated systolic blood pressure and heart rate responses to all stressors and elevated diastolic blood pressure to stressors requiring active coping. These results support the role of behavioral stress in the initiation of the reactivity response.

However, Pickering and Gerin[13] contend that there is no strong evidence for the relationship of laboratory reactivity to the blood pressure variability observed in the field, which would empirically link blood pressure reactivity and hypertension development. This conclusion has been generally supported by van Egeren and Sparrow,[60] who reviewed 11 major studies that showed a weak relationship between resting blood pressure and reactivity status in genetically predisposed normotensives and borderline hypertensives. The strongest relationship appeared to be between diastolic reactivity in the laboratory, using the cold pressor test, and diastolic blood pressure variability observed during ambulatory monitoring.[60]

Part of the problems with both reliability and validity of reactivity tests may be related to the way reactivity is defined, which requires the measurement of change from baseline.[13] Peak blood pressure during dynamic exercise is a strong predictor of average ambulatory blood pressure, whereas the change in pressure from baseline is not.[13] In an attempt to correct this definitional problem, Rose and Fogg[61] provided a mathematical model to adjust for baseline contributions to the measure of reactivity. This measure of blood pressure reactivity is more robust in predicting outcome than a simple change variable.[62] It may be unrealistic to expect that a dynamic response adheres to the same absolute reliability standards of measurements made under resting conditions. Future work should attempt to evaluate categoric reliability of the classification of individuals into reactivity groups.

Pickering and Gerin[13] point out the lack of prospective evidence that hyperreactivity is an independent predictor of hypertension development. Prospective studies of this nature, which would require years of longitudinal data, have not seemed justified so far. However, Frederickson and Matthews[1] argue that there is a need for such prospective studies, which would confirm the independent role of reactivity in hypertension development, given the suggestive empiric evidence that such a link exists.

In conclusion, the empiric evidence for an etiologic role of behaviorally initiated cardiovascular hyperreactivity in hypertension is not definitive. Evidence is stronger that reactivity is a trait marker of preclinical or pathophysiologic phases of hypertension.

Several possible mechanisms have been proposed that may influence the reactivity response. It is plausible that behavioral stresses play a role in the expression of reactivity, particularly in hypertensive people. Although contrary to the reactivity hypothesis, physical stimuli also produce individual differences in reactivity response. Although some argue that every physical stimulus has a behavioral component, the controlled conditions of the laboratory tend to obfuscate this influence. Future research is needed to further explicate the role of behavioral stress, if one exists, in the initiation or maintenance (or both) of reactivity and the eventual pathogenesis of hypertension.

REFERENCES

1. Frederickson M, Matthews K. Cardiovascular responses to behavioral stress and hypertension: a meta-analytic review. *Ann Behav Med.* 1990;12:30–39.

2. Molineux D, Steptoe A. Exaggerated blood pressure responses to submaximal exercise in normotensive adolescents with a family history of hypertension. *J Hypertens.* 1988;6:361–365.

3. Light K. Psychosocial precursors of hypertension: experimental evidence. *Circulation.* 1987;76(suppl I):I67–I75.

4. Jones NL. *Clinical Exercise Testing.* Philadelphia, Pa: W.B. Saunders; 1991.

5. Astrand P-O, Cuddy T, Saltin B, Stenberg J. Cardiac output during submaximal and maximal work. *J Appl Physiol.* 1964;19:268–274.

6. Obrist P. *Cardiovascular Psychophysiology: A Perspective.* New York, NY: Plenum; 1981.

7. Turner J, Carroll D, Courtney H. Cardiac and metabolic responses to "space invaders": an instance of metabolically-exaggerated cardiac adjustment? *Psychophysiology.* 1983;20:544–549.

8. Turner J, Carroll D, Hanson J, Sims J. A comparison of additional heart rate during active psychological challenge calculated from upper and lower body dynamic exercise. *Psychophysiology.* 1988;25:209–216.

9. Sherwood A, Allen M, Obrist P, Langer A. Evaluation of beta-adrenergic influences on cardiovascular and metabolic adjustments to physical and psychological stress. *Psychophysiology.* 1986;23:89–104.

10. Cannon W. *Bodily Changes in Pain, Hunger, Fear and Rage.* New York, NY: Appleton; 1915.

11. Guyton A, Coleman T, Granger H. Circulation: overall regulation. *Annu Rev Physiol.* 1972;34:13–46.

12. Sherwood A, Turner J. A conceptual and methodological overview of cardiovascular reactivity research. In: Turner J, Sherwood A, Light K, eds. *Individual Differences in Cardiovascular Responses to Stress.* New York, NY: Plenum; 1992.

13. Pickering T, Gerin W. Cardiovascular reactivity in the laboratory and the role of behavioral factors in hypertension: a critical review. *Ann Behav Med.* 1990;12:3–16.

14. Folkow B, Hallback M, Weiss L. Cardiovascular responses to acute mental "stress" in spontaneously hypertensive rats. *Clin Sci Mol Med.* 1978;45:1,315–1,335.

15. Sannerstedt R. Hemodynamic response to exercise in patients with arterial hypertension. *Acta Med Scand.* 1966;458(suppl):1s–83s.

16. Amery A, Julius S, Whitlock L, Conway J. Influence of hypertension on the hemodynamic response to exercise. *Circulation.* 1967;36: 231–237.

17. Hallback M, Folkow B. Cardiovascular responses to acute mental stress in spontaneously hypertensive rats. *Acta Physiol Scand.* 1974;90:684–698.

18. Lundin S, Thoren P. Renal function and sympathetic activity during mental stress in normotensive and spontaneously hypertensive rats. *Acta Physiol Scand.* 1982;115:115.

19. Koepke J, Dibona G. High sodium intake enhances renal nerve and antinatriuretic responses to stress in SHR. *Hypertension.* 1985;7:357.

20. Matthews K, Rakaczky C. Familial aspects of the type A behavior pattern and physiologic reactivity to stress. In: Schmidt T, Dembroski T, Blumchen G, eds. *Biological and Psychological Factors in Cardiovascular Diseases.* New York, NY: Springer-Verlag; 1986.

21. Lawler J, Barker G, Hubbard J, Schaub R. Effects of stress on blood pressure and cardiac pathology in rats with borderline hypertension. *Hypertension.* 1981;3:496–505.

22. VanEgeren L, Geilman M. Cardiovascular reactivity to everyday events. In: Johnson E, Gentry W, Julius S, eds. *Personality, Elevated Blood Pressure, and Essential Hypertension.* Washington, DC: Hemisphere; 1992.

23. Julius S. Relationship between the sympathetic tone and cardiovascular responsiveness in the course of hypertension. In: Johnson E, Gentry W, Julius S, eds. *Personality, Elevated Blood Pressure, and Essential Hypertension.* Washington, DC: Hemisphere; 1992.

24. Holaday J. Cardiovascular effects of endogenous opiate systems. *Annu Rev Pharmacol Toxicol.* 1983;23:541–594.

25. McCubbin J, Cheung R, Montgomery T, Bulbulian R, Wilson J. Endogenous opioids and stress reactivity in the development of essential hypertension. In: Johnson E, Gentry W, Julius S, eds. *Personality, Elevated Blood Pressure, and Essential Hypertension.* Washington, DC: Hemisphere; 1992.

26. Egan B, Panis R, Hinderliter A, Schork N, Julius S. Mechanism of increased alpha adrenergic vasoconstriction in human essential hypertension. *J Clin Invest.* 1991;4:924–931.

27. Anderson E, Sinkey C, Lawton W, Mark A. Elevated sympathetic nerve activity in borderline hypertensive humans: evidence from direct intraneural recordings. *Hypertension.* 1989;14:177–183.

28. Yamada Y, Miayajima E, Tochikubo O, Matsukawa T, Ishii M. Age-related changes in muscle sympathetic nerve activity in essential hypertension. *Hypertension.* 1989;13:870–877.

29. Julius S, Pascual A, London R. Role of parasympathetic inhibition in the hyperkinetic type of borderline hypertension. *Circulation.* 1971;44:413–418.

30. Manuck S, Krantz D. Reactivity, hyperreactivity and cardiovascular disease. In: Weiss K, Matthews K, Detre R, Graeff J, eds. *Stress, Reactivity, and Cardiovascular Disease.* Washington, DC: Government Printing Office; 1984. NIH publication 84–2698.

31. Alexander N, Velasquez M. Blood pressure and plasma catecholamines in arterial baroreceptor denervated rats. In: Sleight P, ed. *Arterial Baroreceptors and Hypertension.* London, England: Oxford University Press; 1980.

32. Bristow J, Brown E, Cunningham D, et al. Effect of bicycling on the baroreflex regulation of heart rate. *Acta Physiol Scand.* 1972;86: 582–592.

33. Cunningham D, Strange Peterson E, Peto R, Pickering T, Sleight P. Comparison of the effects of different types of exercise on the baroreflex regulation of heart rate. *Acta Physiol Scand.* 1972;86: 444–455.

34. Sleight P, Fox P. Lopez R, Brooks D. The effect of mental arithmetic on blood pressure variability and baroreflex sensitivity in man. *Clin Sci.* 1978;55:381s–382s.

35. Iwase N, Takata S, Okuwa H, Ogawa J, Ikeda T, Haton N. Abnormal baroreflex control of heart rate in normotensive young subjects with a family history of essential hypertension. *J Hypertens.* 1984; 2(suppl 3):409–411.

36. Conway J, Boon J, Floras J, Vann Jones J, Sleight P. Impaired control of heart rate leads to increased blood pressure variability. *J Hypertens.* 1984;2(suppl 3):395–396.

37. Holaday J, Damato R, Ruvio B, Faden A. Action of nalaxone and TRH on the autonomic regulation of circulation. In: Cost E, Trabucchi M. eds. *Regulatory Peptides from Molecular Biology to Function.* New York, NY: Raven Press; 1983.

38. Mastrianni J, Palkovits M, Kunos G. Activation of brainstem endorphinergic neurons causes cardiovascular depression and facilitates baroreflex bradycardia. *Neuroscience.* 1989;33:559–566.

39. Esler M, Julius S, Zweifler A, et al. Mild high-renin essential hypertension. Neurogenic human hypertension? *N Engl J Med.* 1977;296:405–411.

40. Phillip T, Distler A, Cordes U. Sympathetic nervous system and blood pressure control in essential hypertension. *Lancet.* 1978;4: 939–963.

41. Weidmann P, Grimm M, Meier A, et al. Pathogenic and therapeutic significance of cardiovascular pressor activity as related to plasma catecholamines in borderline and established essential hypertension. *Clin Exp Hypertens [A].* 1980;2:427–449.

42. Egan B. Vascular reactivity, sympathetic tone, and stress. In: Johnson E, Gentry W, Julius S, eds. *Personality, Elevated Blood Pressure, and Essential Hypertension.* Washington, DC: Hemisphere; 1992.

43. Light K. Differential responses to salt-intake-stress interactions. In: Turner J, Sherwood A, Light K, eds. *Individual Differences in Cardiovascular Responses to Stress.* New York, NY: Plenum; 1992.

44. Tobian L, Hanlon S. High sodium chloride diets injure arteries and raise mortality without changing blood pressure. *Hypertension.* 1990;25:900–903.

45. MacGregor G. Sodium and potassium intake and blood pressure. *Hypertension.* 1983;5(suppl III):III79–III84.

46. Egan B, Petrin J, Hoffmann F. NaCl induces differential changes of regional vascular reactivity in salt-sensitive vs salt-resistant man. *Am J Hypertens.* 1991;4:924–931.

47. Takeshita A, Imaizumi T, Ashihara T, Nakamura M. Characteristics of responses to salt loading and deprivation in hypertensive subjects. *Christian Res.* 1982;51:457–464.

48. Luscher T, Raij L, Vanhoutte P. Endothelium-dependent vascular responses in normotensive and hypertensive Dahl rats. *Hypertension.* 1987;9:157–163.

49. Koepke J, Grignolo A, Light K, Obrist P. Central beta-adrenoceptor mediation of the antinatriuretic response to behavioral stress in conscious dogs. *J Pharmacol Exp Ther.* 1983;227:73–77.

50. DiBona G, Jones S. Renal manifestations of NaCl sensitivity in borderline hypertensive rats. *Hypertension.* 1991;17:44–53.

51. Lawler W, Sinkey C, Fitz A, Mark A. Dietary salt produces abnormal renal vasoconstrictor responses to upright posture in borderline hypertensive subjects. *Hypertension.* 1988;11:529–536.

52. Sanders B, Cox R, Lawler J. Cardiovascular and renal responses to stress in border-line hypertensive rat. *Am J Physiol.* 1988;255: R431–R438.

53. Dimsdale J, Ziegler M, Mills P, Delehanty S, Berry C. Effects of salt, race, and hypertension on reactivity to stressors. *Hypertension.* 1990:16:573–580.

54. Dimsdale J, Ziegler M, Mills P, Berry C. Prediction of salt sensitivity. *Am J Hypertens.* 1990;3:429–435.

55. Stem M, Morales P, Haffner S, Valdez R. Hyperdynamic circulation and the insulin resistance syndrome (syndrome "x"). *Hypertension.* 1992:20:802–808.

56. Reaven G. Insulin resistance, hyperinsulinemia, hypertriglyceridemia, and hypertension. *Diabetes Care.* 1991;14:195–202.

57. DeFronzo R, Ferrarmini E. Insulin resistance: a multifaceted syndrome responsible for NIDDM, obesity, hypertension, dyslipidemia, and atherosclerotic cardiovascular disease. *Diabetes Care.* 1991:14:173–194.

58. Skyler J, Donahue R, Marks J, Thompson N, Schneiderman N. Insulin: a determinant of blood pressure? In: Johnson E, Gentry W,

Julius S, eds. *Personality, Elevated Blood Pressure, and Essential Hypertension.* Washington, DC: Hemisphere; 1992.

59. Rose RJ. Familial influences on cardiovascular reactivity to stress. In: Matthews KA, Weiss SM, Detre T, et al, eds. *Handbook of Stress, Reactivity, and Cardiovascular Disease.* New York, NY: Wiley; 1986:259–272.

60. van Egeren L, Sparrow A. Ambulatory monitoring to assess real-life cardiovascular reactivity in type A and type B subjects. *Psychosom Med.* 1990:52:297–306.

61. Rose R, Fogg L. Definition of a responder: analysis of behavior, cardiovascular and endocrine responses to varied workload in air traffic controllers. *J Psychosom Med.* 1993;55:325–338.

62. Potempa K, Folta A, Braun L, Szidon P. The relationship of resting and exercise blood pressure in subjects with essential hypertension before and after drug treatment with propranolol. *Heart Lung.* 1992;21:509–514.

3. Managing Hypertension in the Elderly

THERAPY*

General Considerations

Blood pressure should be reduced slowly and cautiously in the elderly. The goal of treatment for diastolic hypertension is the same as in younger patients (below 90 mm Hg). As for those with high SBP or those with isolated systolic hypertension (ISH), the goal in the Systolic Hypertension in the Elderly Program (SHEP) was to reduce SBP below 160 mm Hg for those with an initial SBP of 180 mm Hg or greater and to reduce SBP by 20 mm Hg or more for those with an initial SBP below 180 mm Hg. For those with stage 2, 3, or 4 systolic hypertension, it would seem prudent to aim to reduce SBP to the range achieved in the SHEP. For older individuals with stage 1 systolic hypertension, SBP in the normal range (below 140 mm Hg) would be appropriate.

Lifestyle modifications should be tried first as an alternative to drug therapy for most elderly patients with hypertension. A weight reduction program that includes judicious, regular, aerobic physical activity and restriction of dietary calories is suitable for elderly individuals who weigh more than approximately 10 percent above their ideal body weight.

The *Fifth Report of the Joint National Committee on Detection, Evaluation, and Treatment of High Blood Pressure (JNC V)* recommends restricting dietary salt intake to less than 6 grams of sodium chloride (2.3 grams of sodium) per day. This guideline may be particularly important for the elderly because they, especially African-Americans and obese individuals, are more likely to be salt-sensitive. However, many have subtle or overt renal damage and may have difficulty maintaining sodium balance, thus risking volume depletion if they restrict their sodium intake excessively. Daily alcohol intake should be limited to no more than two glasses of wine (8 ounces), two beers (24 ounces), or two shots of whiskey (2 ounces). Even though cigarette smoking and dietary saturated fat and cholesterol are not directly implicated in raising blood pressure, elderly patients with hypertension also should be advised to avoid cigarette smoking and to reduce dietary intake of saturated fat and cholesterol, especially if they have dyslipidemia. These measures will optimize CVD prevention. Adequate dietary intake of potassium, calcium, and magnesium should be maintained for general health, even though reduced intake of these

minerals may not lower blood pressure per se. If lifestyle modifications are unsuccessful in achieving goal blood pressure, antihypertensive drug therapy should be added.

Antihypertensive Drug Therapy

Antihypertensive drug therapy should be prescribed carefully in older patients. The elderly often have impaired baroreceptor sensitivity and renal damage, increasing their risk of postural hypotension and volume depletion. Consequently, in older patients, blood pressure should be reduced gradually, treatment should be initiated with smaller than typical doses, and dose titration should be slower than is standard practice in younger patients.

In general, adverse drug reactions are two to three times more common in older patients, although, for antihypertensives, there is no evidence that any drug or class of drugs is less well tolerated in the elderly than in younger patients, especially when used in appropriate doses. In fact, the opposite may be true. For example, the Hypertension Detection and Follow-Up Program noted fewer adverse drug reactions in participants age 60 to 69 than in those under age 50.

Adverse effects of antihypertensive drugs in the elderly are qualitatively similar to those observed in younger patients. Certain specific adverse reactions are likely to occur more often in the elderly as a result of circulatory abnormalities seen with aging and, perhaps, occult or manifest target organ damage.

Until recently, accurate assessments of the frequency and severity of clinical and metabolic adverse drug reactions in the elderly were unavailable. Most of our knowledge came from small and short-term studies of individual agents because, with the exception of the European Working Party on High Blood Pressure in the Elderly (EWPHE), very few large and long-term clinical trials included adequate numbers of older persons. The recent results of the SHEP, the Swedish Trial in Old Patients with Hypertension (STOP-Hypertension), and the Medical Research Council (MRC) trial, plus a more detailed analysis of the EWPHE, now make it possible to better understand the adverse effects of antihypertensives in the elderly, both compared to placebo and, to some degree, to each other. Because most data were obtained with patients on diuretics, β-blockers, other sympatholytics, and hydralazine, we are still lacking adequate comparative data on the adverse effects of ACE inhibitors, calcium antagonists, and α_1-receptor blockers in older subjects.

The Veterans Administration Cooperative Study Group on Antihypertensive Agents recently compared the one-year blood pressure efficacy and tolerance of representatives of six antihypertensive drug classes—thiazide diuretics, β-blockers, ACE inhibitors, calcium antagonists, centrally acting α_2-agonists, and α_1-blockers. A large number of the

---

*Source: *Working Group Report on Hypertension in the Elderly*, National Heart, Lung, and Blood Institute, NIH Publication 94-3527, July 1994.

1,292 patients randomized in this placebo-controlled, parallel, double-blind trial were elderly (26% were African Americans over age 60, and 32% were whites over age 60). Thiazide diuretics (hydrochlorothiazide), β-blockers (atenolol), ACE inhibitors (captopril), and calcium antagonists (diltiazem) were as well tolerated as placebo, but the centrally acting α_2-agonists (clonidine) and the α_1-blockers (prazosin) were responsible for significantly more adverse reactions than the other drugs.

Specific Classes of Antihypertensive Drugs

Virtually all classes of antihypertensive drugs are effective in lowering blood pressure in older individuals. Using the one-year DBP of 95 mm Hg or lower as the criterion for "success," the recent Department of Veterans Affairs Cooperative Trial showed that diltiazem (64%) and hydrochlorothiazide (58%) were the most effective in African Americans over age 60; clonidine (45%), prazosin (38%), and atenolol (33%) were not as effective. Captopril (20%) was less effective than placebo (24%). In whites over age 60, atenolol (68%) was most effective, followed by diltiazem (64%), captopril (60%), clonidine (58%), hydrochlorothiazide (52%), prazosin (48%), and placebo (32%).

Nonetheless, only diuretics and a combination of diuretics and β-blockers have been used in controlled trials that have documented a reduction in cardiovascular morbidity and mortality. The SHEP, the STOP-Hypertension, and the MRC trial in the elderly, all of which showed significant benefit in the elderly, used low doses of thiazide or related diuretics with potassium-sparing diuretics or paid careful attention to supplement potassium and avoid hypokalemia, or used β-blockers.

Diuretics

Initial diuretic therapy should begin with low doses, equivalent to no more than 12.5 mg of hydrochlorothiazide daily. If the serum creatinine ranges between 115 μmol/L and 177 μmol/L (1.3 and 2.0 mg/dL) and blood pressure remains uncontrolled on thiazide-like diuretics, it is sometimes useful to switch to low doses of a loop diuretic such as furosemide (20 mg twice a day) or bumetanide (0.5 mg once a day). Otherwise, loop diuretics should be avoided because they impart a greater risk of volume depletion than thiazides.

Advantages of diuretic therapy. Diuretics have been used in many large trials that have documented a reduction in cardiovascular morbidity and mortality. Diuretics are also the only class of antihypertensive drug currently recommended for initial therapy that tends to cause a disproportionately greater reduction in SBP compared with DBP. They are the least expensive of the various classes of antihypertensive drugs that are effective as monotherapy.

Disadvantages of diuretic therapy. Diuretic therapy requires monitoring for adverse effects on serum potassium, glucose, or lipid levels. Because renal function declines with age in a substantial number of the elderly, more older patients treated with diuretics are at risk of developing clinically significant reductions in glomerular filtration rate. The elderly are more likely to develop hyponatremia. Glucose intolerance and Type II diabetes mellitus are increasingly common with aging; therefore, more elderly persons are at risk of developing hyperglycemia and other metabolic abnormalities associated with the syndrome of insulin resistance (including hypertriglyceridemia and a low high-density lipoprotein cholesterol concentration) than would be expected in younger people. However, there is no proof yet from clinical trials that the use of diuretics has resulted in any increase in drug-induced diabetes mellitus.

In the SHEP, persons with diabetes derived as much benefit in end points for stroke and coronary heart disease as did those without diabetes. Of the SHEP volunteers randomized to either active diuretic-based therapy or placebo, 20.8% developed problems characterized as "intolerable." Overall, 90.1% in the active group and 89.4% in the placebo group complained of a symptom at least once during the trial. This prevalence of complaints was viewed by some as high, but it is hardly surprising considering that all subjects were specifically questioned about problems at least four times per year for an average of 4.5 years. The pattern of symptoms was similar in both groups, and there was little evidence to suggest that any substantial proportion of these problems resulted from adverse drug reactions. Thirteen percent of the patients randomized to active therapy and 7% of those randomized to placebo had their medication stopped due to "side effects." The interpretation is somewhat complicated by the fact that 44% of the placebo group received active antihypertensive therapy by the end of the trial. Dementia and depression were unusual and did not appear to be related to treatment (1.6% of the active group and 1.9% of the placebo group developed dementia, and 4.4% of the active group and 4.2% of the placebo group developed depression).

In the SHEP, the metabolic changes were also minimal, although significantly different between the active and placebo groups. In the EWPHE, gout was more likely to occur with active therapy (hydrochlorothiazide and triamterene). Diabetes also occurred more often with active treatment than with placebo, but the difference was not significant (29 versus 20 cases, respectively); 28 actively treated patients needed oral hypoglycemic agents compared to 18 on placebo. In the STOP-Hypertension, the adverse clinical and biochemical events were minor and not substantively different from those treated with diuretics or β-blockers. In the MRC trial, diuretics were better tolerated than β-blockers.

b-Blockers

Advantages of β-blocker therapy. β-blockers, like thiazide diuretics, have been used in large clinical trials that have documented that active antihypertensive therapy can reduce cardiovascular events. However, in the MRC trial, the group given a β-blocker as initial therapy showed no significant reduction in events when compared to those receiving placebo. β-blockers that do not contain intrinsic sympathomimetic activity (ISA) are the drugs of choice for elderly individuals with hypertension who have had a myocardial infarction. In addition to lowering blood pressure, they reduce the risk of a subsequent event and sudden death.

Disadvantages of β-blocker therapy. Agents that act in the central nervous system, such as β-blockers, may not be tolerated as well in older patients who are more likely to have subtle and otherwise mild cognitive dysfunction. But a Department of Veterans Affairs trial failed to note substantial differences in cognitive function when older men received either metoprolol, reserpine, α-methyldopa, or hydralazine added to thiazide diuretic therapy. β-blockers without ISA may not be as effective in smokers as they are in nonsmokers. β-blockers also have adverse metabolic effects. They worsen insulin sensitivity and can cause glucose intolerance, and β-blockers without ISA raise serum triglycerides and lower high-density lipoprotein cholesterol levels. Those with ISA do not adversely affect serum lipid levels to the same degree but have not been shown to reduce the risk of recurrent myocardial infarction or sudden death. Patients with asthma and chronic obstructive pulmonary disease should not be given β-blockers except with extreme caution.

Calcium Antagonists

Advantages of calcium antagonist therapy. Several calcium antagonists are useful in older patients with angina pectoris as well as in those with relative contraindications (eg, chronic airway disease, gout) to some of the other classes of antihypertensive drugs.

Disadvantages of calcium antagonist therapy. Cardiac abnormalities, such as conduction defects, bradycardia, and systolic or diastolic dysfunction are more common in the elderly and may be more likely to occur when β-blockers and nondihydropyridine calcium antagonists are used. A study reported a high prevalence of first-degree atrioventricular block with diltiazem and bradycardia with atenolol; however, a placebo group was not included in this trial, and similar effects were seen in patients treated with enalapril. Dihydropyridine calcium antagonists cause edema, which may be confused with congestive heart failure; and some calcium antagonists, particularly verapamil, can cause constipation, which is a common problem in the elderly.

ACE Inhibitors

Advantages of ACE inhibitor therapy. ACE inhibitors are the drugs of choice when hypertension is complicated by congestive heart failure caused by systolic dysfunction or if given shortly after a myocardial infarction if ejection fraction is low.

Disadvantages of ACE inhibitor therapy. The major adverse effect of ACE inhibitor therapy is a bothersome dry cough, especially prevalent in women and older individuals. Hyperkalemia, rash, and reversible acute renal failure (which may be more common in the elderly because of a higher prevalence of bilateral renal artery stenosis) are relatively infrequent. Dosage reductions are necessary for most ACE inhibitors when the level of serum creatinine is 220 μmol/L (2.5 mg/dL) or greater.

a-Blockers

Advantages of α-blocker therapy. α-blockers may be useful in elderly individuals with hypertension and dyslipidemia because these agents tend to have either a neutral or beneficial effect on plasma lipid levels. They also are useful in patients with prostatism, a very common problem in elderly men.

Disadvantages of α-blocker therapy. Because baroreceptor function is often abnormal in older persons, drugs that may lower upright blood pressure dramatically, such as α-blockers, can exacerbate orthostatic changes and cause excessive dizziness and syncope in older patients treated with these agents.

Other Drugs

Although central α_2-agonists and other sympatholytics such as reserpine lower blood pressure in older persons, they are generally not tolerated as well as other classes of antihypertensive agents and are not as effective as single-drug therapy in most patients. There is very little information on combination α-β-blockers, but, just as with younger patients with hypertension, they are an appropriate choice in some elderly patients.

MANAGEMENT CONSIDERATIONS*

Psychosocial Factors

Elderly individuals with hypertension are more likely to be aware of their condition and in treatment than are younger persons. They also are more likely to adhere to therapy and to achieve better control of DBP than are younger partici-

---

*Source: *Working Group Report on Hypertension in the Elderly*, National Heart, Lung, and Blood Institute, NIH Publication 94-3527, July 1994.

pants. Nonetheless, practitioners need to be aware of certain physical, medical, psychological, and social factors among elderly patients that may affect adherence to treatment or present other problems.

Physical and Medical Factors

As indicated, a number of physical and medical factors may adversely affect hypertension treatment and control among elderly patients.

- Elderly patients are more likely than younger patients to take multiple prescription and over-the-counter medications, posing a greater risk of *drug interactions*.
- *Impediments in hearing or eyesight* may make instructions difficult for some elderly patients to understand and carry out.
- *Diets* of elderly people are frequently deficient in fresh fruits and vegetables, a problem noted in 75% of adult Americans. Further, nutritional guidance may be needed for elderly individuals who have special nutritional needs or who are limited in their ability to procure, prepare, or consume food.
- *Dementia or even mild cognitive dysfunction or depression* are important considerations in determining the appropriate antihypertensive therapy because patients must be able to cooperate if long-term treatment is to be practical, safe, and effective. Evaluation of the patients' ability to understand and participate in treatment may be accomplished through a simple test such as the Folstein Mini-Mental State. Evidence now shows that treatment can be initiated and maintained without an increase in dementia or depression and without any significant negative effect on cognitive, emotional, physical, or social function.
- Elderly patients often have great *difficulty in opening safety caps*, thus hindering adherence.

Psychological and Social Factors

In addition, a number of psychological and social factors may improve adherence to therapy among older individuals.

- In many older *married couples*, the wife is the medical caregiver. Older men, particularly widowers, take very little responsibility for their own health and for seeking or maintaining medical care.
- Many elderly people *live alone*. Having little contact with family or friends who ask about health and treatment can hinder adherence to therapy.
- *Low and fixed income* and limitations of health insurance benefits can discourage elderly patients from acquiring prescribed medications, keeping appointments, or obtaining routine or special laboratory tests.

- *Transportation problems*, particularly during the colder months and often coupled with a fear of crime, keep many older patients away from sources of medical care.

Flexibility in *scheduling visits and reminders* about visits will help many elderly persons achieve better control of their hypertension. A little extra time and attention to the elderly living alone may increase adherence to treatment. The number of follow-up visits needed to stabilize blood pressure may have to be balanced against financial and transportation problems of older patients. The frequency of office visits sometimes can be reduced by taking advantage of home care services, community blood pressure programs, local health departments, or public health nursing facilities. Professionals should be sensitive to the fact that most health care financing mechanisms do not yet reimburse disadvantaged elderly patients for prescribed medications or health education services. For institutionalized elderly patients, the decision whether or not to treat should depend on the supervision available as well as the *overall condition* and mental status of each individual.

Quality of Life

Until recently, little information has been available about the effect of antihypertensive agents on the quality of life of older patients. Although a recent meta-analysis of nine published trials of 27 population groups (n = 1,620) using 14 antihypertensive drugs reported no evidence of negative effects on physical, social, intellectual, or emotional function, the authors point out that information specific to the elderly had not yet been published. Since then, however, considerable new information has come to light. The SHEP used low doses of diuretics and then β-blockers, and the Department of Veterans Affairs Cooperative Study indicated similar effects on quality of life of hydralazine, metoprolol, methyldopa, or reserpine added to a diuretic. A recent randomized trial compared the effects of atenolol, diltiazem, and enalapril on quality of life in 242 elderly women with hypertension. This trial found no significant differences in measures of cognition, function, or mood in the presence of effective lowering of DBP.

RECOMMENDATIONS*

The National High Blood Pressure Education Program Coordinating Committee recommends the following actions and approaches for both diastolic hypertension and isolated systolic hypertension in the elderly.

---

*Source: *Working Group Report on Hypertension in the Elderly*, National Heart, Lung, and Blood Institute, NIH Publication 94-3527, July 1994.

Detection, Evaluation, and Diagnosis

Health care professionals, irrespective of specialty, should measure blood pressure at each encounter and should inquire about a history of hypertension and any past or present treatment for high blood pressure in new patients.

- Blood pressure should be measured with patients in the sitting and standing positions at every visit before and during treatment. If standing blood pressure is consistently much lower than sitting blood pressure, the standing blood pressure should be used to titrate drug dosages during treatment.
- The diagnosis of hypertension should be made in the presence of an average SBP of 140 mm Hg or greater or average DBP of 90 mm Hg or greater on three consecutive visits.
- Initial evaluation should be designed to discover whether target organ damage or other cardiovascular risk factors are present and to guide therapy. More extensive evaluation should be reserved for abrupt exacerbation of stable hypertension or new onset of DBP greater than 110 mm Hg or SBP greater than 180 mm Hg after age 55; this raises the level of suspicion that an identifiable cause of hypertension, especially renal artery stenosis of the atherosclerotic type, may be present. Patients with hypertension—especially whites with a current or past history of heavy cigarette smoking; clinical evidence of atherosclerosis in the cerebral, coronary, or peripheral vascular circulation; or renal insufficiency of unknown cause—also are more likely to have atherosclerotic renal artery stenosis.
- DBP greater than 100 mm Hg despite triple-drug therapy, resistance to a regimen that has been previously effective, accelerated hypertension, spontaneous hypokalemia, or symptoms suggesting pheochromocytoma warrant thorough evaluation for a secondary cause of the patient's hypertension.
- In some elderly individuals, blood pressure, especially DBP, is falsely high when measured with a standard cuff (pseudohypertension). The excessive calcification and sclerosis present in the large arteries in these individuals require a higher occlusion pressure; therefore, Korotkoff sounds do not accurately reflect intra-arterial blood pressure. Typically, patients with pseudohypertension appear refractory to antihypertensive therapy and often have symptoms suggesting hypotension when their measured blood pressure is high.
- On physical examination, the use of a simple test, the Osler maneuver, to distinguish elderly patients with pseudohypertension has proved to be disappointing. Patients who have a positive Osler maneuver continue to have a palpable (though not pulsatile) radial artery after the sphygmomanometer has been inflated to levels above measured SBP; those who have a negative Osler maneuver do not. Several recent studies have shown substantial intraobserver and interobserver variability (even when the test has been performed by trained observers) and considerable inaccuracy in predicting who did or did not have pseudohypertension. If this condition is suspected on clinical grounds, direct intra-arterial measurement of blood pressure may be necessary.

Treatment

The objective of hypertension therapy is to reduce the cardiovascular risk associated with high blood pressure. Both lifestyle modification and pharmacologic therapy should be employed in treating the elderly. Weight loss, dietary sodium restriction, alcohol reduction, nutrition therapy, and exercise can be used with some elderly patients as either definitive therapy or adjunctive therapy to drug treatment. Care should be taken to ensure that prescribed diets are nutritionally adequate to meet nutrient requirements as recommended by the Food and Nutrition Board of the National Academy of Sciences.

Practitioners should be alert to the hazards of adverse drug interactions in older persons who may be on multiple medications. Over-the-counter preparations also may increase this hazard. Patients on multiple medications may require additional counseling to deal with special adherence problems.

Follow-up visits should be scheduled every two to four weeks until antihypertensive therapy—whether nonpharmacologic or pharmacologic—has stabilized blood pressure. After control has been established, visits may be required no more frequently than every three to four months. Medical treatment may be preferred in managing some elderly patients with secondary hypertension, such as renovascular hypertension and primary aldosteronism.

- For therapeutic purposes, ISH should be approached with the same strategies used for diastolic hypertension.
- Unless there is a reason to favor another agent, diuretics are the preferred initial drug in treating elderly patients with diastolic hypertension. Diuretics are the only class of antihypertensive agents that has been shown to reduce morbidity and mortality reliably in older persons. However, such issues as a cormorbid condition, target organ damage, or other risk factors may make the choice of another drug class more appropriate. Serum sodium, potassium, and creatinine should be measured before diuretic treatment is started and every three or four

months during the first year of treatment. Serum glucose should be measured annually unless the patient develops signs or symptoms suggesting clinical diabetes mellitus. Lipid levels should be checked once a year.

- The initial dose of drug for elderly patients should be one half that prescribed for young and middle-aged adults.
- As stated in the *JNC V*, if there is an inadequate response, the drug dose should be increased, another drug should be substituted, or a second agent from a different class should be added.
- Antihypertensive agents known to produce severe orthostatic hypotension, such as the peripheral-acting adrenergic antagonists, should be used cautiously.

Patient Education and Adherence

Special adherence problems can result from the physical, psychological, and social limitations of elderly people. Professionals counseling elderly patients with high blood pressure may have to innovate, using existing skills and available materials and resources, to help these patients achieve and maintain hypertension control. Strategies for enhanced adherence to treatment are provided in the *JNC V*. The following strategies are more specific for older persons.

- Discussions with patients should include specific information about what to do and how and when to do it.
- Each visit should include adequate time to review adherence to the treatment regimen. Specific questioning, and listening to the patient's answers for clues, can identify problems such as forgetting medication, adverse medication effects, inappropriate food selection, poor eating habits, or financial difficulties with acquiring needed medication or health services.
- Referral to a dietitian should be made to ensure understanding of and adherence to the dietary regimen.
- All health care professionals can and should foster adherence by reinforcing high blood pressure control messages during patient visits. Educational materials that provide hypertension control information are available from the National High Blood Pressure Education Program, National Heart, Lung, and Blood Institute Information Center, P.O. Box 30105, Bethesda, MD 20824-0105.
- Patients should be encouraged to bring *all* their medications (prescription and over-the-counter) at each visit for identification and review. Drug interactions that can contribute to poor response to antihypertensive therapy often can be identified in medication review sessions.

- Insofar as possible, providers should ensure that patients acquire and refill prescribed medications. Nursing and pharmacy personnel can help monitor adherence.
- Pharmacists can promote adherence to treatment by keeping reminder or tickler files that indicate when patients will run out of medication. When pharmacists fill prescriptions for antihypertensive medication, they should emphasize that treatment is usually lifelong and should not be interrupted, and they should provide information about the benefits of treatment and adverse effects of medications.
- Schedules for taking medications should be as simple as possible to encourage adherence. Adherence improves substantially as prescribed dose frequency decreases. Both verbal and written instructions about medications should be provided if feasible; if available, printed materials should be given to patients and family members for home use. Other memory aids reinforcing verbal instructions, such as refillable unit dose dispensers, are often helpful. Selection of these aids should include consideration of hearing and vision impairments, educational background, and present mental status of individual patients.
- A portion of one or more patient visits spent with the patient's spouse, other close relative, neighbor, or other friend can build support for the treatment regimen. Patients living alone should be encouraged to identify one person who can offer reinforcement of the care regimen (even by telephone), assist with medications (such as refilling the unit dose dispenser), or provide transportation to office visits.
- Elderly patients or their physicians should request that pharmacists dispense their medications in containers without childproof safety caps, especially to older persons with arthritis. Large print on container labels may be helpful to many patients with vision impairments.
- Prescribing new medications in small quantities until the drug of choice is determined is helpful to patients with limited financial resources. For those patients with established regimens, a three- to four-month supply may be prescribed, based on patient finances, mental acuity, and scheduled follow-up visits. Because some elderly persons have difficulty swallowing, pill or capsule size should be considered when prescribing medications.
- When appropriate, social service agencies, community or public health departments, and senior citizen programs should be identified to assist elderly patients with special needs, including assistance with filling prescriptions, claiming insurance benefits, preparing meals, arranging home nursing visits, securing transportation, and other services, some of which may be reimbursable through third-party payers or public assistance.

SCREENING ALERTS IN OLDER PERSONS WITH HYPERTENSION

An older person who has hypertension (HTN) is more likely to indicate that the following items listed on the Checklist, Level I and II Screens are descriptive of their condition or life situation. Those with HTN are more likely to experience the types of problems listed below. Of course, anyone with HTN scoring "at risk" on the screens listed may benefit from nutrition and lifestyle interventions to prevent further deterioration or to improve their medical condition.

DETERMINE YOUR NUTRITIONAL HEALTH

Checklist Alerts

- I have an illness or condition that made me change the kind or amount of food I eat.
- I eat few fruits or vegetables, or milk products.
- I have 3 or more drinks of beer, liquor, or wine almost every day.
- I take 3 or more different prescribed or over-the-counter drugs a day.
- Without wanting to, I have lost or gained 10 pounds in the last 6 months.

Level I Screen Alerts

- Body Mass Index >27.
- Has gained more than 10 pounds in the last 6 months.
- Is on a special diet.
- Eats vegetables two or fewer times daily.
- Eats milk or milk products once or not at all daily.
- Eats fruit or drinks fruit juice once or not at all daily.
- Has more than one alcoholic beverage per day (if woman), more than two drinks per day (if man).
- Is housebound.
- Needs assistance with self care.

Level II Screen Alerts

- Body Mass Index >27.
- Serum cholesterol above 240 mg/dl.
- Takes three or more prescription drugs, OTC medications, and/or vitamin/mineral supplements daily.
- Has gained more than 10 pounds in the last 6 months.
- Is on a special diet.
- Eats vegetables two or fewer times daily.
- Eats milk or milk products once or not at all daily.
- Eats fruit or drinks fruit juice once or not at all daily.
- Has more than one alcoholic beverage per day (if woman), more than two drinks per day (if man).
- Is housebound.
- Needs assistance with self care.

Source: Reprinted with permission by The Nutrition Screening Initiative, a project of the American Academy of Family Physicians, The American Dietetic Association, and The National Council on Aging, Inc., and funded in part by a grant from Ross Products Division, Abbott Laboratories, Inc.

4. Clinical Pathway and Care Planning Forms

Hypertension, Borderline—Provider Pathway

	First Visit	Second Visit 2 Weeks Later	Third Visit Week 4	Fourth Visit Week 12	Fifth Visit Month 5	Sixth Visit Month 8 and Every 3 Months or PRN
Date						
Assessment	Vital signs including averages of two successive BPs in each arm Inquire whether patient has recently exercised, smoked a cigarette, or drank coffee Perform funduscopic exam	Focused physical exam including BP measurements as described on first visit	Vital signs including BP measurements as described on first visit Obtain history of cardiovascular risk factors: Smoking, high serum cholesterol, glucose intolerance, ECG evidence of left ventricular hypertrophy, gender, race, age	Vital signs Nonpharmacological treatment compliance or problems Patient's personal record of BP since previous visit	Vital signs Compliance with pharmacological or nonpharmacological treatment plans Patient's personal BP records	Vital signs Treatment plan compliance Patient's personal BP records
Diagnostics and Treatments		If BP is still elevated, CBC; SMA with BUN, creatinine, glucose, potassium, lipid profile	ECG Begin nonpharmacological treatments: Exercise, weight reduction, decreased ETOH (if necessary), decreased sodium intake, smoking cessation Or, if a secondary cause was found, begin treatment of this problem	Begin pharmacological treatment if patient has multiple cardiovascular risk factors, otherwise continue nonpharmacological measures	Pharmacological treatment if with multiple cardiovascular risk factors and BP still >140/90 Nonpharmacological if with few cardiovascular risk factors CBC, SMA with potassium, lipids	Pharmacological if with multiple cardiovascular risk factors; otherwise, nonpharmacological measures (exercise, no smoking, etc)

continues

Hypertension, Borderline continued

	First Visit	Second Visit 2 Weeks Later	Third Visit Week 4	Fourth Visit Week 12	Fifth Visit Month 5	Sixth Visit Month 8 and Every 3 Months or PRN
Date						
Teaching and Counseling	Teach patient that hypertension cannot be established by one episode of elevated BP; subsequent visits are necessary to establish the diagnosis	Explain complications of hypertension and how and when the condition is treated. Explain the need to determine if the hypertension has a secondary cause	Explain risk factors and the need for more vigorous treatment of individuals with more cardiovascular risk factors. Teach walking regimen, smoking cessation. Teach patient to take own BP and keep records		Modify and review treatment plan. Teach purpose and side effects of meds	Modify and review treatment plan as needed
Medications				β-Blocker or diuretic for patients with multiple cardiovascular risk factors	Increase meds dosages if necessary	Consider increasing dosage, adding second line of meds, or changing to a different med if current regimen is not working
Consults/Referrals			Nutrition evaluation and counseling: Low-fat diet, low-sodium diet			
Physiological Outcomes	140/90<BP<160/100	140/90<BP<160/100	140/90<BP<160/100	BP is 5 mm Hg less than original measurements	BP decreased 10 mm Hg from original value	BP remains below 140/90 if patient has multiple cardiovascular risk factors, or below 160/100 if with few risk factors

continues

Hypertension, Borderline continued

	First Visit	Second Visit 2 Weeks Later	Third Visit Week 4	Fourth Visit Week 12	Fifth Visit Month 5	Sixth Visit Month 8 and Every 3 Months or PRN
Date						
Educational Outcomes		Patient knowledge-able of how and when hypertension is treated	Patient understands need to treat high BP Patient understands nonpharmacological treatment measures Patient can take own BP and keep records	Patient knowledge-able of medication dosage, frequency, and side effects	Patient knowledge-able of treatment changes	Patient knowledge-able of disease process, end-organ effects of disease, pharmacological and nonpharma-cological treat-ment regimens, side effects of meds
Psychosocial Outcomes	Patient understands that one mildly elevated BP is insufficient to establish the diagnosis of hypertension, but that it is important to diagnose hypertension if it is present					
Medication Outcomes				No meds or single-agent therapy		Least expense and adverse effects from meds if meds are necessary
Comments						
Initials/Date						

Source: Rufus S. Howe, *Clinical Pathways for Ambulatory Care Case Management*, Aspen Publishers, Inc., © 1996.

Hypertension, Males Older Than 40 Years—Provider Pathway

	First Visit after Diagnosis Established	Second Visit 2 Weeks Later	Third Visit 2 Weeks Later	Fourth Visit 2 Weeks Later	Monthly for 3 Months Then Every 2 Months
Date					
Assessment	BP sitting, standing Fundi Heart sounds Lungs Edema Accurate weight	BP sitting, standing Heart sounds Lungs Edema Accurate weight	BP sitting, standing Heart sounds Lungs Edema Accurate weight	BP Accurate weight	BP Weight
Diagnostics and Treatments	ECG Chest X-ray Lab tests: • UA • BUN • Creatinine • CBC • Potassium • FBS • Cholesterol/HDL • Thyroid function • Uric acid Begin diuretic	Review ECG, chest X-ray, and lab tests with patient	Repeat lab tests: • Potassium • Cholesterol • UA If BP not WNL, add second antihypertensive (β-blockers or angiotensin-converting enzyme inhibitors)	Repeat ECG If BP stable, begin graduated exercise program	Advance to aerobic exercise
Teaching and Counseling	Importance of follow-up Compliance with meds Sodium avoidance Weight loss Stress control	Reinforce need for compliance Review sodium intake Diet review Decrease alcohol	Significance of second antihypertensive Encourage weight loss Check compliance Maintain K+, Ca++, Mg+ levels within expected range	Review meds Stress lifelong need for taking blood pressure medicine Diet review Hints for dining out	Review compliance at each visit
Medications	Diuretic or angiotensin-converting enzyme inhibitors		β-Blocker		Adjust meds PRN

continues

Hypertension, Males Older Than 40 Years continued

	First Visit after Diagnosis Established	Second Visit 2 Weeks Later	Third Visit 2 Weeks Later	Fourth Visit 2 Weeks Later	Monthly for 3 Months Then Every 2 Months
Date					
Consults/Referrals	Ophthalmology				
Physiological Outcomes	Decrease BP to <140/90 No heart or lung dysfunction No edema	Further decrease of BP Heart and lungs okay Excessive diuresis diminished	Normal BP Stable urine output	Normal BP Decreased weight (by diet)	Normal BP maintained Weight at ideal level
Educational Outcomes	Understands hypertension Understands role of sodium	Spouse understands role of sodium in diet	Avoids high sodium intake while dining out	Accepts need for graduated exercise program	
Psychosocial Outcomes	Reassured that hypertension is treatable Fears are allayed	Patient and family understand the disease	Family understands and reinforces need for compliance	Medication becomes part of daily routine	
Medication Outcomes	Daily diuretic in A.M. without fail	Daily medication	Takes both medications daily	Daily medication	Daily medication
Comments					
Initials/Date					

Source: Rufus S. Howe, *Clinical Pathways for Ambulatory Care Case Management*, Aspen Publishers, Inc., © 1996.

Adult Hypertensive on Medications—Provider Pathway

	First Visit after Initial Event	Second Visit Week 2	Third Visit Week 4	Fourth Visit Week 8	Fifth Visit 3 Months and Then Every 3 Months
Date					
Assessment	Cardiac, chest, neck pulses, bruits, extremities, neuro, eyes, orthostatic BP, weight	Orthostatic BP, cardiac, chest, extremities, neuro, pulses	Orthostatic BP, cardiac, chest, extremities, neuro, weight	Orthostatic BP, cardiac, chest, extremities, neuro, weight	Orthostatic BP, cardiac, chest, extremities, neuro, weight
Diagnostics and Treatments	Lipids, BUN, creatinine, chemistry, thyroid UA, ECG, chest X-ray	Follow-up of abnormal results	Follow-up of abnormal results	Follow-up of abnormal results	Follow-up chemistry, lipids, ECG, Pneumovax Age 50: Flu shot in October
Counseling and Teaching	Assess patient's risk factors and family history Need for regular follow-up Meds use and side effects ETOH <1 oz/day	Assess for meds and side effects Review benefits of exercise Review labs	Review exercise plans Review stressors	Assess exercise progress, diet, stress Home BP monitoring unit if willing	Counseling for smoking Review BP log, stress, diet
Consults	Dietitian for 2-g Na diet Consider weight loss	Schedule cardiac stress test if over age 40	Exercise physiologist Cardiac rehab	Stress counselor	Stress management Smoke stoppers
Medications	β-Blocker, calcium channel blocker, ACE inhibitor, or diuretic	Assess compliance	Assess compliance Adjust dose or change to new agent	Assess compliance, side effects	Nicotine patch Assess compliance, side effects Add second med or change if diastolic BP not <90

continues

Adult Hypertensive on Medications continued

	First Visit after Initial Event	Second Visit Week 2	Third Visit Week 4	Fourth Visit Week 8	Fifth Visit 3 Months and Then Every 3 Months
Date					
Physiological Outcomes	Lungs clear, RR normal BS normal No cough, no CHF Neg bruits, no bradycardia, no tachycardia, S_1S_2, neg murmur Neg syncope, neg gout, normal electrolytes No postural hypertension, normal lipids, neg depression, pulses = bilateral × 4, neg DNV, neg pedal edema, minimal med SE, normal kidney and liver function, normal optic disc and vessels Diastolic BP <90	Same as first visit plus minimal med SE	Same as first visit plus minimal med SE	Same as first visit plus minimal med SE Good exercise tolerance	Same as first visit plus weight maintenance or continue weight loss or increase to goal No ED visits No decreased exercise tolerance
Educational Outcomes	Begin patient knowledge base of cardiovascular risk factors, disease treatment, and meds	Discuss med SE Discuss cardiovascular risk factors	Discuss exercise potential and options	Able to discuss diet principles, exercise program Instruct in use of home BP monitoring unit	Brings in BP log Maintains exercise log and 3-day diet record Discusses life stressors Discusses smoking effects on cardiovascular risk
Psychosocial Outcomes	Evaluate for depression, sexual dysfunction, fatigue, beliefs about hypertension, and med SE	Family involved regarding diet and med compliance	Family and patient discuss stressors	Family involved with exercise program Family assists with evaluation of life stressors	Family helping with diet and with decreasing life stressors Developing plan for smoking cessation with patient

continues

Adult Hypertensive on Medications continued

	First Visit after Initial Event	Second Visit Week 2	Third Visit Week 4	Fourth Visit Week 8	Fifth Visit 3 Months and Then Every 3 Months
Date					
Medication Outcomes	Review meds, maintain or modify	Review meds, maintain or modify	Reviews meds and SE, maintain or modify	Review meds, SE, compliance Maintain or modify meds as necessary	Medication compliance with least number of SE
Comments					
Initials/Date					

Source: Rufus S. Howe, *Clinical Pathways for Ambulatory Care Case Management*, Aspen Publishers, Inc., © 1996.

Newly Diagnosed Hypertension—Provider Pathway

	Initial Episode	Second Week	Third to Fourth Weeks	Fifth to Seventh Weeks	Monthly for 3 Months or PRN
Date					
Assessment	PMH: Meds, lifestyle, current diseases PE: Height, weight, orthostatic BP, pulse, fundoscopic exam, heart, lungs, carotids, renal arteries, extremities) ? Any headaches, chest pain, dyspnea	? Any change in lifestyle Review daily BP Vitals, weight, heart, lungs, eyes, carotids, renal arteries, and extremities Review previous week's test results	? Following lifestyle changes ? Any headaches, chest pain, dyspnea Review daily BP Vitals, weight, heart, lungs, eyes, carotids, renal arteries, and extremities	Vitals, weight, heart, lungs, eyes, carotids, renal arteries, and extremities	Vitals, weight, heart, lungs, eyes, carotids, renal arteries, and extremities
Diagnostics and Treatments	Blood chem: Glucose, creatinine, BUN, Na$^+$, K$^+$, lipid profile CBC + DIFF Urine: Protein and glucose ECG Chest X-ray			Serum creatinine, BUN, Na$^+$, K$^+$, glucose, lipids	Serum creatinine, BUN, Na$^+$, K$^+$, glucose, lipids
Teaching and Counseling	Importance of follow-up Stop smoking, ↓ ETOH, ↓ salt, ↓ stress Home monitoring Impending warning signs and symptoms Daily BP—keep diary	Reinforce lifestyle changes Warn about secondary complications of hypertension Advise of need to take meds if BP does not ↓	Reinforce lifestyle changes Instruct about side effects of hydrochlorothiazide	Reinforce lifestyle changes	Advise that if lifestyle changes are followed and BP ↓, then can stop taking diuretic
Medications					Hydrochlorothiazide if BP not under control
Consults/Referrals					

Note: PMH, past medical history.

continues

Newly Diagnosed Hypertension continued

	Initial Episode	Second Week	Third to Fourth Weeks	Fifth to Seventh Weeks	Monthly for 3 Months or PRN
Date					
Physiological Outcomes	BP: Sys <210, dias <120 No chest pain No SOB Diagnostics and treatments within normal limits	BP ↓ as per patient's weekly diary No chest pain No SOB Diagnostics and treatments within normal limits	BP ↓ as per patient's weekly diary Rest of exam negative No symptoms of danger	BP ↓ as per patient's weekly diary Rest of exam negative No symptoms of danger	BP ↓ and remains within normal limits No symptoms of danger
Educational Outcomes	Patient understands importance of lifestyle change Patient agrees to monitor BP at home Patient understands warning signs	Patient has been monitoring BP daily Patient has ↓ number of cigarettes smoked daily Patient has ↓ ETOH, salt, and fat intake	Patient understands more about disease control and treatment	Patient has stopped smoking or decreased number of cigarettes smoked ↓ ETOH intake ↓ salt and fat intake ↑ physical activity	Patient adhering to lifestyle change recommendations
Psychosocial Outcomes	Begin patient knowledge of control of disease and treatment	Patient knowledge about dangers of hypertension increased	Patient incorporating lifestyle changes slowly into own life Patient understands he/she will need meds if BP continues to be uncontrolled	Patient continuing to incorporate changes into lifestyle	Patient continues to follow lifestyle change recommendations
Medication Outcomes	Patient understands that if sys BP is 180–209, and/or dias BP 110–119, may need to begin meds If sys BP is ≥210 or dias BP is ≥120, STAT treatment	Medications started if sys BP is 180–209 and/or dias BP is 110–119 and if patient is without understanding of importance of lifestyle change	Medication use stressed with patient if BP still very elevated	Medications if BP still very elevated	Medications started if lifestyle changes fail or not adhered to Begin with hydrochlorothiazide diuretics if no contraindications
Comments					
Initials/Date					

Source: Rufus S. Howe, *Clinical Pathways for Ambulatory Care Case Management*, Aspen Publishers, Inc., © 1996.

Newly Diagnosed (Mild) Hypertension, 140–159/95–99 mm Hg—Provider Pathway, Office Setting

	First Visit with Increased BP	Second Visit after 1 Week (2 Weeks)	Third Visit after 2 Weeks (1 Month)	Fourth Visit after 4 Weeks (2 Months)	Fifth Visit after 1 Month (3 Months)	Sixth Visit after 3 Months or PRN (6 Months)	Visit Every 6 Months to 1 Year or PRN
Date							
Assessment	PE, including skin, extremities, funduscopy, thyroid, pulses and carotid/ femoral, auscultation and palpation of lungs, heart, peripheral vasculature, neurological exam	Repeat same	Repeat same	Repeat same	Repeat same	Repeat same	Repeat same
Diagnostics and Treatments	BP/postural bilaterally 2× CBC, electrolyte panel, renal function tests, urinalysis, FBS, serum cholesterol, TFTs R/O secondary causes of hypertension	BP bilaterally 2× If BP still high advise: • Salt restriction • Decrease excess weight • Decrease excess ETOH • Increase exercise • Decrease fat in diet and cholesterol	Repeat second visit if BP still high	Repeat second visit if BP still high Consider instituting medication	Repeat second visit if BP still high Institute medication	Repeat second visit if BP still high Continue medical intervention	Repeat second visit if BP still high or change medication Repeat lab work

continues

Newly Diagnosed (Mild) Hypertension continued

	First Visit with Increased BP	Second Visit after 1 Week (2 Weeks)	Third Visit after 2 Weeks (1 Month)	Fourth Visit after 4 Weeks (2 Months)	Fifth Visit after 1 Month (3 Months)	Sixth Visit after 3 Months or PRN (6 Months)	Visit Every 6 Months to 1 Year or PRN
Date							
Teaching and Counseling	Discuss risks of cardiovascular disease: MI, stroke, and organ disease. Discuss possibility of home monitoring. Answer questions	Discuss relaxation techniques PRN. Review lab data. Review risks and warning signs. Recommend lifestyle modifications to avoid medicinal intervention and increased regular office visits for medicines. Answer questions	Review relaxation techniques PRN. Review lifestyle modification success/failure. Answer questions	Discuss medical intervention and begin or hold for 1 month or sooner PRN. Answer questions	Discuss medication administration, SE, discontinue PRN, interactions, warning signs. Answer questions	Discuss necessity to continue lifestyle changes with medical intervention. Answer questions	Repeat same
Medications	None at present	None at present	Discuss first-line treatment	Consider treatment	Individualize first line of therapy: • Thiazide diuretic, or • β-Blocker, or • Ace inhibitor, or • Calcium channel blocker, or • α-Blocker	Increase PRN. Discuss SE. Review warning signs	May add second line of therapy if needed. Discuss SE and warning signs
Consults/Referrals	Refer as necessary with secondary HTN	As per request: • Nutritional advisement • ETOH abuse counseling • Health club or trainer					

continues

Newly Diagnosed (Mild) Hypertension continued

	First Visit with Increased BP	Second Visit after 1 Week (2 Weeks)	Third Visit after 2 Weeks (1 Month)	Fourth Visit after 4 Weeks (2 Months)	Fifth Visit after 1 Month (3 Months)	Sixth Visit after 3 Months or PRN (6 Months)	Visit Every 6 Months to 1 Year or PRN
Date							
Physiological Outcomes	Mild or no symptoms RSR S_1, S_2 without stigmata or edema No funduscopic changes No enlarged nodular thyroid No bruits, diminished pulses Normal DTRs	Mild or no symptoms without pathological changes	Mild or no symptoms without pathological changes	Same	Same	Same	No symptoms
Educational Outcomes	Patient is aware of risk factors associated with hypertension Patient can recognize warning signs of high BP	Patient knows lifestyle changes that must be made to avoid medical intervention Patient learns relaxation techniques to demonstrate at next visit (PRN)	Patient knows lifestyle modifications necessary Patient is familiar with relaxation techniques	Patient discusses success/failure with lifestyle modifications Patient can perform return demonstration on relaxation techniques	Patient understands need for medical intervention with uncontrolled hypertension	Patient expresses and understands disease, self-care, and treatment	Patient understands all new treatments and self-care measures
Psychological Outcomes	Begin patient knowledge base about disease	Extend patient knowledge of nonmedical control of disease	Patient knows that without successful nonpharmacological methods to lower BP, pharmacological treatment is unavoidable	Discuss therapeutic intervention for next appointment if without improvement or consider medical intervention PRN	Patient is aware that lifestyle modifications must continue with medical intervention	Patient maintains self-care and management of BP control	Patient maintains self-care regarding BP control

continues

Newly Diagnosed (Mild) Hypertension continued

	First Visit with Increased BP	Second Visit after 1 Week (2 Weeks)	Third Visit after 2 Weeks (1 Month)	Fourth Visit after 4 Weeks (2 Months)	Fifth Visit after 1 Month (3 Months)	Sixth Visit after 3 Months or PRN (6 Months)	Visit Every 6 Months to 1 Year or PRN
Date							
Medication Outcomes		Patient realizes that medical treatment will also necessitate increased visits to monitor treatment	Discussion of first line of therapy to treat uncontrolled hypertension		Patient understands dosing administration and SE, when to discontinue meds, and RTC PRN	Modify meds PRN according to SE and BP stability	Modify PRN
Comments							
Initials/Date							

Note: DTRs, deep tendon reflexes; ETOH, alcohol; FBS, fasting blood sugar; HTN, hypertension; RTC, return to clinic; TFTs, thyroid function tests.

Source: Rufus S. Howe, *Clinical Pathways for Ambulatory Care Case Management*, Aspen Publishers, Inc., © 1996.

Home Health Care Clinical Pathway—Hypertension

Clinical Path—Dx _Hypertension_   **Pt. Name** _____

KEY

✔ = Done	I =	Instructed/
Ø = None		Reinstructed
N/A = Not Applicable		
V = Variance	A =	Achieved
Signature	Initials	

Goals:

To attain and maintain a normotensive status (within three weeks)

To increase understanding of the disease process (within one week)

To become knowledgeable about, and thus compliant with, medication regimen (within three weeks)

To identify overt warning signs (within one week)

To promote optimal lifestyle (within three weeks)

	Date																			
	Initials																			
EVERY VISIT																				
1. Assess vital signs	BP (R)																			
	BP (L)																			
	Apical pulse																			
	Respirations																			
2. Assess lung sounds																				
3. Assess breathing pattern																				
4. Assess skin color																				
5. Assess for symptoms	Headaches																			
	Dizziness																			
	Vertigo																			
	Palpitations																			
	Fatigue																			
	Epistaxis																			
6. Assess for other cardiac-related signs and symptoms	Chest pain																			
	Carotid bruits																			
	Arrhythmias																			
	Diminished pedal pulses																			
	Abdominal masses																			
7. Assess effectiveness of medications																				
8. Assess untoward side effects of medications																				

continues

Hypertension continued

INSTRUCTION	Date																								
1. Patient rights and responsibilities																									
2. Patient financial liability for home care																									
3. Patient/home safety																									
4. Expectations of home care																									
Use of clinical pathway																									
Role of patient																									
Role of significant other																									
Role of home care staff																									
Payer criteria/discharge plans																									
5. Plan for care (discuss/collaborate)																									
6. Written visit schedule																									
7. Medication regimen																									
8. Pertinent telephone numbers																									
Physician																									
Agency																									
Department of Health hotline																									
Pharmacy																									
Durable medical equipment																									
9. Preventive maintenance																									
Diet																									
Daily weights (if applicable)																									
Timely notification of physician																									
Medical appointment follow-through																									
Assessment of edema																									
10. Disease process																									
Definition of hypertension																									
Signs and symptoms of hypertension																									
Risk factors leading to hypertension																									
Stressors and stress reduction factors																									
11. Medications																									
12. Discharge instructions																									

Source: Barbara Stover Gingerich and Deborah Anne Ondeck, *Clinical Pathways for the Multidisciplinary Home Care Team,* Aspen Publishers, Inc., © 1996.

Skilled Nursing Facility Interdisciplinary Plan of Care— Hypertension

PROBLEM	GOALS	INTERVENTIONS	DISCIPLINES
Hypertension (high blood pressure) or Potential for High Blood Pressure	___ Will have BP range of 150/90 mm Hg to 90/60 mm Hg q ___	___ Assess/record/report to MD prn	N
Contributing Factors	through: _____	A. Hypertension s/s ___ Angina pectoris ___ Diaphoresis ___ Dyspnea	
___ African-American heritage ___ Family history	**And/or**	___ Fatigue ___ Headache ___ Hemoptysis	
R/T	___ Will have BP range of ___ mm Hg to ___ mm Hg q ___	___ Muscle cramps ___ Nausea/vomiting ___ Neck stiffness	
___ Alcohol intake ___ Arteriosclerotic heart disease	by/through: ____	___ Nose bleed (epistaxis) ___ Numbness/tingling in extremities	
___ Atherosclerosis ___ Condition that increases systolic pressure (eg, anemia, hyperthyroidism, aortic insufficiency, atherosclerosis):	**And/or**	___ Palpitations ___ Vertigo ___ Visual disturbance ___ Weakness (May have *no* symptoms)	
_____ _____	___ Will be free of hypertension s/s ___ Angina pectoris ___ Diaphoresis ___ Dyspnea	B. Notify MD of BP: ___ Systolic >200, ___ Diastolic >95, or	
___ Diabetes mellitus ___ Drug use ___ Endocrine disorder	___ Fatigue ___ Headache ___ Hemoptysis	___ _____	
___ Essential hypertension ___ High blood pressure Hx	___ Muscle cramps ___ Nausea/ vomiting	___ Provide/serve/monitor intake of diet/fluids: _____ _____	D N NA
___ Kidney disease ___ Lipid abnormalities	___ Neck stiffness ___ Nose bleed (epistaxis)	___ Check all that apply ___ Fat restriction ___ Reduction diet	
___ Overweight ___ Salt intake Hx, excess ___ Sedentary lifestyle	___ Numbness/ tingling in extremities	___ Salt restriction ___ Small/frequent meals	
___ Smoking history ___ Reason unknown	___ Palpitations ___ Vertigo	___ Monitor/record BP q _____	N
___ _____	___ Visual disturbance ___ Weakness	___ Relaxation techniques Describe: _____ _____	S
	by/through:____		

Resident's name: _____   Date: _____

continues

Hypertension continued

PROBLEM	GOALS	INTERVENTIONS	DISCIPLINES
AEB	**And/or**	___ Discuss with resident/family concerns about blood pressure	S N
___ Angina pectoris	___ _____		
___ BP range:	_____		
___ mm Hg to ___ mm Hg	_____	___ Assist in identifying stressors and developing coping skills	S
___ Diaphoresis	by/through:_____		
___ Dyspnea			
___ Fatigue		___ Adjust activity program to accommodate resident's needs:	A
___ Headache			
___ Hemoptysis		_____	
___ Muscle cramps		_____	
___ Nausea/vomiting			
___ Neck stiffness			
___ Nose bleed (epistaxis)		Invite/escort to: _____	
___ Numbness/tingling in extremities		_____	
___ Palpitations		_____	
___ Vertigo		___ Meds: Administer/monitor effectiveness/side effects	N
___ Visual disturbance		___ See physician order sheet, or	
___ Weakness		___ List: _____	
(May have *no* (symptoms)		_____	
		_____	
___ _____			
_____		___ Resident education	N S D
_____		___ Diet	
_____		___ Disease process	
		___ Exercise	
		___ Stress management	
		___ _____	
		___ _____	___ ___
		_____	___ ___
		_____	
		_____	

Source: Janie L. Krechting and Victoria E. Koper, *Interdisciplinary Care Plans for Long-Term Care*, Aspen Publishers, Inc., © 1996.

PART II

Self-Management of Hypertension: Patient Education

5. Diagnosis and Management of Hypertension

Your High Blood Pressure

As many as 50 million Americans, or one in four adults, have high blood pressure, or "hypertension," which is the medical term for it.

In fact, if you have found out about your high blood pressure, you are one step ahead of many Americans. Millions don't know they have high blood pressure.

Because high blood pressure has no warning signs, it is often called the "silent killer." People may not find out they have it until they have trouble with their heart, brain, or kidney.

When high blood pressure is not detected and treated:

- The heart may get larger, which may lead to heart failure.

- Small blisters (aneurysms) may form in the brain's blood vessels, which may cause a stroke.

- Blood vessels in the kidney may narrow, which may cause kidney failure.

- Arteries throughout the body may "harden" faster, especially those in the heart, brain, and kidneys, which can cause a heart attack, stroke, or kidney failure.

In fact, high blood pressure plays a role in about 700,000 deaths a year from stroke, and heart and kidney disease. The illnesses brought on by uncontrolled high blood pressure cost Americans billions of dollars each year. It's easier and wiser to treat your high blood pressure right from the start.

Source: "High Blood Pressure: Treat It for Life," National Heart, Lung, and Blood Institute, NIH Publication No. 94–3312, August 1994.

What Is Blood Pressure?

Blood is carried from the heart to all of your body's tissues and organs in vessels called arteries. Blood pressure is the force of the blood pushing against the walls of those arteries. In fact, each time the heart beats (about 60–70 times a minute at rest), it pumps out blood into the arteries. Your blood pressure is at its greatest when the heart contracts and is pumping the blood. This is called **systolic pressure**. When the heart is at rest, in between beats, your blood pressure falls. This is the **diastolic pressure.**

Blood pressure is always given as these two numbers, the systolic and diastolic pressures. Both are important. Usually they are written one above or before the other, such as 120/80 mm Hg, with the top number being the systolic and the bottom the diastolic.

Blood pressure changes during the day. It is lowest as you sleep and rises when you get up. It also can rise when you are excited, nervous, or active. Throughout the day, blood pressure can vary.

Still, for most of your waking hours, your blood pressure stays pretty much the same. That level should be normal, around 120/80 mm Hg. When the level stays high, 140/90 mm Hg or above, you have high blood pressure. And, with high blood pressure, the heart has to work harder and you are at an increased risk of a stroke, heart attack, and kidney problems.

What Causes High Blood Pressure?

The causes of high blood pressure can vary and, most of the time, the cause is not known. It might be due to a narrowing in the arteries, a greater than normal volume of blood, or the heart beating faster or more forcefully than it should. With any of these conditions, there is always an increased force against the artery walls. This form of the condition is called "essential hypertension."

Sometimes high blood pressure can be caused by another medical problem, such as kidney disease. When this happens, the condition is called "secondary hypertension." As the name indicates, by treating the main problem, the blood pressure goes down.

Source: "High Blood Pressure: Treat It for Life," National Heart, Lung, and Blood Institute, NIH Publication No. 94–3312, August 1994.

Testing for High Blood Pressure

You probably found out about your high blood pressure during a visit to a clinic or doctor. Maybe you went to a doctor for a physical exam. The doctor asked for your medical history and did some simple tests, such as urine and blood tests. And, your blood pressure was measured.

Having your pressure taken is easy. The doctor uses a device called "sphygmomanometer." Here's how it works: A blood pressure cuff is placed around an arm and inflated with air until blood circulation in the artery is temporarily stopped. A valve is opened and some of the air is slowly let out from the cuff, which allows the blood flow to start again. Using a stethoscope, the doctor listens to the blood flow in an artery at the inner elbow. The first sound heard is the heart as it pumps. This is the **systolic pressure**—the maximum pressure in the artery produced as the heart contracts and the blood begins to flow. More air is slowly released from the cuff. When the beating sound is no longer heard, the heart is at rest. The lowest pressure that remains within the artery when the heart is at rest is the **diastolic pressure.**

Blood Pressure Categories for Adults Age 18 and Older*

Category	Systolic (mm Hg)	Diastolic (mm Hg)
Normal	< 130	< 85
High Normal	130–139	85–89
High Blood Pressure		
Stage 1	140–159	90–99
Stage 2	160–179	100–109
Stage 3	180–209	110–119
Stage 4	≥ 210	≥120

*For those not taking medicine for high blood pressure and not having a short-term serious illness. These categories are from the National High Blood Pressure Education Program.
< = less than   ≥ = greater than or equal to

Some blood pressure devices use a column of mercury or a gauge to record the systolic and diastolic sounds. Others use electronic devices or digital readouts. In these cases, the blood pressure reading appears on a small screen or is signaled in beeps, and no stethoscope is used.

It's not unusual to have your blood pressure measured more than once during your doctor or clinic visit. It is often taken twice and then averaged to get a truer picture. Also, the first time your blood

continues

continued

pressure level appears to be high, you will probably need to have it taken again at another time to be sure that the reading is accurate. Your doctor will likely ask you to come back in a week or two in order to check your pressure again.

Where Does Your Reading Fit In?

An *optimal* reading would be less than 120/80 mm Hg. If the systolic and diastolic measurements fall into two different blood pressure categories, the higher category should be used to classify your condition. For example, if your blood pressure is 155/105 mm Hg, you would be classified as Stage 2 diastolic high blood pressure. If your blood pressure tests high, you will likely need to have the level checked further. Your doctor will likely measure it on at least two more occasions. Each time, two or more additional blood pressure readings may be taken.

HOW DO YOU RATE?

Do you know your blood pressure? Ask your doctor to tell you your numbers. Look at the box to see where your reading fits in.

Blood pressure readings below 140/90 mm Hg are considered normal. If the systolic blood pressure stays at 140 mm Hg or greater, or the diastolic blood pressure stays at 90 mm Hg or greater, you have high blood pressure. High blood pressure is categorized into four stages. As blood pressure goes up, the risk of heart attack, stroke, or kidney disease increases. So taking action becomes more important. For instance, as your pressure rises from normal to Stage 1 high blood pressure, your risk of dying from heart disease or stroke doubles; as it rises to Stage 2, your risk triples.

You may be asked to keep track of your blood pressure. There are several reasons for this. Sometimes, because blood pressure changes throughout the day, the doctor needs more readings to see your blood pressure's range and get a better picture. Another reason is that some people become anxious when they visit a doctor and their blood pressure goes up. This is called "white coat hypertension." When your blood pressure is taken at home, you may be more at ease and thus may get a truer reading.

You can keep track of your blood pressure outside of your doctor's office by taking it at home (see below). But, there are also other ways to get your pressure tested. Many company health clinics, community health centers, and hospitals have nurses and trained professionals who often do blood pressure tests. Check with your doctor or nurse.

If these tests are in the normal range most of the time, fewer checks at your doctor's office may be required to monitor your blood pressure.

continues

continued

HOME BLOOD PRESSURE DEVICES

Tests at home can be done with the familiar blood pressure cuff and a stethoscope, or with an electronic monitor, such as a digital readout monitor. Whatever the device, it must be checked for accuracy when you first get it and, later, once a year. This will keep it in good working order. Also, be sure that the person who will use the device is trained to take blood pressure readings. Your doctor, nurse, or pharmacist can help you check the device and teach you how to use it. You may also ask for their help in choosing the right one for you.

Blood pressure devices can be bought at medical products stores and in drugstores. Check your yellow pages telephone book or with your doctor or nurse to find a store. And above all, don't become a nervous "blood-pressure-taker." Testing your blood pressure at home can be helpful if you don't overdo it.

NOTES:

Source: "High Blood Pressure: Treat It for Life," National Heart, Lung, and Blood Institute, NIH Publication No. 94–3312, August 1994.

Using Home Blood Pressure Monitoring Devices

People with hypertension may benefit from using home blood pressure monitoring devices. Measuring blood pressure at home on a regular schedule may:

- help identify people whose blood pressure is high only when taken during a medical visit
- enable people to collaborate with their doctors in controlling their high blood pressure
- reduce the frequency with which a person needs a doctor for blood pressure evaluation

MECHANICAL GAUGES

The mechanical gauge, or sphygmomanometer, is the type of blood pressure equipment most often used in doctors' offices. It consists of an instrument called a manometer to measure the pressure, an inflatable cuff (air bladder), and a pressure bulb with a release valve to pump up the cuff. Some gauges use mercury manometers (the height of a column of mercury indicates blood pressure), while others use aneroid manometers (the pressure is read on a gauge dial).

Mechanical gauges are much less expensive than electronic sets and give more accurate readings when they function properly. When taking your own blood pressure, however, you must pump up the cuff with one hand, read a dial, and listen with a stethoscope. In other words, these devices require dexterity, good eyesight, acute hearing, and some training.

AUTOMATED ELECTRONIC GAUGES

Automated electronic gauges generally measure blood pressure by either the Korotkoff method or the oscillometric technique. Korotkoff devices use a microphone built into the cuff to detect arterial sounds related to blood pressure; they are subject to false readings caused by noises from the patient's surroundings or patient movement. Oscillometric devices measure and analyze the vibrations (oscillations) from the artery to determine blood pressure. Patient movement can cause false readings with these devices as well.

Finger cuff monitors typically are the oscillometric variety. Because they measure blood pressure at the fingers, they tend to have reduced accuracy and increased sensitivity to the effects of temperature and poor blood circulation.

For best results with automated gauges:

- Avoid eating, smoking, or exercising for at least a half hour before measuring your blood pressure.
- Test daily at about the same time; plan ahead to give yourself time to get over feeling angry or anxious.

continues

continued

- When using a finger cuff device, be sure your body temperature is normal; a room colder than 60° F can cause an inaccurate or unreliable reading.
- Sit quietly and eliminate extraneous noise.
- Follow the manufacturer's instructions carefully.
- Position your arm at heart level, palm up. Wrap the cuff just above the elbow—sleeve rolled above the cuff—and be sure it's not too tight. With a finger device, slip the finger fully into the cuff, keeping it level with the heart.
- Be sure the hoses from the cuff aren't tangled or pinched.
- Take care not to move the hoses during the reading.
- Wait at least five minutes with the cuff fully deflated before taking another reading.
- Bring the device along on medical visits once or more a year to check its accuracy against your doctor's measurements.

Also, the standard-size arm cuff on blood pressure monitors fits arms up to 13 inches in diameter. People with larger arms should order a larger cuff.

NOTES:

Source: Dixie Farley, "High Blood Pressure: Controlling the Silent Killer," *FDA Consumer*, U.S. Food and Drug Administration, December 1991.

Record Your Blood Pressure

Keep your blood pressure readings on this form. Carry it with you to your test and have your doctor or nurse write notes.

Name: _____

Date: _____

    Reading 1: _____

    Reading 2: _____

    Average: _____

Notes: _____

_____

_____

● ● ●

Date: _____

    Reading 1: _____

    Reading 2: _____

    Average: _____

Notes: _____

_____

_____

● ● ●

Date: _____

    Reading 1: _____

    Reading 2: _____

    Average: _____

Notes: _____

_____

_____

● ● ●

Source: "High Blood Pressure: Treat It for Life," National Heart, Lung, and Blood Institute, NIH Publication No. 94–3312, August 1994.

High Blood Pressure—What You and Your Family Should Know

DON'T LET HIGH BLOOD PRESSURE FOOL YOU

You can be a calm, relaxed person and still have high blood pressure. Hypertension is the medical term for high blood pressure; it does **not** refer to being nervous or upset or having an emotional condition. You cannot control your high blood pressure just by staying calm and relaxed. But it can be controlled by treatment. If you don't control it, however, one day your high blood pressure could lead to a heart attack, stroke, or kidney failure. Follow your treatment plan daily even when you feel great.

HIGH BLOOD PRESSURE

Blood pressure is the pressure needed to circulate the blood through the body. When too much of this force is pressing against the artery walls, it is called high blood pressure.

No one knows for sure why some people have high blood pressure. But one out of four adults in the United States has it.

HOW TO TELL IF YOU HAVE HIGH BLOOD PRESSURE

You can look and feel terrific and still have high blood pressure. Some people think that when they have a headache or feel dizzy or anxious, their blood pressure is up—and so that's when they take their medicine. They are wrong; they should follow their doctor's advice. Just because a person feels well doesn't mean his or her blood pressure is normal.

HOW TO CONTROL HIGH BLOOD PRESSURE

Most high blood pressure cannot be cured, but it can be controlled. Daily treatment usually must be continued for life in order to get your blood pressure down and keep it down.

Your doctor or nurse will tell you what to do to control your high blood pressure. Follow his or her advice, and feel free to ask questions about your treatment.

PILLS ARE JUST PART OF THE TREATMENT

If your doctor has prescribed medication, you must take it daily to lower your blood pressure. Your doctor may tell you to lose weight and cut down on salt. Or it may be necessary to stop smoking, reduce alcohol intake, or exercise more. For some people, these lifestyle changes help lower blood pressure. But don't try to choose your own treatment. Talk to your doctor about your plan.

continues

continued

If you are on medicine, keep taking it while you follow the other recommendations. Don't let your prescription run out. Get it refilled.

WHEN YOUR DOCTOR PRESCRIBES NONDRUG TREATMENT

Follow his or her advice. Make efforts to lose weight (those extra few pounds may raise your blood pressure). Cut back on salt, and your pressure may fall or help the medication work more effectively. Exercise in moderation may also help you control your blood pressure.

GET YOUR FAMILY TO HELP OUT

Your family needs you. They want to keep you healthy and active. Be sure to tell them about your high blood pressure. Tell them what the doctor said to do. Your family can:

- remind you when to take your pills
- help you lose weight if you need to
- serve meals low in salt

Then you can help your family by having them get their blood pressure checked, the way you did.

SOME THINGS TO REMEMBER

- One out of four adults has high blood pressure.
- A doctor, a nurse, or an assistant at a health clinic can tell you if you have high blood pressure.
- Use less salt in the foods you eat, lose weight, stop smoking, and exercise more.
- If prescribed, take your high blood pressure pills every day.
- Tell your family and friends about your high blood pressure.

Once you have high blood pressure, you will probably need to be under a doctor's care. If you treat it, it can be kept under control. You can be healthy, live a full life, and continue your normal activities even though you are following treatment.

Source: "High Blood Pressure: Things You and Your Family Should Know," National High Blood Pressure Education Program; National Heart, Lung, and Blood Institute; National Institutes of Health; Public Health Service; U.S. Department of Health and Human Services, NIH Publication No. 88–2025, September 1988.

Presión alta: Lo que usted y su familia deben saber

NO DEJE QUE LA PRESION ARTERIAL ALTA LE ENGAÑE

Aunque usted sea una persona tranquila y relajada, puede sufrir de tensión arterial alta. Hipertensión es el término médico usado para referirse a la presión arterial alta; no significa que la persona esté nerviosa, molesta, o inquieta. Usted no puede controlar la presión arterial con sólo relajándose y permaneciendo calmado. Debe controlarla con tratamiento adecuado. Si usted no lo hace, la presión alta puede provocarle algún día un ataque al corazón, un derrame cerebral, o problemas con los riñones. Tome su medicina regularmente aunque se sienta bien.

¿QUÉ ES LA PRESIÓN ARTERIAL ALTA?

Presión arterial es la fuerza que se necesita para que la sangre circule por el cuerpo. Se llama presión arterial alta cuando esta fuerza ejerce demasiada presión contra las paredes de las arterias.

No se sabe con seguridad por qué algunas personas sufren de presión arterial alta, pero en los Estados Unidos, uno de cada cuatro adultos padece de ella.

CÓMO SABER SI SU PRESIÓN ARTERIAL ES ALTA

Usted puede tener la presión alta aunque se vea y se sienta muy bien. Algunas personas creen que su presión ha subido cuando tienen dolor de cabeza, o se sienten mareados o nerviosos. . . . Y ese es el momento en que se toman la medicina! Esto es una equivocación. Las medicinas deben ser tomadas de acuerdo a las instrucciones que le ha dado su médico. Recuerde que el sólo hecho de que usted se sienta bien no demuestra que su presión arterial sea normal.

CÓMO CONTROLAR LA PRESIÓN ARTERIAL ALTA

La presión arterial no se puede curar en la mayoría de los casos, pero se puede controlar. Generalmente debe seguirse un tratamiento regular de por vida para bajar la presión y mantenerla estable.

Su médico o enfermera le explicará qué debe hacer para controlar su presión arterial alta. Siga sus recomendaciones y pregúnteles acerca de su tratamiento.

LAS PASTILLAS SON SÓLO UNA PARTE DEL TRATAMIENTO

Si su médico le ha recetado medicinas para bajar la presión, debe tomarlas regularmente. Es posible que el médico le recomiende también que pierda peso y use menos sal. Podría ser

continúa

continuación

necesario dejar de fumar, reducir el consumo de alcohol, o hacer más ejercicio. Estos cambios en el sistema de vida pueden ser útiles para que baje la presión arterial en algunas personas. Pero no trate de determinar cuál es su propio tratamiento. Hable con su médico acerca de su plan. Si le han recetado medicinas, tómelas mientras sigue las otras recomendaciones. No espere a que la medicina se acabe para renovar su receta. Hágalo con tiempo.

CUANDO EL MÉDICO RECETA UN TRATAMIENTO SIN DROGAS

Siga las instrucciones del médico. Trate de perder peso (esas libras de más pueden subir su presión arterial). Es posible que su presión baje si usa menos sal, o que por lo menos ésto ayude para que las medicinas sean más efectivas. El ejercicio moderado puede servirle para bajar de peso.

HAGA QUE SU FAMILIA LE AYUDE

Su familia le necesita. Ellos desean que usted permanezca saludable y activo. Hable con ellos de su presión arterial alta. Dígales cuáles han sido las recomendaciones del médico.

Su familia puede:

- recordarle que tome sus pastillas
- ayudarle a que pierda peso, si lo necesita
- servir comida baja en sal

Por su parte, usted puede ayudar a su familia haciendo que ellos se examinen la presión arterial, de la misma manera que usted se examinó.

ALGUNAS COSAS QUE DEBE RECORDAR

- Uno de cada cuatro adultos sufre de presión arterial alta.
- El médico, la enfermera, o el asistente de una clínica de salud puede decirle si tiene la presión arterial alta.
- Use menos sal en sus alimentos; baje de peso; deje de fumar; y haga más ejercicio.
- Si se lo recetan, tome todo los días las pastillas para bajar la presión arterial alta.
- Hable con sus familiares y amigos acerca de su presión arterial alta.

Es posible que si usted sufre de presión arterial alta, necesite estar bajo supervisión médica. Si usted se pone en tratamiento, podrá mantenerla controlada; y además, gozar de buena salud, vivir una vida plena, y continuar con sus actividades normales.

Source: "High Blood Pressure: Things You and Your Family Should Know," National High Blood Pressure Education Program; National Heart, Lung, and Blood Institute; National Institutes of Health; Public Health Service; U.S. Department of Health and Human Services, NIH Publication No. 88–2025, September 1988.

Taking Action To Control High Blood Pressure

Having high blood pressure means that you must make some changes in your life. You'll need to do some or all of the following:

- Lose weight if you're overweight.

- Be physically active.

- Choose foods low in salt and sodium.

- Limit your alcohol intake.

- Take your high blood pressure pills.

You don't have to try to make all of the changes necessary right off the bat. The key is to focus on one or two at a time. Once they become part of your normal routine, you can go on to the next change. Sometimes one change leads naturally to another. For example, increasing physical activity will help you lose weight.

The first four steps can also help prevent many people from developing high blood pressure. So you can follow them with your family to keep everyone healthy.

Source: "High Blood Pressure: Treat It for Life," National Heart, Lung, and Blood Institute, NIH Publication No. 94–3312, August 1994.

Tips for Reaching Your Blood Pressure Goal

WORKING FOR CONTROL

If you have high blood pressure, ask your doctor exactly what you can do to control it and what your blood pressure goal should be for your age and medical condition. By working toward this goal, you can take an active role in your own health care. Reaching your goal can mean reducing your chances of having a stroke, heart disease, and kidney damage.

TEAMING UP WITH YOUR DOCTOR

Controlling your high blood pressure calls for teamwork between you and your doctor. Here are ways you can work with your doctor to treat and control your high blood pressure:

- Keep your doctor's appointments. If you must cancel an appointment, be sure to schedule another visit as soon as possible. Mark your appointment dates on your calendar. Ask the doctor's office staff to remind you of your appointment. Ask about evening and weekend hours if necessary.
- Prepare for doctor visits. Make notes of the problems you are having. Keep a list of all the medicines you are taking, including nonprescription drugs. Write down all the questions you have for your doctor.
- Talk to your doctor. Ask any questions you have about your doctor's instructions, and ask for these instructions to be written down. Describe any problems you are having following your doctor's advice. Discuss any concerns or fears you have about your condition and treatment. Ask about your latest blood pressure measurement, ask what the numbers are and what they mean, and talk about the progress you are making toward your blood pressure goal.
- If your doctor prescribes medicine, ask about the name and purpose of the drug; how and when to take it; possible side effects and what to do if they occur; and what foods, drinks, and other medicines to avoid while you are taking your prescription. Ask for written information on the medicine you are taking.
- Ask about generic drugs, which are often much cheaper than brand name drugs.
- Give your doctor time to find the treatment that works best for you—the one that lowers your blood pressure with the fewest side effects.

TAKING YOUR MEDICINE

If medicine is prescribed for you to control your high blood pressure, you must take it every day according to your doctor's instructions. This means building new habits. Here are tips to help you take your medicine properly:

continues

continued

- Try to take your medicine at the same time each day. Combine this activity with daily routines. If you take one pill a day, keep your medicine near something that is part of your morning routine, such as your toothbrush. If you take several pills a day, ask your doctor if you can take them with meals. If so, keep your medicine on the dining table.
- If you take more than one medicine, count out the day's pills in advance and keep them in separate containers that are labeled with the time you should take the pills.
- Keep a medication calendar that you can mark each time you take a dose of your medicine. Also mark when you will need to refill your prescription.
- Carry a pillbox with a one-day supply of your medicine in your pocket or purse when you leave your house. If you are traveling, be sure to carry your medicine in your hand luggage. Refill prescriptions before going on out-of-town trips.
- Don't skip taking your medicine because you feel good. If you miss a dose, call your doctor for instructions to get back on schedule. Do not take an extra dose for ones you've missed. If you notice any side effects, tell your doctor. Do not change dosages or stop taking your medicine without your doctor's specific instructions.
- Always refill your prescription **before** you run out of pills. Keep almost-empty medicine bottles handy and in the open as a reminder to get prescriptions refilled. Ask your pharmacist if there is a system for reminding you to refill your prescription, such as receiving a postcard or telephone call from the pharmacy.
- If you have trouble reading medicine labels, ask your pharmacist for large type on the label. Some people color code their medicine bottles and write dosage information on a piece of paper the same color as the bottle.
- If child-proof safety caps are hard for you to remove, ask your pharmacist for easy-to-open caps. Ask your doctor to write on your prescription that you need easy-off caps.

ASKING OTHERS TO HELP

Your family, friends, and community service organizations can be part of your high blood pressure control team. Here are some ways you can ask others to help you reach your blood pressure goal:

- Ask your spouse or another close relative to go with you to the doctor. He or she can ask questions and learn what to do to help you reach and maintain your blood pressure goal.
- Ask your spouse, another family member, or a neighbor to remind you to take your medicine, refill your prescriptions, keep your doctor's appointments, and follow your diet.
- It is easier to make diet changes if the whole household is on the same diet plan. If you are cutting calories and reducing salt and alcohol in your diet, ask your spouse and other household members to join you in this healthy habit.
- If transportation is a problem, ask a relative or neighbor to drive you to doctor's appointments. Try to find a drugstore that delivers prescriptions.

continues

continued

- Ask social service agencies and public health departments about special programs that might offer assistance for prescription costs, insurance questions, transportation, and other problems.

STAYING IN CONTROL

Once you have started to work toward your blood pressure goal, you may be surprised to find it easier and less complicated than you thought it would be. A good way to see progress toward your goal is to keep your own record of your blood pressure measurements. After each doctor's visit, write down your measurement on a chart and see how close you are getting toward your goal.

Remember, because high blood pressure cannot be cured, you must control it for the rest of your life. Once you have reached your goal and your blood pressure is controlled, you must continue to follow your prescribed treatment. If you stop treatment, your blood pressure may rise again, increasing your chances of stroke, heart disease, and kidney damage. See your doctor for regular checkups, and continue to follow his or her advice. Meet the challenge of high blood pressure control!

NOTES:

Source: *Go for Your Goal: Be a Champion of Control*, National Blood Pressure Education Program; National Heart, Lung, and Blood Institute, National Institutes of Health; Public Health Service; U.S. Department of Health and Human Services.

Diabetes and High Blood Pressure

There are two types of diabetes: non-insulin-dependent diabetes mellitus (NIDDM) and insulin-dependent diabetes mellitus (IDDM). NIDDM is the most common form. It can often be controlled by following a specific meal plan and increasing physical activity. In some cases insulin or a pill may also be needed. IDDM is controlled by injecting insulin as well as following a specific eating and activity plan.

People who have high blood pressure and either form of diabetes also have an increased risk of heart and kidney problems and stroke. They usually have high blood cholesterol too.

To treat both your high blood pressure and your diabetes, you'll probably be asked to make some changes in what you eat:

- You'll have to eat foods low in salt and sodium, saturated fat, and cholesterol.

- Your specific meal plan will include eating small portions of poultry, fish, and lean meats, more fruits and vegetables, as well as low-fat or nonfat dairy products and whole grain breads and cereals.

- If you are overweight, you'll need to watch your calories as well.

If your blood pressure doesn't lower to 130/85 mm Hg, you probably also will need to take some medicine.

NOTES:

Source: "High Blood Pressure: Treat It for Life," National Heart, Lung, and Blood Institute, NIH Publication No. 94–3312, August 1994.

High Blood Pressure Glossary

Aneurysms Small blister-like outpouchings of blood vessel walls. They can rupture, causing bleeding.

Blood Pressure Pressure of blood against artery walls. Recorded as two numbers: systolic is written before or over diastolic.

- **Systolic:** maximum pressure in the artery produced as the heart contracts and blood begins to flow.
- **Diastolic:** minimum pressure that remains within the artery when the heart is at rest.

Cardiovascular Term that describes the heart and blood vessels.

Cholesterol A waxy substance produced by the body and taken in with food. The body needs cholesterol for functions such as making hormones. When too much cholesterol circulates in the blood, it speeds arteriosclerosis, or "hardening of the arteries."

Generic Drug A medicine that has the same active drug as a trademarked brand-named version. Generic drugs usually cost less than their brand-name versions.

Hypertension The medical term for high blood pressure.

mm Hg Abbreviation for millimeters of mercury. It is used to express measures of blood pressure. It refers to the height to which the pressure in your blood vessels would push a column of mercury.

Potassium A mineral in the body's cells necessary for maintaining fluid balance. Good sources of potassium are bananas and orange juice. "Salt substitutes" usually contain potassium.

Salt Common table salt or sodium chloride.

Sodium A mineral that can contribute to high blood pressure in some people. It is found in baking soda, some antacids, the food preservative MSG (monosodium glutamate), among other items.

Sphygmomanometer A device used to measure blood pressure.

Stroke Sudden loss of function of part of the brain because of loss of blood flow. Stroke may be caused by a clot (thrombosis) or rupture (hemorrhage) of a blood vessel to the brain.

Vascular A term to describe blood vessels.

Source: "High Blood Pressure: Treat It for Life," National Heart, Lung, and Blood Institute, NIH Publication No. 94–3312, August 1994.

Check Your Healthy Heart IQ

Answer "true" or "false" to the following questions to test your knowledge of heart disease and its risk factors. Be sure to check the answers and explanations on the back of this sheet to see how well you do.

1. The risk factors for heart disease that you *can do something about* are: high blood pressure, high blood cholesterol, smoking, obesity, and physical inactivity.   T   F

2. A stroke is often the first symptom of high blood pressure, and a heart attack is often the first symptom of high blood cholesterol.   T   F

3. A blood pressure greater than or equal to 140/90 mm Hg is generally considered to be high.   T   F

4. High blood pressure affects the same number of blacks as it does whites.   T   F

5. The best ways to treat and control high blood pressure are to control your weight, exercise, eat less salt (sodium), restrict your intake of alcohol, and take your high blood pressure medicine, if prescribed by your doctor.   T   F

6. A blood cholesterol level of 240 mg/dL is desirable for adults.   T   F

7. The most effective dietary way to lower the level of your blood cholesterol is to eat foods low in cholesterol.   T   F

8. Lowering blood cholesterol levels can help people who have already had a heart attack.   T   F

9. Only children from families at high risk of heart disease need to have their blood cholesterol levels checked.   T   F

10. Smoking is a major risk factor for four of the five leading causes of death including heart attack, stroke, cancer, and lung diseases such as emphysema and bronchitis.   T   F

11. If you have had a heart attack, quitting smoking can help reduce your chances of having a second attack.   T   F

12. Someone who has smoked for 30 to 40 years probably will not be able to quit smoking.   T   F

13. The best way to lose weight is to increase physical activity and eat fewer calories.   T   F

14. Heart disease is the leading killer of men and women in the United States.   T   F

continues

continued

1. TRUE   High blood pressure, smoking, and high blood cholesterol are the three most important risk factors for heart disease. On the average, each one doubles your chance of developing heart disease. So a person who has all three of these risk factors is 8 times more likely to develop heart disease than someone who has none. Obesity increases the likelihood of developing high blood cholesterol and high blood pressure, which increase your risk for heart disease. Physical inactivity increases your risk of heart attack. Regular exercise and good nutrition are essential to reducing high blood pressure, high blood cholesterol, and over-weight. People who exercise are also more likely to cut down or stop smoking.

2. TRUE   A person with high blood pressure or high blood cholesterol may feel fine and look great; there are often no signs that anything is wrong until a stroke or heart attack occurs. To find out if you have high blood pressure or high blood cholesterol, you should be tested by a doctor, nurse, or other health professional.

3. TRUE   A blood pressure of 140/90 mm Hg or greater is generally classified as high blood pressure. However, blood pressures that fall below 140/90 mm Hg can sometimes be a problem. If the diastolic pressure, the second or lower number is between 85–89, a person is at increased risk for heart disease or stroke and should have his/her blood pressure checked at least once a year by a health professional. The higher your blood pressure, the greater your risk of developing heart disease or stroke. Controlling high blood pressure reduces your risk.

4. FALSE   High blood pressure is more common in blacks than in whites. It affects 29 out of every 100 black adults compared to 26 out of every 100 white adults. Also, with aging, high blood pressure is generally more severe among blacks than among whites, and therefore causes more strokes, heart disease, and kidney failure.

5. TRUE   Recent studies show that lifestyle changes can help keep blood pressure levels normal even into advanced age and are important in treating and preventing high blood pressure. Limit high-salt foods which include many snack foods, such as potato chips, salted pretzels, and salted crackers; processed foods, such as canned soups; and condiments, such as ketchup and soy sauce. Also, it is extremely important to take blood pressure medication, if prescribed by your doctor to make sure your blood pressure stays under control.

continues

continued

6. FALSE   A total blood cholesterol level of under 200 mg/dL is desirable and usually puts you at a lower risk for heart disease. A blood cholesterol level of 240 mg/dL or above is high and increases your risk of heart disease. If your cholesterol level is high, your doctor will want to check your levels of LDL-cholesterol ("bad" cholesterol) and HDL-cholesterol ("good" cholesterol). A HIGH level of LDL-cholesterol increases your risk of heart disease, as does a LOW level of HDL-cholesterol. A cholesterol level of 200–239 mg/dL is considered borderline-high and usually increases your risk for heart disease. If your cholesterol is borderline-high, you should speak to your doctor to see if additional cholesterol tests are needed. All adults 20 years of age or older should have their blood cholesterol level checked at least once every 5 years.

7. FALSE   Reducing the amount of cholesterol in your diet is important; however, eating foods low in saturated fat is the most effective dietary way to lower blood cholesterol levels, along with eating less total fat and cholesterol. Choose low-saturated fat foods, such as grains, fruits, and vegetables; low-fat or skim milk and milk products; lean cuts of meat; fish; and chicken. Trim fat from meat before cooking; bake or broil meat rather than fry; use less fat and oil; and take the skin off chicken and turkey. Reducing overweight will also help lower your level of LDL-cholesterol as well as increase your level of HDL-cholesterol.

8. TRUE   People who have had one heart attack are at much higher risk for a second attack. Reducing blood cholesterol levels can greatly slow down (and, in some people, even reverse) the buildup of cholesterol and fat in the walls of the coronary arteries and significantly reduce the chances of a second heart attack.

9. TRUE   Children from "high risk" families in which a parent has high blood cholesterol (240 mg/dL or above), or in which a parent or grandparent has had heart disease at an early age (at 55 years of age or younger), should have their cholesterol levels tested. If a child from such a family has a cholesterol level that is high, it should be lowered under medical supervision, primarily with diet, to reduce the risk of developing heart disease as an adult. For most children who are not from high-risk families, the best way to reduce the risk of adult heart disease is to follow a low-saturated fat, low cholesterol eating pattern. All children over the age of 2 years and all adults should adopt a heart-healthy eating pattern as a principal way of reducing coronary heart disease.

continues

continued

10. TRUE   Heavy smokers are 2 to 4 times more likely to have a heart attack than nonsmokers, and the heart attack death rate among all smokers is 70 percent greater than that of nonsmokers. Older male smokers are also nearly twice as likely to die from stroke than older men who do not smoke, and these odds are nearly as high for older female smokers. Further, the risk of dying of lung cancer is 22 times higher for male smokers than male nonsmokers and 12 times higher for female smokers than female nonsmokers. Finally, 80 percent of all deaths from emphysema and bronchitis are directly due to smoking.

11. TRUE   One year after quitting, ex-smokers cut their extra risk for heart attack by about half or more, and eventually the risk will return to normal in healthy ex-smokers. Even if you have already had a heart attack, you can reduce your chances of having a second attack if you quit smoking. Ex-smokers can also reduce their risk of stroke and cancer, improve blood flow and lung function, and help stop diseases like emphysema and bronchitis from getting worse.

12. FALSE   Older smokers are more likely to succeed at quitting smoking than younger smokers. Quitting helps relieve smoking-related symptoms like shortness of breath, coughing, and chest pain. Many quit to avoid further health problems and take control of their lives.

13. TRUE   Weight control is a question of balance. You get calories from the food you eat. You burn off calories by exercising. Cutting down on calories, especially calories from fat, is key to losing weight. Combining this with a regular physical activity, like walking, cycling, jogging, or swimming, not only can help in losing weight but also in maintaining weight loss. A steady weight loss of ½ to 1 pounds a week is safe for most adults, and the weight is more likely to stay off over the long run. Losing weight, if you are overweight, may also help reduce your blood pressure, lower your LDL-cholesterol, and raise your HDL-cholesterol. Being physically active and eating fewer calories will also help you control your weight if you quit smoking.

14. TRUE   Coronary heart disease is the #1 killer in the United States. Approximately 489,000 Americans died of coronary heart disease in 1990, and approximately half of these deaths were women.

Source: Reprinted from *Check Your Healthy Heart IQ.* National Heart, Lung, and Blood Institute, National Institutes of Health. Publication No. 92-2724, October 1992.

Prevent High Blood Pressure

If your blood pressure is not high now, take steps to prevent it from becoming high. Here's how:

Aim for a Healthy Weight

- Choose foods lower in fat and calories.
- Eat smaller portions.
- Try not to gain extra weight. Lose weight if you are overweight. Try losing weight slowly, about ½ to 1 pound each week until you reach a healthy weight.
- Be physically active every day.

Eat Less Salt and Sodium

- Read the food label. Choose foods with less salt and sodium.
- Prepare lower sodium meals from scratch instead of using convenience foods that are high in sodium.
- Use spices, herbs, and salt-free seasoning blends instead of salt.
- Use only small amounts of cured or smoked meats for flavor.
- Use less salt when cooking.

What Else Can You Do? Add Spice to Your Life

When you cook, try adding herbs and spices instead of salt.

Poultry, Fish, Meat	
Poultry	Ginger, rosemary, thyme, curry powder, dill, sage, tarragon, oregano, cloves, orange rind
Fish	Curry powder, pepper, lemon juice, ginger, marjoram, onion, paprika
Pork	Garlic, onion, sage, ginger, curry, cloves, bay leaf, oregano
Vegetables	
Greens	Thyme, ginger, onion, dill, garlic
Potatoes	Garlic, pepper, paprika, thyme, onion, sage
Beans	Thyme, onion, dill, cumin, oregano, garlic, tarragon, rosemary
Okra	Garlic, pepper, thyme, onion

continues

continued

Eat More Fruits and Vegetables

- Eat more fruits and vegetables in meals and as snacks.
- Add more vegetables to stews and casseroles.
- Serve fruit as a dessert more often.

Be Active Every Day

- Walk a little further each day or walk to the bus stop.
- Dance, skip, jump, run . . . take every opportunity to move your body.
- Use the stairs instead of the elevator.

Cut Back on Alcoholic Beverages

- Alcohol raises blood pressure. Alcohol also adds calories and may make it harder to lose weight. Men who drink should have no more than two drinks a day. Women who drink should have no more than one drink a day. Pregnant women should not drink any alcohol.

LOWER YOUR HIGH BLOOD PRESSURE

If you have high blood pressure, you may be able to lower or keep your high blood pressure down. Practice these steps.

- Maintain a healthy weight.
- Be more active every day.
- Eat fewer foods high in salt and sodium.
- Cut back on alcoholic beverages.

You may also need medicine to lower your high blood pressure. Tell your doctor about any medicine you are already taking.

Follow these tips if you take medicine:

- Take your medicine the way your doctor tells you. To help you remember, plan to take your medicine at the same time every day.
- Tell the doctor right away if the medicine makes you feel strange or sick. The doctor may make changes in your medicine.
- Make sure you don't miss any days. Refill your prescription before you use up your medicine.
- Have your blood pressure checked often to be sure your medicine is working the way you and your doctor planned.
- Don't stop taking your medicine if your blood pressure is okay—that means the medicine is working.

continues

continued

Check what you will do to prevent or lower your high blood pressure. Try to do them all.

☐ Maintain a healthy weight.

☐ Be more active every day.

☐ Eat fewer foods high in salt and sodium.

☐ Eat more fruits and vegetables.

☐ Cut back on the number of alcoholic beverages, if you drink.

☐ Have blood pressure checked.

☐ Take medicine the way the doctor says.

Empower Yourself!

Keep a record of your blood pressure.

Date

Reading

Goal _____

Source: "Protect Your Heart," NIH Publication No. 97-4062, National Heart, Lung, and Blood Institute, National Institutes of Health, September 1997.

What Else Might Prevent High Blood Pressure?

Other things also may help prevent blood pressure. Here's a roundup of what's being said about them—and whether it's true or false.

DIETARY SUPPLEMENTS—POTASSIUM, CALCIUM, MAGNESIUM, FISH OILS

- **Potassium.** Eating foods rich in potassium appears to protect some people from developing high blood pressure. You probably can get enough potassium from your diet, so a supplement isn't necessary. Many fruits, vegetables, dairy foods, and fish are good sources of potassium (see box for examples).
- **Calcium.** Populations with low calcium intakes have rates of high blood pressure. However, it has not been proven that taking calcium tablets will prevent high blood pressure. But it is important to be sure to get at least the recommended amount of calcium—800 milligrams per day for adults (pregnant and breastfeeding women need more)—from the foods you eat. Dairy foods like low fat selections of milk, yogurt, and cheese are good sources of calcium. Low fat and nonfat dairy products have even more calcium than the high fat types.
- **Magnesium.** A diet low in magnesium may make your blood pressure rise. But doctors don't recommend taking extra magnesium to help prevent high blood pressure—the amount you get in a healthy diet is enough. Magnesium is found in whole grains, green leafy vegetables, nuts, seeds, and dry peas and beans.

Good Sources of Potassium

• Catfish	• Bananas
• Lean pork	• Prunes and
• Lean veal	prune juice
• Cod	• Orange juice
• Flounder	• Lima beans
• Trout	• Stewed tomatoes
• Milk	• Spinach
• Yogurt	• Plantain
• Dry peas and beans	• Sweet potatoes
• Green beans	• Pumpkin
• Apricots	• Potatoes
• Peaches	• Winter squash

Source: Adapted from "Good Sources of Nutrients, Potassium," U.S. Department of Agriculture, 1990.

- **Fish Oils.** A type of fat called "omega-3 fatty acids" is found in fatty fish like mackerel and salmon. Large amounts of fish oils may help reduce high blood pressure, but their role in prevention is unclear. But taking fish oil pills is not recommended because high doses can cause unpleasant side effects. The pills are also high in fat and calories. Of course, most fish if not fried or made with added fat are low in saturated fat and calories and can be eaten often.

continues

continued

OTHER FACTORS

- **Fats, Carbohydrates, and Protein.** Varying the amount and type of fats, carbohydrates, and protein in the diet has little, if any, effect on blood pressure. But for overall heart health, it is crucial to limit the amount of fat in your diet, especially the saturated fat found in foods like fatty meats and whole milk dairy foods. Saturated fats raise your blood cholesterol level, and a high blood cholesterol level is another risk factor for heart disease. Foods high in fat are also high in calories. Remember, foods high in complex carbohydrates (starch and fiber) are low in fat and calories—so eating these foods in moderate amounts instead of high fat foods can help you lose weight if you are overweight or to prevent you from gaining weight.
- **Caffeine.** The caffeine in drinks like coffee, tea, and sodas my cause blood pressure to go up, but only temporarily. In a short time your blood pressure will go back down. Unless you are sensitive to caffeine and your blood pressure does not go down, you do not have to limit caffeine to prevent developing high blood pressure.
- **Garlic or Onions.** Increased amounts of garlic and onions have not been found to affect blood pressure. Of course, they are tasty substitutes for salty seasonings and can be used often.
- **Stress Management.** Stress can make blood pressure go up for a while and over time may contribute to the cause of high blood pressure. So it's natural to think that stress management techniques like biofeedback, meditation, and relaxation would help prevent high blood pressure. But this doesn't seem to be the case: the few studies that have looked at this have not shown that stress management helps to prevent high blood pressure. Of course, stress management techniques are helpful if they help you feel better or stick to a weight-loss and/or exercise program.

Source: "Facts About How To Prevent High Blood Pressure," NIH Publication No. 96-3281, National, Heart, Lung, and Blood Institute, National Institutes of Health, October 1996.

¡Póngase en acción—Prevenga la presión alta!

LA PRESIÓN ALTA SE CONOCE COMO "EL ASESINO SILENCIOSO." ES UNA ENFERMEDAD QUE NO DA SÍNTOMAS.

¿Por qué es peligrosa la presión arterial alta?

La presión alta es una enfermedad grave. Cuando su presión está alta, su corazón trabaja más fuerte de lo necesario para circular sangre a todas las partes del cuerpo. Sin tratamiento, la presión alta aumenta sus riesgos de:

- derrame cerebral
- ataque al corazón
- problemas en los riñones
- problemas en los ojos
- muerte

Está en sus manos un corazón sano. . .

1. Mida su presión arterial. Su médico le dirá si su presión está alta. Está alta si es 140/90 ó más. La presión deseable es 120/80. ¡Aunque su presión esté en un nivel deseable, mídasela una vez al año!
2. ¡Está en sus manos. . .! Lea este folleto y ponga en práctica los consejos para *prevenir* la presión alta. Siga los consejos de este folleto para *bajar* su presión si la tiene alta.

TOME ACCIÓN HOY PARA ESTAR SALUDABLE Y NO SUFRIR DE PRESIÓN ALTA MÁS TARDE

Para prevenir la presión alta

- Trate de mantener un peso saludable. Si tiene sobrepeso, trate de no aumentarlo. Baje de peso si tiene sobrepeso. Trate de perder peso poco a poco, de media libra a una libra por semana, hasta lograr un peso saludable.
- Manténgase activo todos los días. Puede caminar, bailar, practicar deportes, usar las escaleras o hacer otras actividades que disfrute.
- Disminuya la cantidad de sal y sodio al cocinar. Compre alimentos marcados en la etiqueta como "sin sodio," "bajo en sodio" o "sodio reducido". Quite el salero de la mesa.
- Reduzca el consumo de bebidas alcohólicas. Los hombres no deben tomar más de uno o dos tragos al día. Las mujeres no deben tomar más de un trago al día. Las mujeres embarazadas no deben tomar nada de alcohol.

continúa

continuación

NO SE DESANIME SI TIENE LA PRESIÓN ALTA. SIGA LOS CONSEJOS Y PODRÁ CONTROLAR O BAJAR LA PRESIÓN ALTA

Para *bajar* su presión alta

1. Siga estos consejos
   - trate de mantener un peso saludable.
   - manténgase activo todo los días.
   - disminuya el uso de alimentos que tengan alto contenido de sal y sodio.
   - reduzca el consumo de bebidas alcohólicas.
2. Tome su medicina como lo indica el médico.
3. Mídase la presión arterial con frecuencia.

Source: "Póngase en acción—Prevenga la presión alta," NIH Publication No. 96-4041, National Heart, Lung, and Blood Institute, National Institutes of Health, September 1996.

High Blood Pressure Prevention IQ

Test your knowledge of high blood pressure with the following questions. Circle each true or false. The answers are given on the following pages.

1. There is nothing you can do to prevent high blood pressure.   T   F

2. If your mother or father has high blood pressure, you'll get it.   T   F

3. Young adults don't get high blood pressure.   T   F

4. High blood pressure has no symptoms.   T   F

5. Stress causes high blood pressure.   T   F

6. High blood pressure is not life-threatening.   T   F

7. Blood pressure is high when it's at or over 140/90 mm Hg.   T   F

8. If you're overweight, you are two to six times more likely to develop high blood pressure.   T   F

9. You have to exercise vigorously every day to improve your blood pressure and heart health.   T   F

10. Americans eat two to three times more salt and sodium than they need.   T   F

11. Drinking alcohol lowers blood pressure.   T   F

12. High blood pressure has no cure.   T   F

How well did you do? →

continues

continued

ANSWERS TO THE HIGH BLOOD PRESSURE PREVENTION IQ QUIZ

1. FALSE. High blood pressure can be prevented with four steps: keep a healthy weight; become physically active; limit your salt and sodium use; and, if you drink alcoholic beverages, do so in moderation.

2. FALSE. You are more likely to get high blood pressure if it runs in your family, but that doesn't mean you must get it. Your chance of getting high blood pressure is also greater if you're older or an African American. But high blood pressure is NOT an inevitable part of aging and everyone can take steps to prevent the disease—the steps are given in answer 1.

3. FALSE. About 15 percent of those ages 18–39 are among the 50 million Americans with high blood pressure. Once you have high blood pressure, you have it for the rest of your life. So start now to prevent it.

4. TRUE. High blood pressure, or "hypertension," usually has no symptoms. In fact, it is often called the "silent killer." You can have high blood pressure and feel fine. That's why it's important to have your blood pressure checked—it's a simple test.

5. FALSE. Stress does make blood pressure go up, but only temporarily. Ups and downs in blood pressure are normal. Run for a bus and your pressure rises; sleep and it drops. Blood pressure is the force of blood against the walls of arteries. Blood pressure becomes dangerous when it's always high. That harms your heart and blood vessels. So what does cause high blood pressure? In the vast majority of cases, a single cause is never found.

6. FALSE. High blood pressure is the main cause of stroke and a factor in the development of heart disease and kidney failure.

7. TRUE. But even blood pressures slightly under 140/90 mm Hg can increase your risk of heart disease or stroke.

8. TRUE. As weight increases, so does blood pressure. It's important to stay at a healthy weight. If you need to reduce, try to lose ½ to 1 pound a week. Choose foods low in fat (especially saturated fat), since fat is high in calories. Even if you're at a good weight, the healthiest way to eat is low fat, low cholesterol.

continues

continued

9. FALSE. Studies show that even a little physical activity helps prevent high blood pressure and strengthens your heart. Even among the overweight, those who are active have lower blood pressures than those who aren't. It's best to do some activity for 30 minutes, most days. Walk, garden, or bowl. If you don't have a 30-minute period, do something for 15 minutes, twice a day. Every bit helps—so make activity part of your daily routine.

10. TRUE. Americans eat way too much salt and sodium. And some people, such as many African Americans, are especially sensitive to salt. Salt is made of sodium and chloride, and it's mostly the sodium that affects blood pressure. Salt is only one form of sodium—there are others. So you need to watch your use of both salt and sodium. That includes what's added to foods at the table and in cooking, and what's already in processed foods and snacks. Americans, especially people with high blood pressure, should eat no more than about 6 grams of salt a day, which equals about 2,400 milligrams of sodium.

11. FALSE. Drinking too much alcohol can raise blood pressure. If you drink, have no more than two drinks a day. The "Dietary Guidelines" recommend that for overall health, women should limit their alcohol to no more than one drink a day. A drink would be 1.5 ounces of 80 proof whiskey, or 5 ounces of wine, or 12 ounces of beer.

12. TRUE. But high blood pressure can be treated and controlled. Treatment usually includes lifestyle changes—losing weight, if overweight; becoming physically active; limiting salt and sodium; and avoiding drinking excess alcohol—and, if needed, medication. But the best way to avoid the dangers of high blood pressure is to prevent the condition.

For more information on high blood pressure,
call 1-800-575-WELL,
or write to the
National Heart, Lung, and Blood Institute Information Center,
P.O. Box 30105,
Bethesda, MD 20824-0105.

Source: Reprinted from *Check Your High Blood Pressure Prevention IQ.* National Heart, Lung, and Blood Institute, National Institutes of Health, Publication No. 94-3671, September 1994.

Exercise and High Blood Pressure

Be physically active. Regular activity does more than help you lose weight: It makes you feel and look better, helps lower high blood pressure, and can reduce your risk of having a heart attack.

You don't have to run marathons to benefit from physical activity. Any activity, if done at least 30 minutes a day over the course of most days, can help. Look at the box for ideas to get you moving.

Certain forms of activity are best for conditioning your heart and lungs. Called "aerobic," they cause the body to use oxygen more efficiently. Examples include brisk walking, swimming, bicycling, and running. The activity should be done for at least 30 minutes, three or four times a week.

Whatever the activity, if you don't have 30 minutes, try two 15-minute periods or even three 10-minute sessions. But do something!

Many people are able to start an activity without seeing a doctor first. However, before beginning an activity, check with a doctor if you are taking high blood pressure medicine, have heart disease, have had a heart attack or a stroke, or have any other serious health problem.

Otherwise, get out and get active. Start slowly, if necessary, and work up to a comfortable pace and schedule. You may want to start doing an activity only twice a week. Then build to three or four times a week. The key is to begin and stay with it.

And have your family join in—regular physical activity is one of the best steps to prevent high blood pressure.

Active Ideas

Take a walk
Use the stairs
Get off the bus one or two stops early and walk the rest of the way
Park further away from the store or office
Ride a bike
Work in the yard or garden
Go dancing
Go bowling
Carry your own groceries

---

continues

continued

CALORIES BURNED DURING PHYSICAL ACTIVITIES

Activity	Calories Burned Per Hour
Bicycling, 6 mph	240
Bicycling, 12 mph	410
Cross-country skiing	700
Jogging, 5½ mph	740
Jogging, 7 mph	920
Jumping rope	750
Running in place	650
Running, 10 mph	1,280
Swimming, 25 yds/min	275
Swimming, 50 yds/min	500
Tennis-singles	400
Walking, 2 mph	240
Walking, 3 mph	320
Walking, 4½ mph	440

Note: These figures are for a 150-pound person. The amount of calories you burn depends on how much you weigh. The more you weigh, the more calories you burn. To find the number of calories you would burn in any activity, divide your weight by 150 and multiply that result by the number of calories for an activity. For example, how much would a 100-pound person burn in 1 hour of bicycling at 6 mph? First divide 100 by 150 to get 0.67. Then multiply 0.67 by 240 calories. That equals 160 calories. A 200-pound person bicycling for 1 hour at 6 mph would burn 320 calories— 200/150 multiplied by 240.

Source: "High Blood Pressure: Treat It for Life," National Heart, Lung, and Blood Institute, NIH Publication No. 94–3312, August 1994.

A Sample Walking Program

	Warm up	Target zone* exercising	Cool down	Total
Week 1				
Session A	Walk normally 5 min.	Then walk briskly 5 min.	Then walk normally 5 min.	15 min.
Session B	Repeat above pattern			
Session C	Repeat above pattern			
	Continue with at least three exercise sessions during each week of the program. If you find a particular week's pattern tiring, repeat it before going on to the next pattern. You do not have to complete the walking program in 12 weeks.			
Week 2	Walk 5 min.	Walk briskly 7 min.	Walk 5 min.	17 min.
Week 3	Walk 5 min.	Walk briskly 9 min.	Walk 5 min.	19 min.
Week 4	Walk 5 min.	Walk briskly 11 min.	Walk 5 min.	21 min.
Week 5	Walk 5 min.	Walk briskly 13 min.	Walk 5 min.	23 min.
Week 6	Walk 5 min.	Walk briskly 15 min.	Walk 5 min.	25 min.
Week 7	Walk 5 min.	Walk briskly 18 min.	Walk 5 min.	28 min.
Week 8	Walk 5 min.	Walk briskly 20 min.	Walk 5 min.	30 min.
Week 9	Walk 5 min.	Walk briskly 23 min.	Walk 5 min.	33 min.
Week 10	Walk 5 min.	Walk briskly 26 min.	Walk 5 min.	36 min.
Week 11	Walk 5 min.	Walk briskly 28 min.	Walk 5 min.	38 min.
Week 12	Walk 5 min.	Walk briskly 30 min.	Walk 5 min.	40 min.

Week 13 on: Check your pulse periodically to see if you are exercising within your target zone (*see following page). As you get more in shape, try exercising within the upper range of your target zone. Gradually increase your brisk walking time to 30 to 60 minutes, three or four times a week. But don't push too hard. Remember that your goal is to get the benefits you are seeking and enjoy your activity. The most important thing is to stick with it.

Source: "High Blood Pressure: Treat It for Life," National Heart, Lung, and Blood Institute, NIH Publication No. 94–3312, August 1994.

Check Your Target Heart Rate

1 Right after you stop exercising, take your pulse: Place the tips of your first two fingers lightly over one of the blood vessels on your neck, just to the left or right of your Adam's apple. Or try the pulse spot inside your wrist just below the base of your thumb.

2 Count your pulse for 10 seconds and multiply the number by 6.

3 Compare the number to the right grouping below: Look for the age grouping that is closest to your age and read the line across. For example, if you are 43, the closest age on the chart is 45; the target zone is 88–131 beats per minute.

Age	Target Heart Rate Zone	
20 years	100–150	beats per minute
25 years	98–146	beats per minute
30 years	95–142	beats per minute
35 years	93–138	beats per minute
40 years	90–135	beats per minute
45 years	88–131	beats per minute
50 years	85–127	beats per minute
55 years	83–123	beats per minute
60 years	80–120	beats per minute
65 years	78–116	beats per minute
70 years	75–113	beats per minute

Source: *Exercise and Your Heart*, National Heart, Lung, and Blood Institute and the American Heart Association, NIH Publication No. 93–1677.

Losing Weight

Lose weight if you are overweight. Losing extra pounds is a very important step that you can take to reduce your high blood pressure. Losing just a small amount of weight can help lower your blood pressure. For some people—those with less severe high blood pressure—losing weight may be all that's needed to control their hypertension. For others, losing weight may reduce the medication they need to take for their high blood pressure.

Try These Low-Fat Foods

- Baked, broiled, or poached:
  - Chicken and turkey (without the skin)
  - Fish
  - Lean cuts of meat (like round or sirloin)
- Skim or 1% milk, evaporated skimmed milk
- Lower-fat, low-sodium cheeses
- Low-fat yogurt, ice milk
- Fresh, frozen, or canned fruit
- Fresh, frozen, or no salt added canned vegetables (without cream or cheese sauces)
- Plain rice and pasta
- English muffins, bagels, breads, and soft tortillas
- Cold (ready-to-eat) cereals lower in sodium
- Cooked hot cereals (not instant, which are high in sodium)

Note: Read the food label and choose cheeses, breads, and cereals lower in fat and sodium.

ABOUT WEIGHT

Two things count about weight (1) how much and (2) where.

How Much—

As your body weight increases over your desirable weight, your blood pressure goes up.

Where—

Extra pounds are bad enough, but it also matters where those pounds are stored. If they are around your belly, you are "apple-shaped." If they are around your hips and thighs, you are "pear-

continues

---

continued

shaped." Where you store weight is for the most part inherited from your parents, just like the color of your eyes or hair, although men tend to be "apple-shaped," and women "pear-shaped." If you are apple-shaped, you are at a greater risk for heart disease. But whether you are an "apple" or a "pear," you should take steps to lose extra pounds.

And by losing excess weight, you will not only help to reduce your blood pressure but also feel better, be more able to exercise, and reduce your chance of having a heart attack.

To help you lose weight: Eat fewer calories than you burn. *Don't* try to see how fast you can lose weight. It's best to do it slowly. "Fad" diets do not work over the long haul because they cannot be followed for life. When people go back to their old way of eating, they usually regain the weight, leading to cycles of weight loss and gain.

A Word about Fats

While fats do not directly raise blood pressure, they do affect the health of your heart and blood vessels. Fats, especially "saturated fat," play a role in raising the cholesterol in your bloodstream. A high blood cholesterol level is a risk factor that increases your chance of developing heart disease.

Saturated fat is often found in foods from animals. This includes fatty meats, the skin of poultry, and whole-milk dairy products, such as butter, cheese, cream, and ice cream. It is also in coconut, palm kernel, and palm oils. These oils are found mostly in processed foods, such as baked goods, snack foods, and crackers. If you use saturated fat, keep the amount small. Instead of saturated fat, try soft or liquid margarine and such oils as canola, safflower, and olive. However, all kinds of fats have the same amount of calories and need to be limited to help you lose weight.

Try to lose about ½ to 1 pound a week. This isn't as hard as it sounds. One pound equals 3,500 calories—or 7 times 500. So if you cut 500 calories a day by eating less and being more active, you should lose about 1 pound in a week. For example in one day if you replace a chocolate candy bar at lunch with a small apple, have a piece of baked chicken instead of fried chicken at dinner, and then take a 15-minute brisk walk after lunch and dinner instead of lingering at the table, you can cut your calories by 500. Making these kind of changes every day will help you to lose about a pound a week.

continues

continued

DIET

Choose Foods Low in Calories and Fat

Low-calorie foods are great for losing weight. But you may not know that healthy low-fat foods can also be low in calories. Fat, no matter what kind it is, saturated or unsaturated (see above), is a concentrated source of calories. So if you replace fatty foods with less fatty foods, but keep the same portion sizes, you'll eat fewer calories. For example, save calories by eating baked fish instead of fried fish or low-fat yogurt instead of ice cream.

Foods High in Starch and/or Fiber

Fruits	Whole-grain cereals
Vegetables	Pasta and rice
Whole-grain bread	Dry peas and beans

Note: Use the food label to choose breads and cereals lower in sodium.

Fatty foods to cut down on include: butter and margarine, fatty meats, whole-milk dairy foods (such as cheese), fried foods, and many sweets and snacks. Try some of the enjoyable low-fat alternatives for fatty foods.

Foods low in fat also include those high in starch and fiber. These foods also are good sources of vitamins and minerals. Some foods high in starch and/or fiber are listed above. Try to replace foods higher in fat with these kinds of items.

Limit Your Serving Size

To reduce your daily calorie intake, you'll need to watch how much you eat, not just what. This means cutting down on portion sizes.

Try to take only mid-sized helpings of foods high in starch and fiber, and only small helpings of fatty foods, such as cheese and high-fat meats. And don't go back for seconds.

Keep a Food Diary

One good way to change what and how much you eat is with a food diary. For 2–3 days, record what you eat, when you eat it, and why. Try to include one weekend day. Be sure to include snacks. This will tell you what food habits you have—and what bad habits may be causing you to be overweight.

continues

continued

Once you understand your habits, you can set goals to change them. For example, you may find you often snack on fatty, high-calorie foods while watching television. Change this habit by having fresh fruit, unsalted popcorn, or unsalted pretzels handy as you watch TV. Or, you may find that you skip breakfast and then eat a very large lunch. Perhaps you picked up the habit because you don't have enough time in the mornings to eat breakfast at home. Instead of eating too much at lunch, take a low-fat muffin, bagel, or cereal with you and eat breakfast at work.

EXERCISE

The other part of using more calories than you eat is being physically active. Regular activity helps you lose weight—and keep it off—and improves the health of your heart and lungs.

NOTES:

Source: "High Blood Pressure: Treat It for Life," National Heart, Lung, and Blood Institute, NIH Publication No. 94–3312, August 1994.

Hypertension and Your Diet

NUTRITIONAL GOALS

As part of your medical therapy, your physician has ordered a sodium-controlled (2–3 g) diet to reduce cardiovascular stress and fluid retention. In addition, eating a variety of foods that have been divided into small meals and snacks will help ensure adequate vitamin and mineral intake. This restricted-sodium diet is intended to prevent any increased fluid accumulation. It is also desirable that you maintain your ideal body weight to help reduce cardiovascular stress. Therefore, it is very important to follow your diet carefully. If you have not received an individualized sodium-controlled diet plan, please request one from your nurse or home care dietitian.

Sodium comes in many forms. Table salt is one of the more prevalent forms of sodium. It is important to read food labels carefully and avoid foods that list "salt" or "sodium compounds" as one of the first three ingredients. There are four general guidelines for reducing sodium intake.

1. Do not add salt in cooking or to any foods once prepared.
2. Avoid regular processed products (i.e., >250 mg sodium/serving); choose reduced-sodium products (<250 mg sodium/serving), for example
   - luncheon meats (e.g., salami, corned beef, pastrami), cured meats (e.g., bacon, smoked ham)
   - processed cheeses
   - salted potato chips, pretzels, and other visibly salted snacks
   - canned soups, meats, and vegetables
   - sodium-containing condiments (e.g., soy sauce and many other condiments)
3. Avoid or minimize caffeine and alcohol as directed by your physician.
4. There are many foods that can be included in your diet.
   - freshly prepared meats, poultry, or fish
   - fresh or canned fruits
   - fresh, frozen, or low-sodium canned vegetables
   - reduced-sodium cheeses
   - unsalted snack foods

Be sure to check with your physician or nurse if you need to restrict your fluid intake.

Source: Barbara Stover Gingerich and Deborah Anne Ondeck, *Clinical pathways for the Multidisciplinary Home Care Team,* Aspen Publishers. Inc., © 1996.

Choose Low-Salt Foods

Choose foods low in salt and sodium. Americans eat more salt (sodium chloride) and other forms of sodium than they need. And guess what? They also have high rates of high blood pressure.

Studies show that when some people cut back on salt and sodium, their blood pressure drops. It happens particularly among African Americans and the elderly.

Sodium occurs naturally in foods. It also is added to food in various ways: during processing, cooking, or at the table.

People with high blood pressure should eat no more than about 2.4 grams (2,400 milligrams) of sodium a day. That equals 6 grams or 1 teaspoon of table salt. But remember that the 6 grams includes ALL salt eaten—including that in processed foods and added during cooking or at the table. And for people with high normal blood pressure, cutting back on salt and sodium is also a good way to prevent blood pressure from rising.

These days, it's easier than ever to keep track of how much salt and sodium you eat. Information on salt and sodium is available on new food labels.

Pork

Many people think that pork should not be eaten when trying to cut back on sodium. But fresh pork usually has no more sodium than do beef and poultry. Here are a few principles to help you keep pork dishes low in sodium:

- Choose fresh lean pork like pork chops, pork loin, or pork roast. Fresh pork has about the same amount of sodium as any other fresh cut of meat.
- Take care of how the pork is prepared. Spice it up with some of the low sodium seasonings listed on page 181. Also try the recipe for baked pork chops on page 191.
- Cut back on cured and processed pork like bacon, ham, sausage, and luncheon meats. Such products are very high in sodium.

LEARNING THE CLAIMS ON NUTRITION LABELS

Just what does "sodium-free" or "low-sodium" mean? Here are the answers:

- **Sodium-free** = less than 5 mg of sodium in a serving
- **Low-sodium** = 140 mg or less of sodium in a serving
- **Very low sodium** = 35 mg or less of sodium in a serving

continues

continued

- **Reduced or less sodium** = sodium at least 25 percent less per serving than the regular version of that food
- **Light or light in sodium** = sodium at least 50 percent less per serving than the regular version of that food
- **No salt added** = no salt is added during processing in a food that usually has salt added

GETTING THE LOWDOWN ON LOW-SODIUM PRODUCTS

Many food products come in "low" or "reduced sodium" versions. Among these are:

convenience foods (such as frozen dinners)

mixed dishes (such as pizza)

packaged mixes

salad dressings

vegetable juices

canned vegetables

soups (including dried soup mixes and bouillon)

condiments (such as catsup and soy sauce)

snack foods (such as chips, pretzels, and nuts)

crackers

baked goods

cheeses

butter and margarine

processed meats

TIPS ON REDUCING SALT AND SODIUM

- Add less salt at the table and in cooking. Reduce the amount a little each day until none is used. Try spices and herbs instead (see page 181).
- Cook with low-salt ingredients. Remove salt from recipes whenever possible—rice, pasta, and hot cereals can be cooked with little or no salt.
- Use fewer sauces, mixes, and "instant" products—this includes flavored rices, pasta, and cereal, since they usually have salt added.
- Use fresh, frozen, or canned fruits.
- Use vegetables that are fresh, frozen without sauce, or canned with no salt added.
- Check nutrition labels for the amount of sodium in foods. Look for products that say "sodium-free," "very low sodium," "low-sodium," "reduced or less sodium," "light in sodium," or "unsalted," especially on cans, boxes, bottles, and bags.
- Rinse salt from canned foods.
- Limit smoked, cured, or processed beef, pork, or poultry.
- Watch out for sodium in medicines—for instance some antacids contain sodium.

Source: "High Blood Pressure: Treat It for Life," National Heart, Lung, and Blood Institute, NIH Publication No. 94–3312, August 1994.

Cut Down on Salt and Sodium

EATING LESS SALT AND SODIUM HELPS YOU PREVENT OR LOWER HIGH BLOOD PRESSURE

"I want to keep my blood pressure under control, so I cut back on salt and sodium. I took my salt shaker off the table and use less salt in my cooking. My doctor said to eat fewer regular canned soups and lunch meats because they have too much sodium and salt. After making my own homemade soups again, my family won't even eat canned soups. Too salty—and not as good as mine!"

—Christina López

Sodium is a part of salt. It also is a part of mixtures used to flavor and preserve foods. You can make a few simple changes to help you and your family eat less salt and sodium.

When You Shop

- Buy fruits and vegetables for snacks instead of salty chips and salty crackers.
- Read food labels. Buy foods that say "reduced sodium," "low in sodium," "sodium free," or "no salt added."
- Choose fewer regular canned and processed foods like sausage, bologna, pepperoni, salami, ham, canned or dried soups, pickles, and olives.

When You Cook

- Each day cut back a little on the amount of salt you add to foods. You will soon get used to eating less salt.
- Use spices instead of salt. Season your food with herbs and spices such as pepper, cumin, mint, or cilantro.
- Use garlic *powder* and onion *powder* instead of garlic salt and onion salt.
- Use less bouillon cubes, soy sauce, and ketchup.

When You Are at the Table

- Take the salt shaker off the table.

Try These Spices Instead of Salt to Season Food

For beef. . .   Try bay leaf, garlic, marjoram, basil, pepper, thyme, cilantro.

For chicken. . . Try marjoram, oregano, rosemary, sage, tarragon.

For fish. . .   Try curry powder, dill, parsley

You will be amazed at how good your food will taste!

---

continues

continued

Choose Two or Three Things You Will Do To Eat Less Salt and Sodium

☐ Make homemade soups with less salt.
☐ Check food labels when you shop. Buy foods marked "low sodium," "reduced sodium," "sodium free," or "no salt added."
☐ Season your foods with spices instead of seasoned salt and bouillon cubes.
☐ Take the salt shaker off your table.
☐ Eat fruits like mango and orange without adding any salt.

Source: "Cut Down on Salt and Sodium," NIH Publication No. 96-4042. U.S. Department of Health and Human Services, National Heart, Lung, and Blood Institute, National Institutes of Health, September 1996.

¡Coma menos sal y sodio!

COMER MENOS SAL Y SODIO LE AYUDA A PREVENIR O BAJAR LA PRESIÓN ALTA.

"Yo quiero tener la presión bajo control, por eso uso menos sal y sodio. Quité el salero de la mesa y ahora uso menos sal cuando cocino. Mi médico me dijo que comiera menos sopas enlatadas y carnes procesadas porque tienen mucha sal y sodio. Desde que comencé a hacer mis sopitas caseras, a mi familia ya no le gustó las sopas enlatadas. ¡Muy saladas y no tan sabrosas como las que yo hago!"

—Cristina López

El sodio es parte de la sal. También es parte de otras mezclas usadas para dar sabor y preservar los alimentos. Usted puede hacer algunos cambios sencillos que le ayuden a usted y a su familia a comer menos sal y sodio.

Cuando compre

- Escoja frutas y vegetales para comer como bocadillos en vez de papas fritas saladas y galletas saladas.
- Lea las etiquetas de los alimentos. Compre los que tienen marcado "reducido en sodio," "bajo en sodio" o "sin sodio".
- Reduzca el consumo de alimentos enlatados y procesados, como chorizo, mortadela, peperoni, salami, jamón, sopas enlatadas o de sobre, pepino encurtido y aceitunas.

Cuando cocine

- Cada día disminuya un poco la cantidad de sal que usa. Con el tiempo se acostumbrará a comer menos sal.
- Use especias en vez de sal. Déle sabor a sus comidas con hierbas y especias tales como pimienta, comino, menta o cilantro.
- Use ajo en *polvo* y cebolla en *polvo* en vez de sal de ajo o sal de cebolla.
- Disminuya el uso de cubitos de caldo, salsa de soya y salsa de tomate (ketchup).

En la mesa

- Quite el salero de la mesa.

continúa

continuación

Para sazonar sus comidas pruebe estas especias en vez de sal

Con carne de res. . .   Pruebe hoja de laurel, ajo, mejorana, albahaca, pimienta, tomillo, cilantro.

Con pollo. . .   Pruebe mejorana, orégano, romero, salvia, tarragón.

Con pescado. . .   Pruebe curry en polvo, eneldo, perejil.

¡Se sorprenderá con el buen sabor de su comida!

Escoja dos o tres cosas que hará para comer menos sal y sodio.

☐ Preparar las sopas caseras con menos sal.
☐ Leer las etiquetas de los alimentos al hacer las compras. Comprar los que están marcados como "bajo en sodio", "reducido en sodio" o "sin sodio".
☐ Sazonar las comidas con especias en vez de condimentos con sal y cubos de caldo.
☐ Quitar el salero de la mesa.
☐ Comer las frutas como el mango y la naranja sin sal.

Source: "Coma menos sal y sodio!" NIH Publication No. 96-4042, U.S. Department of Health and Human Services, National Heart, Lung, and Blood Institute, National Institutes of Health, September 1996.

No Added Salt Diet

Reduced sodium (salt) is suggested for those with certain medical conditions.

- Limit prepared foods such as packaged casserole or stuffing mixes, frozen dinners, and canned soups and stews.
- Select meals with less than 800 milligrams (mg) of sodium per serving, such as frozen entrees.
- Do not use the salt shaker. Use salt sparingly in cooking, if at all.
- Use the following guidelines to plan your food choices.

Food Group	Good Low-Sodium Choices	Avoid
Dairy	Milk, yogurt, regular cheese, ricotta, and cream cheese (2 oz daily); low-sodium cheese as desired	Blue cheese, cheese spreads, processed cheese, Romano, Parmesan
Meat or Substitute	Fresh or frozen beef, chicken, lamb, veal, pork, turkey, fish, or shellfish; dried beans, peas, eggs, unsalted peanut butter, low-sodium water packed tuna; kosher poultry	Smoked, dried, or cured meat such as ham, bacon, sausage, cold cuts, hot dogs, corned beef, kosher meats; fish such as anchovies, sardines, salted cod, smoked herring
Fruits and Vegetables	Fresh, dried, frozen, or canned fruit and juices; fresh or frozen vegetables; low-sodium canned vegetables; low-sodium tomato or vegetable juice	Regular tomato or vegetable juice, sauerkraut, pickled beets, "boil in bag" vegetables, sauce-covered vegetables, regular canned vegetables
Soups	Homemade or low-sodium soups or stew, low-sodium bouillon or broth, low-sodium canned soups	Canned, frozen, dried or condensed soups, bouillon, or broth
Potatoes and Potato Substitutes	White or sweet potatoes; squash; enriched rice, barley, noodles, spaghetti, macaroni, and other pastas; homemade bread stuffing	Commercially prepared potato, rice, or pasta mixes; commercial bread stuffing
Breads and Cereals	Enriched white, wheat, rye, and pumpernickel breads and rolls; biscuits, muffins, cornbread, pancakes, waffles, and most dry cereals and cold cereals; unsalted crackers and bread sticks	Breads, rolls, and crackers with salted tops; instant hot cereals; instant potato and rice mixes

continues

continued

Seasonings, Sauces, Condiments	Mayonnaise, catsup, salad dressings (in limited amounts), mustard, hot pepper sauce, herbs and spices such as bay leaf, fresh garlic, lemon, parsley, pepper, onion or garlic powder, oregano, rosemary, sage, thyme, vinegar	Miso, monosodium glutamate (MSG), meat tenderizers, olives, packaged or canned sauces or gravies, pickles, soy sauce, steak sauce, tamari
Snacks	Unsalted nuts, unsalted popcorn, and other unsalted snack food items	Salted potato chips, salted pretzels, salted nuts, corn curls, salted popcorn, and other salted snacks

- **Dining out:** Order individually prepared food items and ask for no salt, etc., in the preparation. (Check table above for condiments to avoid.)
- **Air travel:** Request low-sodium (low-salt) meals when reserving your flight.
- **Medications:** Avoid medications that are high in sodium, such as Alka Seltzer, Brioschi, Bromo Seltzer, and Rolaids. Discuss a low-sodium alternative medication with your health care provider.

NOTES:

Courtesy of Youville Lifecare, Cambridge, Massachusetts.

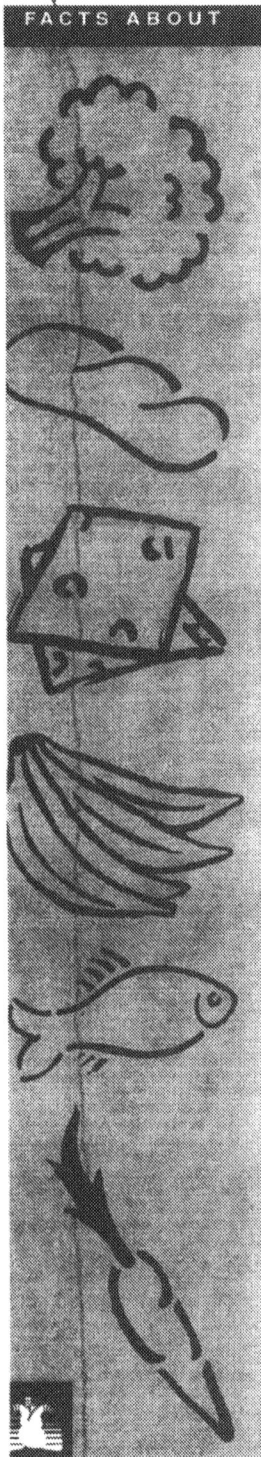

FACTS ABOUT

The DASH Diet

Research has shown that diet affects the development of high blood pressure, or hypertension (the medical term). Recently, a study found that a particular eating plan can lower elevated blood pressure.

This fact sheet tells what high blood pressure is and how you can follow the eating plan. It offers tips on how to start and stay on the plan, as well as a week of menus and recipes for some of the dishes.

The eating plan is meant for those with elevated blood pressure. It also is a heart-healthy plan that you can share with your family.

WHAT IS HIGH BLOOD PRESSURE?

Blood pressure is the force of blood against artery walls. It is measured in millimeters of mercury (mm Hg) and recorded as two numbers—systolic pressure (as the heart beats) over diastolic pressure (between heartbeats). Both numbers are important (see chart on page 2).

When blood pressure is too high, the heart is working harder than it should.

Once developed, high blood pressure lasts a lifetime. It is a dangerous condition, which often has no warning signs or symptoms. If uncontrolled, it can lead to heart and kidney disease, and stroke.

High blood pressure affects about 50 million—or one in four—adult Americans. High blood pressure is especially common among African Americans, who tend to develop it earlier and more often than whites. Many Americans also tend to develop high blood pressure as they age. About half of all Americans age 60 and older have high blood pressure.

High blood pressure can be controlled by the following steps: lose weight, if overweight; become physically active; eat healthy, including choosing foods lower in salt and sodium; limit alcohol intake; and, if prescribed, take high blood pressure pills. All steps but the last also help prevent high blood pressure.

WHAT IS THE DASH DIET?

Even slight elevations of blood pressure above the optimal level of less than 120/80 mm Hg are unhealthy. The higher the blood pressure above normal, the greater the health risk.

continues

BLOOD PRESSURE CATEGORIES FOR ADULTS*			
	Systolic**		**Diastolic****
Optimal	<120 mm Hg	and	<80 mm Hg
Normal	<130 mm Hg	and	<85 mm Hg
High-Normal	130–139 mm Hg	or	85–89 mm Hg
High			
Stage 1	140–159 mm Hg	or	90–99 mm Hg
Stage 2	160–179 mm Hg	or	100–109 mm Hg
Stage 3	≥180 mm Hg	or	≥110 mm Hg

*Categories are for those age 18 and older and come from the National High Blood Pressure Education Program. The categories are for those not on a high blood pressure drug and who have no short-term serious illness.

** If your systolic and diastolic pressures fall into different categories, your overall status is the higher category.

< means less than, and ≥ means greater than or equal to

In the past, researchers had tested various single nutrients, such as calcium and magnesium, to find clues about what affects blood pressure. These studies were done mostly with dietary supplements and their findings were not conclusive.

Then, scientists supported by the National Heart, Lung, and Blood Institute (NHLBI) tested nutrients as they occur together in food. The results were dramatic. The clinical study, called "DASH" for Dietary Approaches to Stop Hypertension, found that elevated blood pressures can be reduced with an eating plan low in saturated fat, total fat, and cholesterol, and rich in fruits, vegetables, and lowfat dairy foods. The plan is rich in magnesium, potassium, and calcium, as well as protein and fiber.

DASH involved 459 adults with systolic blood pressures of less than 160 mm Hg and diastolic pressures of 80–95 mm Hg. About half of the participants were women and 60 percent were African Americans.

DASH compared three eating plans:

- A plan similar in nutrients to what many Americans consume
- A plan similar to what Americans consume but higher in fruits and vegetables
- A "combination" plan— the DASH diet—lower in saturated fat, total fat, and cholesterol, and rich in fruits, vegetables, and lowfat dairy foods

All three plans used about 3,000 milligrams of sodium daily— about 20 percent below the U.S. average for adults. None of the plans was vegetarian or used specialty foods.

Results showed that both the fruit/vegetable and combination plans reduced blood pressure, but the combination plan had the greatest effect. The DASH eating plan reduced blood pressure by an average of about 6 mm Hg for systolic and 3 mm Hg for diastolic. It worked even better for those with high blood pressure—the systolic dropped on average about 11 mm Hg and the diastolic about 6 mm Hg. Further, the reductions came fast—within 2 weeks of starting the eating plan.

HOW DO I MAKE THE DASH?

"Following the DASH Diet" on page 4 gives the servings . and food groups for the DASH eating plan. The number of servings you need may vary, depending on your caloric need.

You should be aware that the DASH plan has more daily servings of fruits, vegetables, and grains than you may be used to eating. This makes it high in fiber, which can cause bloating and diarrhea. To get used to the new eating plan, gradually increase your servings of fruits, vegetables, and grains.

continues

GET THOSE NUTRIENTS

The DASH eating plan is rich in various nutrients believed to benefit blood pressure and in other factors involved in good health. The amounts of the nutrients vary by how much you eat. If you eat about 2,000 calories a day on the plan, the nutrients you get will include:

4,700 milligrams of potassium

500 milligrams of magnesium

1,240 milligrams of calcium

Those totals are about two to three times the amounts most Americans get.

The menus and recipes in this fact sheet also have slightly less salt and sodium than were in the DASH study's meals. These average about 2,400 milligrams of sodium per day, compared with about 3,000 milligrams in the DASH study meals. Twenty-four hundred milligrams of sodium equals about 6 grams, or 1 teaspoon, of table salt (sodium chloride). This amount follows the current recommendation of both the Federal Government's Dietary Guidelines for Americans and the NHLBI's National High Blood Pressure Education Program. The DASH eating plan makes it easier to consume less salt and sodium, because it is rich in fruits and vegetables, which are lower in sodium than many other foods. You can also keep salt and sodium down by using fewer already prepared foods and less salt at the table and in cooking. The next phase of the study—

called DASH2—is examining the relationship between blood pressure, eating patterns, and a reduced sodium intake. It should yield important findings about how much sodium and salt is advisable to prevent or control high blood pressure when using the DASH eating plan.

How can you get started on DASH? It's easy. The DASH plan requires no special foods and has no hard-to-follow recipes. One way to begin is by seeing how DASH compares with your current food habits. Use the "What's On Your Plate?" form on page 5. Fill it in for 1–2 days and see how it compares with the DASH plan. This will help you see what you need to change.

Remember that some days you may eat more than what's recommended from one food group and less of another. But don't worry. Just be sure that the average of several days or a week comes close to what's recommended.

Then, check the "Getting Started" suggestions on page 6 and the "Tips on Eating the DASH Way" listed in the box on the right. Finally, use the menus that begin on page 7—or make up your own—and you're all set.

One note: It's important that, if you have high blood pressure and take a medication, you should not stop your therapy. Use the DASH diet and talk about your drug treatment with your doctor.

TIPS ON EATING THE DASH DIET WAY

- Make it easier to increase your servings of fruits and vegetables to eight a day by trying to have two servings of fruits and/or vegetables at each meal. For instance, for lunch have one fruit and one vegetable. Then add one fruit and one vegetable as snacks.

- To increase your dairy servings to three a day, try to have one lowfat or fat free dairy serving at each meal. If you have trouble digesting dairy products, try taking lactase enzyme pills or drops (available at drugstores and groceries) with the dairy foods. Or, buy lactose free milk or milk with lactase enzyme added to it.

- Choose whole grain foods to get added nutrients, especially the B vitamins. For example, choose whole wheat bread or whole grain cereals.

- Use the percent Daily Value on food labels to compare products and choose those lowest in saturated fat, total fat, cholesterol, and sodium.

- Feed your craving for sweets with fresh or dried fruit or fruit-flavored gelatin.

- Use fresh, frozen, canned, or dried fruits.

- Use fresh, frozen, or no-salt-added canned vegetables.

continues

FOLLOWING THE DASH DIET

The DASH eating plan shown below is based on 2,000 calories a day. The number of daily servings in a food group may vary from those listed depending on your caloric needs.

Use this chart to help you plan your menus or take it with you when you go to the store.

FOOD GROUP	DAILY SERVINGS (except as noted)	SERVING SIZES	EXAMPLES AND NOTES	SIGNIFICANCE OF EACH FOOD GROUP TO THE DASH EATING PLAN
Grains & grain products	7–8	1 slice bread 1 cup dry cereal* 1/2 cup cooked rice, pasta, or cereal	whole wheat bread, English muffin, pita bread, bagel, cereals. grits, oatmeal. crackers, unsalted pretzels and popcorn	major sources of energy and fiber
Vegetables	4–5	1 cup raw leafy vegetable 1/2 cup cooked vegetable 6 oz vegetable juice	tomatoes. potatoes, carrots, green peas, squash, broccoli, turnip greens, collards, kale, spinach, artichokes. green beans, lima beans. sweet potatoes	rich sources of potassium, magnesium, and fiber
Fruits	4–5	6 oz fruit juice 1 medium fruit 1/4 cup dried fruit 1/2 cup fresh, frozen, or canned fruit	apricots, bananas, dates, grapes, oranges, orange juice, grapefruit, grapefruit juice, mangoes, melons, peaches, pineapples, prunes, raisins, strawberries, tangerines	important sources of potassium, magnesium, and fiber
Lowfat or fat free dairy foods	2–3	8 oz milk 1 cup yogurt 1 1/2 oz cheese	fat free (skim) or lowfat (1%) milk, fat free or lowfat buttermilk, fat free or lowfat regular or frozen yogurt, lowfat and fat free cheese	major sources of calcium and protein
Meats, poultry, and fish	2 or less	3 oz cooked meats, poultry, or fish	select only lean; trim away visible fats; broil, roast, or boil, instead of frying; remove skin from poultry	rich sources of protein and magnesium
Nuts, seeds, and dry beans	4–5 per week	1/3 cup or 1 1/2 oz nuts 2 Tbsp or 1/2 oz seeds 1/2 cup cooked dry beans	almonds, filberts, mixed nuts, peanuts, walnuts, sunflower seeds, kidney beans, lentils and peas	rich sources of energy, magnesium, potassium, protein, and fiber
Fats & oils**	2–3	1 tsp soft margarine 1 Tbsp lowfat mayonnaise 2 Tbsp light salad dressing 1 tsp vegetable oil	soft margarine. lowfat mayonnaise, light salad dressing. vegetable oil (such as olive, corn, canola, or safflower)	Besides fats added to foods, remember to choose foods that contain less fats
Sweets	5 per week	1 Tbsp sugar 1 Tbsp jelly or jam 1/2 oz jelly beans 8 oz lemonade	maple syrup, sugar, jelly, jam, fruit-flavored gelatin, jelly beans, hard candy, fruit punch, sorbet, ices	Sweets should be low in fat

* Serving sizes vary between 1/2–1 1/4 cups. Check the product's nutrition label
** Fat content changes serving counts for fats and oils: For example, 1 Tbsp of regular salad dressing equals 1 serving; 1 Tbsp of a lowfat dressing equals 1/2 serving; 1 Tbsp of a fat free dressing equals 0 servings

WHAT'S ON YOUR PLATE?

Use this form to track your food habits before you start on the DASH eating plan or to see how you're doing after a few weeks. To record more than 1 day, just copy the form. Total each day's food groups and compare what you ate with the DASH plan. To see how the form looks completed, check the menus, which start on page 7.

Food	Amount (serving size)	Number of servings by DASH food group							
		Grains	Vegetables	Fruits	Dairy foods	Meat, poultry, & fish	Nuts, seeds, & dry beans	Fats and oils	Sweets
Breakfast									
Example: whole wheat bread & soft margarine	2 slices 2 tsp	2						2	
Lunch									
Dinner									
Snacks									
DAY'S TOTAL									
Compare yours with the DASH plan		7–8	4–5	4–5	2–3	2 or less	4–5 a week	2–3	5 a week

continues

GETTING STARTED

It's easy to adopt the DASH eating diet. Here are some ways to get started:

Change gradually.

- If you now eat one or two vegetables a day, add a serving at lunch and another at dinner.
- If you don't eat fruit now or have only juice at breakfast, add a serving to your meals or have it as a snack.
- Use only half the butter, margarine, or salad dressing you do now.
- Try lowfat or fat free condiments, such as fat free salad dressings.
- Gradually increase dairy products to three servings per day. For example, drink milk with lunch or dinner, instead of soda, alcohol, or sugar-sweetened tea. Choose lowfat (1 percent) or fat free (skim) dairy products to reduce total fat intake.

Treat meat as one part of the whole meal, instead of the focus.

- Buy less meat. If it's not there, you won't eat it.
- Limit meat to 6 ounces a day (two servings)—all that's needed. Three to four ounces is about the size of a deck of cards.
- If you now eat large portions of meat, cut them back gradually—by a half or a third at each meal.
- Include two or more vegetarian-style (meatless) meals each week.
- Increase servings of vegetables, rice, pasta, and dry beans in meals. Try casseroles and pasta, and stir-fry dishes, having less meat and more vegetables, grains, and dry beans.

Use fruits or lowfat foods as desserts and snacks.

- Fruits and lowfat foods offer great taste and variety. Use fruits canned in their own juice. Fresh fruits require little or no preparation. Dried fruits are easy to carry with you.
- Try these snack ideas: unsalted pretzels or nuts mixed with raisins; graham crackers; lowfat and fat free yogurt and frozen yogurt; plain popcorn with no salt or butter added; and raw vegetables.

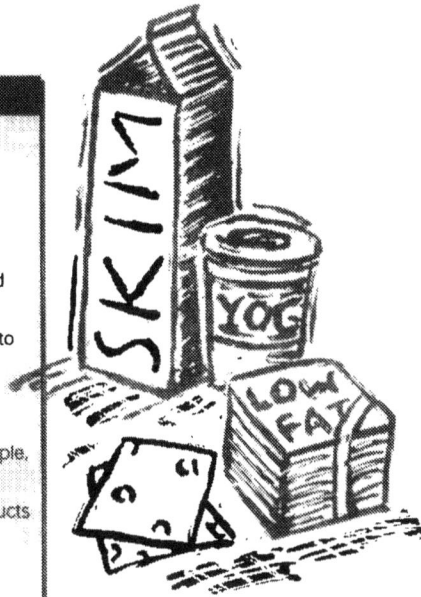

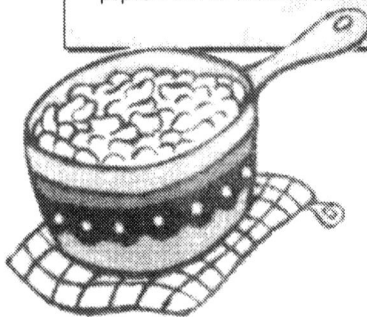

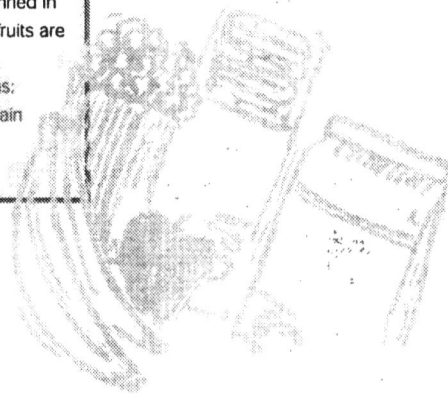

continues

A WEEK WITH THE DASH DIET

Here is a week of menus from the DASH eating plan. The menus are based on 2,000 calories a day—serving sizes should be increased or decreased for other caloric levels. Also, to ease the calculations, some of the serving sizes have been rounded off. Recipes are given for starred items.

DAY 1

Food	Amount		Grains	Vegetables	Fruits	Dairy foods	Meat, poultry, & fish	Nuts, seeds, & dry beans	Fats and oils	Sweets
Breakfast										
apple juice	1	cup			1 1/2					
bran cereal, ready-to-eat	2/3	cup	1							
raisins	2	Tbsp			1/2					
fat free milk	1	cup				1				
whole wheat bread	1	slice	1							
soft margarine	1 1/2	tsp							1 1/2	
Lunch										
chicken sandwich:										
chicken breast, no skin	3	oz					1			
American cheese, reduced fat	2	slices (1 1/2 oz)					1			
loose leaf lettuce	2	large leaves		1/2						
tomato	2	slices (1/4" thick)		1/2						
light mayonnaise	1	Tbsp							1	
whole wheat bread	2	slices	2							
apple	1	medium			1					
Dinner										
vegetarian spaghetti sauce*	3/4	cup		1 1/2						
spaghetti	1	cup	2							
Parmesan cheese	4	Tbsp				1				
green beans	1/2	cup		1						
spinach salad:										
spinach, raw	1	cup		1						
mushrooms, raw	1/4	cup		1/4						
croutons	2	Tbsp	1/4							
Italian dressing, lowfat	2	Tbsp							1	
dinner roll	1	medium	1							
frozen yogurt, lowfat	1/2	cup				1/2				
Snack										
orange juice	1	cup			1 1/2					
banana	1	large			1 1/2					
Totals			7 1/4	4 3/4	6	3 1/2	1	0	3 1/2	0

Per Day:

Calories	1,995	Magnesium	458	mg
Total Fat	50 g**	Potassium	4,254	mg
Saturated Fat	15 g	Calcium	1,384	mg
Cholesterol	124 mg***	Sodium	3,127	mg

* recipe on page 14
** g=gram
*** mg=milligram

DAY 2

Food	Amount		Servings Provided							
			Grains	Vegetables	Fruits	Dairy foods	Meat, poultry, & fish	Nuts, seeds, & dry beans	Fats and oils	Sweets
Breakfast										
prune juice	3/4	cup				1				
oatmeal	1/2	cup	1							
whole wheat bread	1	slice	1							
soft margarine	1	tsp							1	
fat free milk	1	cup				1				
banana	1	medium			1					
Lunch										
BBQ beef sandwich:										
lean beef	2	oz					3/4			
BBQ sauce	1	Tbsp								
roll	1	large	1 1/2							
boiled potatoes	1	cup		2						
cheddar cheese, natural	1 1/2	oz				1				
salad:										
loose leaf lettuce	2	leaves		1/2						
tomato	2	slices (1/4" thick)		1/2						
green pepper	2	strips		1/2						
salad dressing, lowfat	2	tsp							1/3	
cranberry juice	1	cup			1 1/2					
Dinner										
trout, or other fish, baked										
in lemon juice	3	oz					1			
brown rice	1/2	cup	1							
three-bean salad:										
kidney beans	1/2	cup						1		
green beans	1/2	cup		1						
yellow beans	1/4	cup		1/2						
Italian dressing, lowfat	4	tsp							2/3	
corn muffin	1	medium	1							
soft margarine	1	tsp							1	
spinach, cooked	1/2	cup		1						
Snacks										
orange	1	medium			1					
dried fruit mixture	1/4	cup (1 oz)			1					
Totals			5 1/2	6	5 1/2	2	1 3/4	1	3	0

Per Day:

Calories	2,055		Magnesium	456 mg
Total Fat	50 g		Potassium	4,404 mg
Saturated Fat	17 g		Calcium	1,076 mg
Cholesterol	180 mg		Sodium	2,579 mg

continues

DAY 3

Food	Amount		Grains	Vegetables	Fruits	Dairy foods	Meat, poultry, & fish	Nuts, seeds, & dry beans	Fats and oils	Sweets
Breakfast										
orange juice	1	cup			1 1/2					
cornflakes	3/4	cup	1							
whole wheat bread	1	slice	1							
soft margarine	1	tsp							1	
fat free milk	1	cup				1				
Lunch										
sandwich:										
ham, lean, low sodium	2	oz					3/4			
cheese, reduced fat	2	slices (1 1/2 oz)				1				
whole wheat bread	2	slices	2							
loose leaf lettuce	2	leaves		1/2						
tomato	2	slices (1/4" thick)		1/2						
mustard	1	tsp								
apple	1	medium			1					
Dinner										
chicken with Spanish rice*	1 1/2	cup	2	1			1		1/2	
green peas	1/2	cup		1						
corn muffin	1	medium	1							
melon balls	1	cup			2					
fat free milk	1	cup				1				
Snacks										
apricots, dried	1/3	cup (1 1/2 oz)			1 1/2					
almonds	1/3	cup (1 1/2 oz)						1		
orange	1	large			1 1/2					
Totals			7	3	7 1/2	3	1 3/4	1	1 1/2	0

Per Day:

Calories	1,987		Magnesium	469 mg
Total Fat	53 g		Potassium	4,857 mg
Saturated Fat	13 g		Calcium	1,372 mg
Cholesterol	153 mg		Sodium	2,921 mg

recipe on page 14

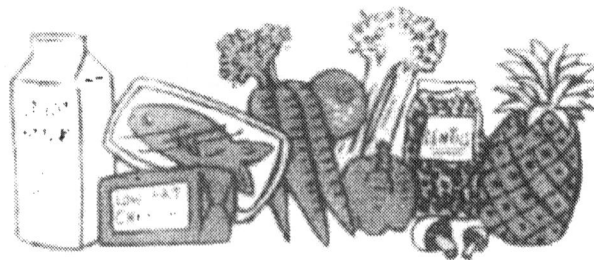

continues

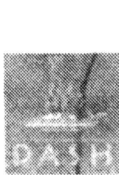

DAY 4 Food	Amount		Grains	Vegetables	Fruits	Dairy foods	Meat, poultry, & fish	Nuts, seeds, & dry beans	Fats and oils	Sweets
Breakfast										
orange juice	1	cup			1 1/2					
English muffin	1	whole	2							
marmalade	2	tsp								2/3
soft margarine	1	tsp							1	
fat free milk	1	cup				1				
Lunch										
sandwich:										
tuna, water-packed (rinsed and drained)	1/4	cup					1/2			
whole wheat bread	2	slices	2							
iceberg lettuce	1/2	cup		1/2						
tomato	2	slices (1/8" thick)		1/4						
light mayonnaise	1	Tbsp							1	
carrot and celery sticks	4	sticks each		1/4						
broccoli	2/3	cup		1 1/2						
cheddar cheese, reduced fat	1	oz				3/4				
cranberry juice cocktail	1/2	cup			3/4					
Dinner										
chicken breast, no skin	3	oz					1			
brown rice	1	cup	2							
stewed tomatoes	1/2	cup		1						
lima beans	1/2	cup		1						
spinach, cooked	1/3	cup		3/4						
dinner roll	1	medium	1							
soft margarine	1	tsp							1	
fat free milk	1	cup				1				
Snacks										
mixed nuts	1/4	cup (1 oz)						3/4		
apricots, dried	1/3	cup (1 1/2 oz)			1 1/2					
pretzels	3/4	cup (1 oz)	1							
orange	1	medium			1					
Totals			8	5 1/4	4 3/4	2 3/4	1 1/2	3/4	3	2/3

Per Day:

Calories	2,007		Calcium	1,391 mg
Total Fat	47 g		Magnesium	506 mg
Saturated Fat	11 g		Potassium	4,243 mg
Cholesterol	108 mg		Sodium	2,074 mg

continues

DAY 5

Food	Amount		Grains	Vegetables	Fruits	Dairy foods	Meat, poultry, & fish	Nuts, seeds, & dry beans	Fats and oils	Sweets
Breakfast										
orange juice	1	cup			1 1/2					
yogurt, fat free	1	cup				1				
fruit granola bars, lowfat	2		2							
fat free milk	1	cup				1				
banana	1	small			1/2					
Lunch										
turkey sandwich:										
turkey breast	3	oz					1			
loose leaf lettuce	1	leaf		1/4						
tomato	2	slices (1/4" thick)		1/2						
light mayonnaise	1	Tbsp							1	
whole wheat bread	2	slices	2							
carrots	7	sticks		1/4						
orange, fresh	1	medium			1					
Dinner										
spicy baked fish*	3	oz					1		3/4	
brown rice	1	cup	2							
spinach, cooked	1	cup		2						
zucchini, cooked	1/2	cup		1						
dinner roll	1	medium	1							
soft margarine	2	tsp							2	
fat free milk	1/2	cup				1/2				
melon balls	1	cup			2					
Snacks										
peanuts	1/4	cup (1 oz)						3/4		
apricots, dried	1/3	cup (1 1/2 oz)			1 1/2					
Totals			7	4	6 1/2	2 1/2	2	3/4	3 3/4	0

Per Day:

Calories	2,028	Magnesium	575 mg
Total Fat	51 g	Potassium	5,265 mg
Saturated Fat	9 g	Calcium	1,364 mg
Cholesterol	115 mg	Sodium	2,411 mg

*recipe on page 15

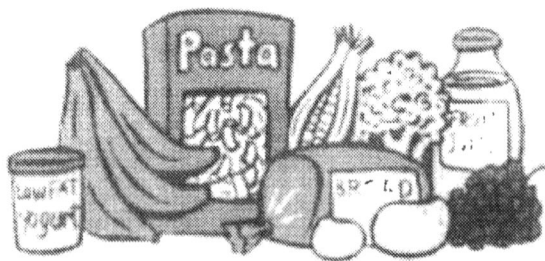

continues

continued

DAY 6

Food	Amount		Grains	Vegetables	Fruits	Dairy foods	Meat, poultry, & fish	Nuts, seeds, & dry beans	Fats and oils	Sweets
Breakfast										
orange juice	1	cup			1 1/2					
bran cereal	2/3	cup	1							
whole wheat bread	1	slice	1							
soft margarine	1	tsp							1	
fat free milk	1	cup				1				
banana	1	small			1/2					
Lunch										
chicken salad sandwich:										
chicken salad*	3/4	cup					1		2	
tomato	2	slices (1/4" thick)		1/2						
whole wheat pita bread	1	small	1							
apple	1	medium			1					
Dinner										
roast beef, lean	3	oz					1			
dinner roll	1	large	1 1/2							
baked potato	1	medium		2						
soft margarine	1	tsp							1	
green beans, cooked	3/4	cup		1 1/2						
frozen peaches	1/2	cup			1					
fat free milk	1	cup				1				
Snacks										
almonds	1/3	cup (1 1/2 oz)						1		
yogurt, lowfat	1	cup				1				
orange juice	1/2	cup			3/4					
Totals			4 1/2	4	4 3/4	3	2	1	4	0

Per Day:

Calories	2,072		Magnesium	508 mg
Total Fat	55 g		Potassium	4,540 mg
Saturated Fat	12 g		Calcium	1,320 mg
Cholesterol	161 mg		Sodium	1,602 mg

*recipe on page 14

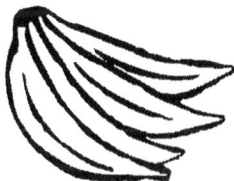

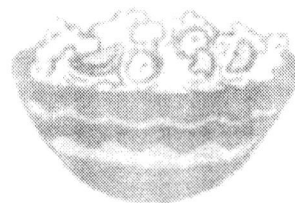

continues

DAY 7

Food	Amount		Grains	Vegetables	Fruits	Dairy foods	Meat, poultry, & fish	Nuts, seeds, & dry beans	Fats and oils	Sweets
Breakfast										
grape juice	1	cup			1 1/2					
bran flakes cereal	3/4	cup	1							
banana	1	medium			1					
whole wheat bread	1	slice	1							
soft margarine	1	tsp							1	
fat free milk	1	cup				1				
Lunch										
tuna salad sandwich:										
tuna	1/2	cup					1			
light mayonnaise	2	tsp							2/3	
iceberg lettuce	3/4	cup		3/4						
whole wheat bread	2	slices	2							
apricot nectar	3/4	cup			1					
apple	1	medium			1					
Dinner										
zucchini lasagna*	1/6	recipe	3	1		1				
spinach salad:										
spinach	1 1/4	cup		1 1/4						
tomato	2	slices (1/2" thick)		1						
Parmesan cheese	4	tsp				1/4				
oil and vinegar salad dressing:										
vegetable oil	2	tsp							2	
vinegar	1	tsp								
dinner roll	1	medium	1							
soft margarine	1	tsp							1	
Snacks										
almonds	2	Tbsp (3/4 oz)						1/2		
raisins	1/3	cup			1 1/2					
yogurt, fat free	1	cup				1				
Totals			8	4	6	3 1/4	1	1/2	4 2/3	0

Per Day:

Calories	1,976		Magnesium	506 mg
Total Fat	47 g		Potassium	4,290 mg
Saturated Fat	10 g		Calcium	1,248 mg
Cholesterol	52 mg		Sodium	1,911 mg

recipe on page 15

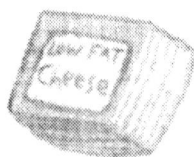

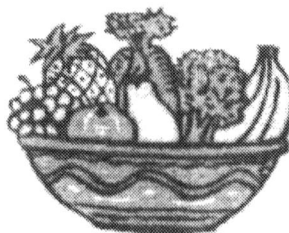

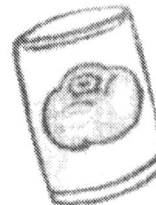

continues

RECIPES FOR HEART HEALTH

Here are some recipes to help you cook up a week of tasty heart healthy meals:

Vegetarian Spaghetti Sauce
(Day 1)

2	Tbsp	olive oil
2	small	onions, chopped
3	cloves	garlic, chopped
1 1/4	cup	zucchini, sliced
1	Tbsp	oregano. dried
1	Tbsp	basil, dried
1	8 oz can	tomato sauce
1	6 oz can	tomato paste
2	medium	tomatoes, chopped
1	cup	water

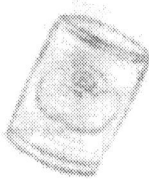

Makes 6 servings.
Serving size: 3/4 cup

Per Serving:

Calories	102		Magnesium	37 mg
Total Fat	5 g		Potassium	623 mg
Saturated Fat	1 g		Calcium	42 mg
Cholesterol	0 mg		Sodium	459 mg

1. In a medium skillet, heat oil. Saute onions, garlic, and zucchini in oil for 5 minutes on medium heat.
2. Add remaining ingredients and simmer covered for 45 minutes. Serve over spaghetti.

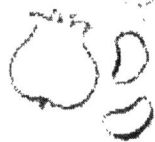

Chicken and Spanish Rice
(Day 3)

1	cup	onions, chopped
3/4	cup	sweet green peppers
2	tsp	vegetable oil
1	cup	tomato sauce
1	tsp	parsley, chopped
1/4	tsp	black pepper
1 1/2	tsp	garlic, minced
5	cup	white rice, cooked in unsalted water
3 1/4	cup	chicken breast, cooked (skin and bone removed), diced

Makes 5 servings.
Serving size: 1 1/2 cup

Per Serving:

Calories	406		Magnesium	57 mg
Total Fat	6 g		Potassium	529 mg
Saturated fat	2 g		Calcium	45 mg
Cholesterol	75 mg		Sodium	367 mg

1. In a large skillet saute onions and green peppers in oil for 5 minutes on medium heat.
2. Add tomato sauce and spices. Heat through.
3. Add cooked rice and chicken and heat through.

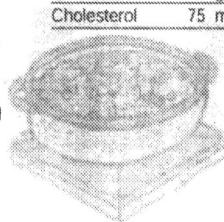

Chicken Salad
(Day 6)

3 1/4	cup	chicken, cooked, cubed, skinless
1/4	cup	celery, chopped
1	Tbsp	lemon juice
1/2	tsp	onion powder
1/8	tsp	salt
3	Tbsp	light mayonnaise

Makes 5 servings.
Serving size: 3/4 cup

Per Serving:

Calories	183		Magnesium	25 mg
Total fat	7 g		Potassium	240 mg
Saturated fat	2 g		Calcium	17 mg
Cholesterol	78 mg		Sodium	201 mg

In a large bowl combine all ingredients. Mix well.

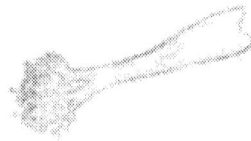

continues

Spicy Baked Fish

(Day 5)

		cooking oil spray
1	lb	cod (or other fish) fillet
1	Tbsp	olive oil
1	tsp	spicy seasoning mix

1. Preheat oven to 350° F. Spray a casserole dish with cooking oil spray.
2. Wash and dry fish. Place in dish and drizzle with oil and seasoning mixture.
3. Bake uncovered for 15 minutes or until fish flakes with fork. Cut into 4 pieces. Serve with rice.

Makes 4 servings.
Serving size: 1 piece (3 oz)

Per Serving:

Calories	134	Magnesium	52 mg
Total Fat	5 g	Potassium	309 mg
Saturated Fat	1 g	Calcium	18 mg
Cholesterol	60 mg	Sodium	93 mg

Spicy seasoning mix

1 1/2	tsp	white pepper
1/2	tsp	cayenne pepper
1/2	tsp	black pepper
1	tsp	onion powder
1 1/4	tsp	garlic powder
1	Tbsp	basil, dried
1 1/2	tsp	thyme, dried

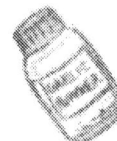

Mix all ingredients together. Store in an airtight container. Use in meat, poultry, fish, or vegetable dishes. Try replacing the salt in the salt shaker and use at the table.

Zucchini Lasagna

(Day 7)

1/2	pound	lasagna noodles, cooked in unsalted water
3/4	cup	mozzarella cheese, part-skim
1 1/2	cup	fat free cottage cheese
1/4	cup	Parmesan cheese
1 1/2	cup	zucchini, raw, sliced
2 1/2	cup	tomato sauce, low sodium
2	tsp	basil, dried
2	tsp	oregano, dried
1/4	cup	onion, chopped
1	clove	garlic
1/8	tsp	black pepper

Makes 6 servings.
Serving size: 1 piece

Per serving:

Calories	276	Magnesium	55 mg
Total Fat	5 g	Potassium	561 mg
Saturated fat	2 g	Calcium	216 mg
Cholesterol	11 mg	Sodium	380 mg

1. Preheat oven to 350° F. Lightly spray a 9 x 13 inch baking dish with vegetable oil spray. Set aside.
2. In a small bowl, combine 1/8 cup mozzarella and 1 Tbsp Parmesan cheese. Mix well and set aside.
3. In a medium bowl, combine remaining mozzarella and Parmesan cheese with all of the cottage cheese. Mix well and set aside.
4. Combine tomato sauce with remaining ingredients. Spread a thin layer of tomato sauce in the bottom of the baking dish. Add about a third of the noodles in a single layer. Spread half of the cottage cheese mixture on top. Add a layer of zucchini. Repeat layering. Add a thin coating of sauce. Top with the noodles, sauce, and reserved cheese mixture. Cover with alumium foil.
5. Bake 30 to 40 minutes. Let stand 10 to 15 minutes. Cut into 6 portions.

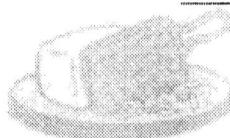

continues

continued

MAKING THE DASH TO GOOD HEALTH

The DASH plan is a new way of eating—for a lifetime. If you slip from the eating plan for a few days, don't let it keep you from reaching your health goals. Get back on track. Here's how:

■ **Ask yourself why you got off-track.**
Was it at a party? Were you feeling stress at home or work? Find out what triggered your sidetrack—and start again with DASH.

■ **Don't worry about a slip.**
Everyone slips—especially when learning something new. Remember that changing your lifestyle is a long-term process.

■ **See if you tried to do too much at once.**
Often, those starting a new lifestyle try to change too much at once. Instead, change one or two things at a time. Slowly but surely is the best way to succeed.

■ **Break the process down into small steps.**
This not only keeps you from trying to do too much at once but also keeps the changes simpler. Break complex goals into smaller, simpler steps, each of which is attainable.

■ **Write it down.**
Use the table on page 5 to keep track of what you eat. This can help you find the problem. Besides noting what you eat, also record: where you are, what you're doing, and how you feel. Keep track for several days. You may find, for instance, that you eat high fat foods while watching television. If so, you could start keeping a substitute snack on hand to eat instead of the high fat foods. This record also helps you be sure you're getting enough of each food group.

■ **Celebrate success.**
Treat yourself to a non-food treat for your accomplishments.

Menus and recipes were analyzed using the Minnesota Data System software—Food Data Base version 29.2; Nutrient Data Base version 29.2—developed by the Nutrition Coordinating Center. University of Minnesota, Minneapolis, MN.

Source: "The DASH Diet," NIH Publication No. 98-4082, U.S. Department of Health and Human Services, National Heart, Lung, and Blood Institute, National Institutes of Health, September 1998.

Reading Nutrition Labels

Nutrition Facts

Serving Size: 1 cup (228 g)
Servings Per Package 2

Amount Per Serving

Calories 260	Calories from Fat 120

	% Daily Value*
Total Fat 13g	**20%**
Saturated Fat 5g	**25%**
Cholesterol 30mg	**10%**
Sodium 600mg	**28%**
Total Carbohydrate 31g	**10%**
Dietary Fiber 0g	**0%**
Sugars 5g	
Protein 5g	

Vitamin A 4%	•	Vitamin C 2%
Calcium 15%	•	Iron 4%

* Percent Daily Values are based on a 2,000 calorie diet. Your Daily Values may be higher or lower depending on your calorie needs:

	Calories:	2,000	2,500
Total Fat	Less than	65g	80g
Sat Fat	Less than	20g	25g
Cholesterol	Less than	300g	300g
Sodium	Less than	2,400mg	2,400mg
Total Carbohydrate		300g	375g
Dietary Fiber		25g	30g

Calories per gram:
Fat 9 • Carbohydrate 4 • Protein 4

Ingredients: water, enriched flour, salt, sodium sulfate, malt, egg white, spices.

READ THE LABEL

Reading food labels will help you choose foods low in calories, total and saturated fat, cholesterol, and sodium. Labels have two important parts: the nutrition information and the ingredients list. Also, some labels have different claims like "reduced" or "light." Here's a closer look at labels.

Read the Nutrition Information

Look for the amount of calories, sodium, and total and saturated fat on a food product's nutrition label, shown at the left. If you have high blood pressure, compare similar products to find the one with the smallest amounts of sodium, as well as fat and calories if you also need to lose weight.

Look at the Ingredients

All food labels list the product's ingredients in descending order by weight. The ingredient in the greatest amount is listed first. The ingredient in the least amount is listed last. So, when watching your sodium look on the label for the words "sodium" or "salt." As you can see from the ingredients box to the left if either word is listed first or more than once on the label, then the food probably has a lot of sodium.

Source: "High Blood Pressure: Treat It for Life," National Heart, Lung, and Blood Institute, NIH Publication No. 94–3312, August 1994.

Using Spices Instead of Salt

SPICY CHOICES

Get out of the salt shaker rut and open your spice rack to lots of new tastes. Here are some great choices—

- Basil
- Cinnamon
- Dill
- Garlic or Garlic powder (NOT garlic SALT)
- Onion or Onion powder (NOT onion SALT)
- Poultry seasoning

- Tarragon
- Bay leaves
- Cumin
- Dry mustard
- Ginger
- Mint
- Oregano
- Parsley
- Rosemary
- Thyme

- Chili powder
- Curry powder
- Fruit juices
- Marjoram
- Nutmeg
- Paprika
- Pepper (black and red)
- Sage
- No-salt spice blends

SPICE IT UP

It's easy to make foods tasty without using salt. Try these foods with the suggested flavorings, spices, and herbs:

Meat

Beef	Bay leaf, garlic, marjoram, nutmeg, onion, pepper, sage, thyme
Lamb	Curry powder, garlic, rosemary, mint
Pork	Garlic, onion, sage, pepper, oregano
Veal	Bay leaf, curry powder, ginger, marjoram, oregano
Chicken	Ginger, lemon juice, lime juice, marjoram, oregano, paprika, poultry seasoning, rosemary, sage, tarragon, thyme
Fish	Curry powder, dill, dry mustard, lemon juice, lime juice, marjoram, paprika, pepper

continues

continued

Vegetables

Carrots	Cinnamon, cloves, marjoram, nutmeg, rosemary, sage
Corn	Cumin, curry powder, onion, paprika, parsley
Green beans	Dill, curry power, lemon juice, marjoram, oregano, tarragon, thyme
Greens	Onion, pepper
Peas	Ginger, marjoram, onion, parsley, sage
Potatoes	Dill, garlic, onion, paprika, parsley, sage
Squash	
Summer	Cloves, curry powder, marjoram, nutmeg, rosemary, sage
Winter	Cinnamon, ginger, nutmeg, onion
Tomatoes	Basil, bay leaf, dill, garlic, marjoram, onion, oregano, parsley, pepper

Source: "High Blood Pressure: Treat It for Life," National Heart, Lung, and Blood Institute, NIH Publication No. 94–3312, August 1994.

Sodium in Foods

TYPE OF FOOD	SODIUM (mg)
Meat, Poultry, Fish, and Shellfish	
Fresh meat (including lean cuts of beef, pork, lamb and veal), poultry, finfish, cooked, 3 oz.	Less than 90
Shellfish, 3 oz.	100–325
Tuna, canned, 3 oz.	300
*Sausage, 2 oz.	515
*Bologna, 2 oz.	535
*Frankfurter, 1½ oz.	560
Boiled ham, 2 oz.	750
Lean ham, 3 oz.	1,025
Eggs	
Egg white, 1	55
*Whole egg, 1	65
Egg substitute, ¼ cup = 1 egg	80–120
Dairy Products	
Milk	
*Whole milk, 1 cup	120
Skim or 1% milk, 1 cup	125
Buttermilk (salt added), 1 cup	260
Cheese	
*Natural cheese:	
*Swiss cheese, 1 oz.	75
*Cheddar cheese, 1 oz.	175
*Blue cheese, 1 oz.	395
Low-fat cheese, 1 oz.	150
*Processed cheese and cheese spreads, 1 oz.	340–450
Lower-sodium and lower-fat versions	Read the label
*Cottage cheese (regular), ½ cup	455
Cottage cheese (low-fat), ½ cup	460
Yogurt	
*Yogurt, whole milk, plain, 8 oz.	105
Yogurt, fruited or flavored, low-fat or nonfat, 8 oz.	120–150

TYPE OF FOOD	SODIUM (mg)
Yogurt, nonfat or low-fat, plain, 8 oz.	160–175
Breads, Cereals, Rice, Pasta, Dry Peas and Beans	
Breads and crackers	
Bread, 1 slice	110–175
English muffin, ½	130
Bagel, ½	190
Cracker, saltine type, 5 squares	195
*Baking powder biscuit, 1	305
Cereals	
Ready-to-eat	
Shredded wheat, ¾ cup	Less than 5
Puffed wheat and rice cereals, 1-½ to 1-⅔ cup	Less than 5
Granola-type cereals, ½ cup	5–25
Ring and nugget cereals, 1 cup	170–310
Flaked cereals, ⅔ to 1 cup	170–360
Cooked	
Cooked cereal (unsalted), ½ cup	Less than 5
Instant cooked cereal, 1 packet = ¾ cup	180
Pasta and rice	
Cooked rice and pasta, (unsalted), ½ cup	Less than 10
*Flavored rice mix, cooked, ½ cup	250–390
Beans and peas	
Peanut butter, unsalted, 2 tbsp.	Less than 5
Peanut butter, 2 tbsp.	150
Dry beans, home cooked, (unsalted), or no salt added canned, ½ cup	Less than 5

continues

continued

TYPE OF FOOD	SODIUM (mg)
Dry beans, plain canned, ½ cup	350–590
*Dry beans, canned in added fat or meat, ½ cup	425–630

Vegetables

Fresh or frozen vegetables, or no salt added canned (cooked without salt), ½ cup	Less than 70
Vegetables, canned, no sauce, ½ cup	55–470
*Vegetables, canned or frozen with sauce, ½ cup	Read the label
Tomato juice, canned, ¾ cup	660

Fruits

Fruits (fresh, frozen, canned), ½ cup	Less than 10

Fats and Oils

Oil, 1 tbsp.	0
*Butter, unsalted, 1 tsp.	1
*Butter, salted, 1 tsp.	25
Margarine, unsalted, 1 tsp.	Less than 5
Margarine, salted, 1 tsp.	50
Imitation mayonnaise, 1 tbsp.	75
*Mayonnaise, 1 tbsp.	80
Prepared salad dressings, low calorie, 2 tbsp.	50–310
*Prepared salad dressings, 2 tbsp.	210–440

Snacks

Popcorn, chips, and nuts

Unsalted nuts, ¼ cup	Less than 5

TYPE OF FOOD	SODIUM (mg)
Salted nuts, ¼ cup	185
*Unsalted potato chips and corn chips, 1 cup	Less than 5
*Salted potato chips and corn chips, 1 cup	170–285
Unsalted popcorn, 2½ cups	Less than 10
Salted popcorn, 2½ cups	330

Candy

Jelly beans, 10 large	5
*Milk chocolate bar, 1 ounce bar	25

Frozen desserts

*Ice cream, ½ cup	35–50
Frozen yogurt, low-fat or nonfat, ½ cup	40–55
Ice milk, ½ cup	55–60

Condiments

Mustard, chili sauce, hot sauce, 1 tsp.	35–65
Catsup, steak sauce, 1 tbsp.	100–230
Salsa, tartar sauce, 2 tbsp.	200–315
Salt, 1/6 tsp.	390
Pickles, 5 slices	280–460
Soy sauce, lower-sodium, 1 tbsp.	600
Soy sauce, 1 tbsp.	1,030

Convenience foods

**Canned and dehydrated soups, 1 cup	600–1,300
**Lower-sodium versions	Read the label
***Canned and frozen main dishes, 8 oz.	500–1,570
***Lower-sodium versions	Read the label

*Choices are higher in saturated fat, cholesterol, or both.
**Creamy soups are higher in saturated fat and cholesterol.
***Limit main dishes that have ingredients high in saturated fat, cholesterol, or both.

continues

continued

Take Care

Some fatty foods contain large amounts of salt. Examples include processed pork, bacon, and corned beef.

Also "fast foods" can contain both salt and fat. At the restaurant, ask that salt not be added to your meal during cooking. To cut down on how much of these foods you have, try eating smaller portions. If possible, choose foods that are baked or grilled—and hold the mayo and special sauces such as barbecue or tartar. These tips are also important for those trying to lose weight.

Source: "High Blood Pressure: Treat It for Life," National Heart, Lung, and Blood Institute, NIH Publication No. 94–3312, August 1994. Adapted from Home and Garden Bulletin 253–7, United States Department of Agriculture, July 1993.

Sodium Intake Information

Food	Amount		Time	Place	Who Present
	In Cooking	At Table			

Source: Linda G. Snetselaar, *Nutrition Counseling Skills for Medical Nutrition Therapy,* Aspen Publishers, Inc., © 1997.

Contract for a Sodium-Modified Diet

I agree to carry out each of the following steps and supply each reinforcer listed as each step is achieved:

Steps	**Reinforcer**
1. Eliminate salting before tasting.	Read a new cookbook.
2. Slowly eat unsalted foods to allow detection of true flavors.	Buy a new scarf.
3. Add new spices to foods in place of salt.	Buy a new pair of shoes.

Signed: _____

Cosigned (nutrition counselor): _____

Date: _____

Source: Linda G. Snetselaar, *Nutrition Counseling Skills for Medical Nutrition Therapy,* Aspen Publishers, Inc., © 1997.

Menu Ideas for People with High Blood Pressure

Here are two days of menus to show you how delicious and satisfying healthy eating can be.

DAY 1

Breakfast

2 large rectangles shredded wheat with
   1 medium banana
½ cup skim or 1% milk
1 slice toast with
1 teaspoon tub margarine
1 cup coffee with
1 tablespoon skim or 1% milk

Lunch—A La Fast Food

1 grilled chicken sandwich
1 tossed salad with
1 tablespoon oil and vinegar dressing
1 low-fat yogurt cone
1 cup lemonade

Snack

1 medium orange

Dinner

2 rolls *autumn stuffed cabbage
½ cup rice with parsley and
1 teaspoon tub margarine
1 cup skim or 1% milk
3 fig bar cookies

Snack

1 English muffin with
2 teaspoons each tub margarine and jelly

Total Nutrients**:

Calories 2,260
Sodium . . . . 2,220 mg
Total fat . . . . 70 g
Saturated fat . . . . . 20 g
Cholesterol . . . . . . 165 mg
% of calories: . . . . 28% from total fat
                8% from saturated fat

*Starred items have recipes given
**Values rounded

DAY 2

Breakfast

1 cup cooked oatmeal
2 tablespoons raisins
½ cup skim or 1% milk
2 slices whole wheat toast with
2 teaspoons tub margarine
6 ounces orange juice
1 cup coffee
1 tablespoon skim or 1% milk

Snack

1 medium banana

Lunch

1 cup *beef and bean chili
4 whole grain crackers, unsalted
1 cup tossed salad with
1 tablespoon low-calorie dressing
1 cup skim or 1% milk

Dinner

1 *baked pork chop made with *hot 'n' spicy
   seasoning
½ cup *garlic mashed potatoes
½ cup *green-bean sauté
1 dinner roll with
1 teaspoon tub margarine
1 cup skim or 1% milk
1 small slice *apple Coffee Cake

Total Nutrients**:

Calories 2,060
Sodium 1,670
Total fat . . . . 60 g
Saturated fat . . . 15 g
Cholesterol . . . . 180 mg
% of calories . . . 26% from total fat
              7% from saturated fat

continues

continued

Autumn Stuffed Cabbage

Don't wait until autumn—these braised, stuffed cabbage leaves will add variety to your menu year-round.

Ingredients

1 head cabbage
½ pound lean ground beef
½ pound ground turkey
1 small onion, minced
1 slice stale whole wheat bread, crumbled (about ⅓ cup)
¼ cup water
⅛ teaspoon freshly ground black pepper
1 16-ounce can whole tomatoes
1 small onion, sliced
1 cup water
1 medium carrot, sliced
1 tablespoon lemon juice
2 tablespoons brown sugar
1 tablespoon corn starch

Preparation

- Rinse and core the cabbage. Carefully remove 10 outer leaves and place in a medium saucepan. Cover with boiling water. Simmer 5 minutes.
- Remove and drain cooked cabbage leaves on paper toweling.
- Shred ½ cup raw cabbage and set aside.
- Brown ground beef and turkey and the minced onion in medium skillet. Drain fat.

- Place the drained meat mixture, bread crumbs, water, and pepper in medium mixing bowl.
- Drain tomatoes, reserving liquid, and add ½ cup tomato juice from can to meat mixture. Mix well; then place ¼ cup filling on each parboiled, drained cabbage leaf. Roll up and secure with toothpick.
- Place folded side down in skillet.
- Add tomatoes, water, ½ cup shredded cabbage, sliced onion and carrot.
- Cover and simmer about 1 hour (or until cabbage is tender), basting occasionally.
- Remove cabbage rolls to serving platter, keep warm.
- Mix lemon juice, brown sugar, and cornstarch together in small bowl.
- Add to vegetables and liquid in skillet and cook, stirring occasionally, until thickened and clear. Serve over cabbage rolls.

Makes 5 servings, 2 rolls each

Nutrients per serving

Calories 257
Total fat . . . . 9 g
Saturated fat . . . . 3 g
Cholesterol . . . . . . 54 mg
Sodium . . . . 266 mg

continues

continued

Beef and Bean Chili

Real Southwest cooking need not be too hot to swallow. Try this version for plenty of flavor.

Ingredients

2 pounds lean stew beef, cut in 1-inch cubes
3 tablespoons vegetable oil
2 cups water
2 cloves garlic, minced
1 large onion, finely chopped
1 tablespoon flour
1 green pepper, chopped
2 pounds fresh tomatoes, seeded and
  chopped
2 teaspoons chili powder
1 tablespoon oregano
1 teaspoon cumin
2 cups kidney beans, cooked without salt (If
  using canned beans, drain and rinse well)

Preparation

- Brown meat in a large skillet with 2 table-spoons vegetable oil. Add water. Simmer covered 1 hour.

- Heat remaining tablespoon of vegetable oil in small skillet. Add garlic and onion and cook over low heat until onion is softened. Add to meat mixture.
- Add flour to meat and cook for 2 minutes. Add green pepper, tomatoes, chili powder, oregano, cumin, and cooked beans to meat. Simmer 1½ hours. Taste for seasoning.

Makes 9 servings

Nutrients per serving

Calories	274
Total fat	10 g
Saturated fat	2 g
Cholesterol	65 mg
Sodium	158 mg

continues

continued

Baked Pork Chops

Spicy and moist—the secret of these chops is in the coating.

Ingredients

6 lean, ½-inch thick center-cut pork chops
1 egg white
1 cup evaporated skim milk
¾ cup cornflake crumbs
¼ cup fine dry bread crumbs
2 tablespoons hot 'n' spicy seasoning
   (see below)
½ teaspoon salt
Nonstick spray coating

Preparation

- Trim all fat from chops.
- Beat egg white with evaporated skim milk. Place chops in milk mixture; let stand for 5 minutes, turning chops once.
- Meanwhile, mix together cornflake crumbs, bread crumbs, hot 'n' spicy seasoning, and salt.
- Remove chops from milk mixture. Coat thoroughly with crumb mixture.
- Spray a 13" x 9" baking pan with nonstick spray coating.
- Place chops in pan and bake in 375 degree oven for 20 minutes. Turn chops and bake 15 minutes longer or until no pink remains.

Note: If desired, substitute skinless, boneless chicken, turkey parts, or fish for pork chops and bake for 20 minutes.

Makes 6 servings

Nutrients per serving

Calories 186
Total fat . . . . 5 g
Saturated fat . . . . 2 g
Cholesterol . . . . . . 31 mg
Sodium . . . . 393 mg

Hot'n Spicy Seasoning

This'll spice up your baked pork chops—and other dishes too.

Ingredients

¼ cup paprika
2 tablespoons dried oregano, crushed
2 teaspoons chili powder
1 teaspoon garlic powder
1 teaspoon black pepper
½ teaspoon red (cayenne) pepper
½ teaspoon dry mustard

Preparation

Mix together all ingredients. Store in airtight container.

Makes about ⅓ cup

continues

continued

Garlic Mashed Potatoes

Potatoes with a whole new flavoring—a marriage made in heaven.

Ingredients

1 pound (about 2 large) potatoes, peeled and quartered
2 cups skim milk
2 large cloves garlic, chopped
½ teaspoon white pepper

Preparation

- Cook potatoes, covered, in a small amount of boiling water for 20–25 minutes or until tender. Remove from heat. Drain and re-cover.
- Meanwhile, in a small saucepan over low heat, cook garlic in milk until garlic is soft, about 30 minutes.
- Add milk-garlic mixture and white pepper to potatoes. Beat with an electric mixer on low speed or mash with a potato masher until smooth.

Microwave Directions

- Scrub potatoes, pat dry, and prick with a fork. On a plate, cook potatoes, uncovered, on 100% (high) power until tender (about 12 minutes), turning potatoes over once. Let stand 5 minutes. Peel and quarter.
- Meanwhile in a 4-cup glass measuring cup, combine milk and garlic. Cook, uncovered, on 50% (medium) power until garlic is soft (about 4 minutes).
- Continue as directed above.

Makes 4 servings

Nutrients per serving

Calories 141
Total fat . . . . <1 g
Saturated fat . . . . <1 g
Cholesterol . . . . . . 2 mg
Sodium . . . . 70 mg

< = less than

continues

continued

Green-Bean Sauté

Fresh green beans cooked lightly and tossed with parsley.

Ingredients

1 pound fresh green beans, cut in 1-inch pieces
1 tablespoon corn oil
1 large yellow onion, halved lengthwise and thinly sliced
⅛ teaspoon freshly ground black pepper
1 tablespoon fresh parsley, minced

Preparation

- Steam or cook green beans in boiling water to cover for 10–12 minutes, or until barely fork tender. Drain well.
- Heat oil in large skillet. Sauté onion until golden.
- Stir in green beans and pepper. Heat through.
- Toss with parsley before serving.

Makes 4 servings

Nutrients per serving

Calories 64
Total fat . . . . 4 g
Saturated fat . . . . <1 g
Cholesterol . . . . . . 0 mg
Sodium . . . . 15 mg

< = less than

continues

continued

Apple Coffee Cake

Chunks of tart apples and heaps of raisins and pecans make this cake sublime.

Ingredients

5 cups tart apples, finely chopped
1 cup sugar
1 cup dark raisins
½ cup pecans, chopped
¼ cup corn oil
2 teaspoons vanilla
1 egg, beaten
2½ cups sifted all-purpose flour
1½ teaspoons baking soda
2 teaspoons ground cinnamon

Preparation

- Preheat oven to 350 degrees.
- Lightly oil a 13" x 9" × 2 pan.
- In large mixing bowl, combine apples with sugar, raisins, and pecans; mix well. Let stand 30 minutes.
- Stir in oil, vanilla, and egg.
- Sift together flour, soda, and cinnamon; stir into apple mixture about a third at a time, just enough to moisten dry ingredients.
- Turn batter into pan. Bake 35–40 minutes. Cool cake slightly before serving.

Makes 20 servings

Nutrients per serving

Calories 188
Total fat . . . . 5 g
Saturated fat . . . . <1 g
Cholesterol . . . . . . 11 mg
Sodium . . . . 68 mg
< = less than

Source: "High Blood Pressure: Treat It for Life," National Heart, Lung, and Blood Institute, NIH Publication No. 94–3312, August 1994.

Alcohol and High Blood Pressure

Limit your alcohol intake. Alcohol can harm the liver, brain, and heart. Drinking too much can raise blood pressure.

Usually, even with high blood pressure, you can have an occasional drink. And those trying to avoid developing high blood pressure can drink, if they do so moderately.

Some evidence suggests that one drink a day may even lower the risk of having a heart attack. But this has yet to be proved, and too much alcohol poses dangers.

Also, if you are trying to lose weight, remember that alcoholic drinks contain calories, about 70–180 calories per drink, depending on the type.

So if you don't drink, it's best not to start. If you drink, limit your daily alcohol intake to no more than two drinks a day. The "Dietary Guidelines for Americans" recommends that for overall health women should limit their alcohol to no more than one drink a day.

One Drink of Alcohol Means

- 1½ ounces of 80-proof or 1 ounce of 100-proof whiskey, or
- 5 ounces of wine, or
- 12 ounces of beer (regular or light)

Source: "High Blood Pressure: Treat It for Life," National Heart, Lung, and Blood Institute, NIH Publication No. 94–3312, August 1994.

Heart Healthy Eating Self-Contract

I, _____, agree with the following small steps to reduce my fat intake.

☐ I pledge to use the Food Guide Pyramid twice a week to choose foods to make a healthy meal.

☐ I pledge to eat a fruit or vegetable for a snack every day.

☐ I pledge to select low fat foods more often & my favorite high fat food, _____, only once a week.

Within the next 4 weeks, by _____, I'll be following these pledges regularly.

If I do, I will reward myself with/by _____

_____.

If I do not, I will *revise the contract and start over*.

_____

Signature   Date

_____

Witness   Date

Source: Gail C. Frank-Spohrer, *Community Nutrition: Applying Epidemiology to Contemporary Practice*, Aspen Publishers, Inc., © 1996.

Types of Medications for High Blood Pressure

Here are the kinds of drugs used most often to lower high blood pressure and how they work.

- **Diuretics** are commonly used for lowering high blood pressure. They're sometimes called "water pills" because they flush excess sodium and water from the body through the urine. This lessens the amount of fluid in the blood. Sodium is also flushed out of the blood vessel walls, allowing the blood vessels to dilate. As a result, there is less pressure on the blood vessels. Diuretics come in different brands, and doctors prescribe different kinds for different people.
- **Beta blockers** reduce the number of nerve impulses that occur in the heart and blood vessels. This reduction slows the heart, which beats less often and with less contracting force—so blood pressure drops and the heart works less hard.
- **ACE inhibitors** block a hormone which is made in the kidney. This hormone narrows the blood vessels and causes blood pressure to rise.
- **Calcium channel blockers** keep calcium from entering the muscle cells of the heart and blood vessels. This causes the blood vessels to relax.
- **Alpha blockers** work on the nervous system to relax the blood vessels, allowing the blood to pass more easily.
- **Alpha-beta blockers** work the same way alpha blockers do but also slow the heartbeat so less blood is pumped through the vessels.
- **Nervous system inhibitors** relax blood vessels by controlling nerve impulses.
- **Vasodilators** open blood vessels by relaxing the muscle in the vessel walls.

POSSIBLE SIDE EFFECTS

Side effects can occur with any drug. Even aspirin sometimes causes stomach problems. Some high blood pressure drugs may make you feel tired or sleepy or cause you to have a rash or a cough.

The important thing is that you pay attention to how you feel. And, if you have a side effect, don't stop taking your medication—that can cause trouble. Tell your doctor about the problem as soon as possible. Sometimes, a change in dosage will stop the difficulty. Or, a different drug may be found that will not produce side effects for you.

A reminder: It is important to take a blood pressure medicine according to its instructions. One or two pills a day control most high blood pressure. Sometimes, however, more than one drug is needed. Taking pills may seem bothersome and costly. But not taking them can lead to illness, disability, or death.

continues

continued

If you are worried about the cost of a drug, talk to your doctor or pharmacist about a less expensive one. For example, your doctor may be able to prescribe a generic drug that has the same effect as a brand name medication, or switch you to another less costly type of drug.

SPEAK UP AND ASK

If your doctor prescribes a drug to treat your high blood pressure, be sure to ask

- when it should be taken
- what you can eat and drink with it, or how long you must wait before and after a meal to take it
- what other drugs can or cannot be taken at the same time
- what to do if you run out of a drug
- what to do if you forget to take a dose
- if there are any special instructions

NOTES:

Source: "High Blood Pressure: Treat It for Life," National Heart, Lung, and Blood Institute, NIH Publication No. 94–3312, August 1994.

Generic Names of High Blood Pressure Medicines

Type of Medicine	Generic Name	Type of Medicine	Generic Name
Diuretics	amiloride bendroflumethiazide benzthiazide	Angiotensin Antagonists	losartan valsartan
	bumetanide chlorothiazide chlorthalidone furosemide hydrochlorothiazide hydroflumethiazide indapamide methyclothiazide metolazone	Calcium Channel Blockers	amlodipine diltiazam felodipine isradipine nicardipine nifedipine nisoldipine verapamil
	polythiazide spironolactone torsemide triamterene	Alpha Blockers	doxazosin prazosin terazosin
	trichlormethiazide	Alpha-Beta Blockers	labetalol carvedilol
Beta Blockers	acebutolol atenolol betaxolol bisoprolol carteolol metoprolol nadolol penbutolol pindolol	Nervous System Inhibitors	clonidine guanabenz guanadrel guanethidine guanfacine methyldopa reserpine
	propranolol timolol	Vasodilators	hydralazine minoxidil
ACE Inhibitors	benazepril captopril enalapril fosinopril lisinopril moexipril quinapril ramipril trandolapril		

Source: "Controlling High Blood Pressure: A Woman's Guide," National Heart, Lung, and Blood Institute, National Institutes of Health.

How To Take Diuretics

This handout is about a particular group of diuretics called potassium-sparing diuretics-hydrochlorothiazide combinations. These drugs are used primarily for treating high blood pressure.

ABOUT DIURETICS

This medicine is a combination of two types of diuretics—potassium-sparing and hydrochlorothiazides—that help decrease the amount of water and sodium in the body by acting on the kidneys to increase the flow of urine. Other diuretics tend to reduce the amount of potassium in the body. But "potassium-sparing" diuretics help retain or "spare" this electrolyte. Potassium is vital to body functions, including muscle contraction.

These drugs come in pill form in three formulations: amiloride and hydrochlorothiazide; spironolactone and hydrochlorothiazide; and triamterene and hydrochlorothiazide, the most frequently prescribed. See box for a list of brand names.

Formulations and Commonly Used Brand Names

Amiloride/hydrochlorothiazide
- Moduretic
- Spironolactone/hydrochlorothiazide
  —Aldactazide
  —Spirozide

- Triamterene/hydrochlorothiazide
  —Diazide
  —Maxzide
  —Co-Triamterzide

CONDITIONS THESE MEDICINES TREAT

Potassium-sparing diuretics hydrochlorothiazide combinations are most commonly used to control high blood pressure (hypertension). Untreated, high blood pressure can cause serious problems such as heart failure, blood vessel disease, stroke, or kidney failure.

People taking this medicine for high blood pressure may have to take it for the rest of their lives, even though they may not feel sick.

In addition to the drug, doctors may also prescribe a low-salt diet to help reduce hypertension. The medicine is usually more effective when the diet is followed properly.

This medicine is also used to reduce swelling, such as in the ankles or lungs, caused by an excessive amount of water in the body. However, it is usually not used for treating the normal swelling of feet and hands that occurs during pregnancy.

continues

continued

HOW TO TAKE

Because this medicine may increase the frequency of urination, it is best to plan your dose or doses so they least affect your daily schedule or sleep. If you are taking only one dose a day, take it in the morning after breakfast. If you are taking more than one dose, take the last dose no later than 6 PM, unless directed otherwise by your doctor. To make it easier to remember to take your medicine, take it at the same time each day.

If the medicine upsets your stomach, it may be taken with meals or a glass of milk. This will help prevent stomach upset.

MISSED DOSES

A missed dose should be taken as soon as possible. However, if it's almost time for your next dose, skip the missed dose and go back to your regular dosing schedule. Do not take double doses.

RELIEF OF SYMPTOMS

If this medicine is being used to control hypertension, there may be no noticeable effects. High blood pressure may not have any outward signs. In fact, most people with high blood pressure feel normal.

It is important to continue to take the medicine exactly as directed and to keep appointments with your doctor even if you feel well.

If this medicine is being used to reduce swelling, its effects should be noticeable in from a few days to a few weeks, depending on the condition it is being used to treat.

SIDE EFFECTS AND RISKS

Initial Effects

Initially, this medicine may cause unusual tiredness and an increase in the amount of urine and frequency of urination. These effects should lessen after you have taken the medicine for a few weeks.

Potassium Level

This medicine also may increase or decrease the amount of potassium in your body, depending on which of the two components of the drug have the predominant effect. For this reason, doctors

continues

continued

ordinarily do blood tests the first few months you're on the drug and periodically thereafter to monitor the amount of potassium in your body. To offset any decrease or increase, your doctor may instruct you to eat or avoid certain foods. For example, you may be advised to eat foods or drink beverages that have a high potassium content (e.g., citrus fruit juices and bananas), use salt substitutes, or take a potassium supplement. However, do not use salt substitutes or low-sodium milk unless your doctor tells you to because they may contain potassium. Too much or too little potassium can be harmful.

The symptoms of an increase in potassium are dry mouth, increased thirst, irregular heartbeat, mood or mental changes, muscle cramps or pain, shortness of breath or difficulty breathing, unusual tiredness or weakness, a weak pulse, and numbness or tingling in hands, feet, or lips. If any of these occurs, check with your doctor as soon as possible.

Blood Sugar

If you are already on a special diet, as for diabetes, tell your doctor. Hydrochlorothiazide can raise your blood sugar.

Sensitivity to Sunlight

This medicine also may cause increased sensitivity to sunlight in a few people. Exposure to sunlight, even for brief periods, may cause severe sunburn, skin rash, redness, itching, discoloration of skin, or change in vision. If you notice an increased sensitivity to sunlight while taking this medicine, it's wise to take precautions to reduce your exposure to direct sunlight. If you have a severe reaction from the sun, discuss it with your doctor.

Other Side Effects

If a pregnant woman takes hydrochlorothiazide, there is a slight chance her newborn infant may have low potassium. For this reason, it is usually not prescribed during pregnancy. The drug has not been shown to cause birth defects.

Rarely, these diuretics may cause a number of other side effects. Check with your doctor as soon as possible if you have any of the following:

- black, tarry stools
- blood in urine or stools
- cough or hoarseness
- fever or chills
- joint pain
- lower back or side pain

continues

continued

- painful or difficult urination
- pinpoint-size red spots on skin
- skin rash or hives
- severe stomach pain with nausea and vomiting
- unusual bleeding or bruising
- yellow eyes or skin

In addition, on rare occasions triamterene may cause a bright red tongue, a burning feeling in the tongue, and cracked corners of the mouth. Check with your doctor as soon as possible if these occur.

As your body adjusts to this medicine, other side effects may occur, but they usually do not require medical attention unless they continue or are bothersome. The most common are loss of appetite, nausea and vomiting, stomach cramps and diarrhea, and upset stomach. Less common are decreased sexual ability, dizziness or light-headedness when getting up from lying down or sitting, and headache.

Spironolactone sometimes causes breast tenderness in women, enlarged breasts in men, clumsiness, deepening of voice in females, increased hair growth in females, irregular menstrual periods, and sweating. These conditions gradually disappear over two or three months after the medicine is stopped.

Amiloride sometimes causes constipation.

Other rarer side effects not listed here may occur in a few people. If you have any new symptoms while taking this medication, check with your doctor.

BEFORE USING THIS MEDICINE

Tell your doctor

- if you have ever had any unusual or allergic reaction to amiloride, spironolactone, triamterene, sulfonamides, bumetanide, furosemide, acetazolamide, dichlorphenamide, methazolamide, hydrochlorothiazide, or any of the other thiazide diuretics
- if you are on a special diet, such as low sodium, because this could affect how the drug works in your body
- if you are allergic to any substance, such as foods, sulfites or other preservatives, or dyes, because these diuretics, like most other medicines that come in pill form, contain preservatives and dyes that may cause an allergic reaction in some people
- if you are pregnant or may become pregnant, because, in general, diuretics should not be taken during pregnancy unless recommended by the doctor

continues

continued

- if you are breastfeeding (Although spironolactone, triamterene, and hydrochlorothiazide may pass into breast milk, they have not been shown to cause problems in nursing babies. It is not known whether amiloride passes into breast milk.)
- if you have any of the following medical problems: sugar diabetes; kidney disease; liver disease; menstrual problems or breast enlargement; inflammation of the pancreas; or a history of gout, kidney stones, or lupus erythematosus

PRECAUTIONS AND WARNINGS

If you get sick and have severe or continuing vomiting or diarrhea while taking this medicine, check with your doctor. These problems may cause you to lose additional water and potassium and lead to low blood pressure.

Before having any kind of surgery (including dental surgery) or emergency treatment, inform the doctor or dentist that you are taking this medicine.

Before taking any medical tests, tell the doctor you are taking this medicine. It may affect the test results.

If you are taking this medicine for high blood pressure, do not take any other medicine unless you have discussed it with your doctor. This includes nonprescription drugs—particularly those for appetite control, asthma, colds, cough, hay fever, or sinus problems—some of which contain ingredients that may increase your blood pressure.

If you are taking triamterene and hydrochlorothiazide, do not change brands without first checking with your doctor. If you refill your medicine and it looks different, check with your pharmacist.

Source: Sharon Snider, "How To Take Your Medicine: Diuretics," *FDA Consumer*, U.S. Food and Drug Administration, October 1990.

How To Take Beta Blocker Medicines

GENERIC NAMES OF BETA BLOCKERS

Beta blocker medicines are available under the following generic names

- acebutolol
- atenolol
- betaxolol
- carteolol
- labetalol
- metoprolol

- nadolol
- penbutolol
- pindolol
- propranolol
- timolol

CONDITIONS THESE MEDICINES TREAT

All beta blockers are used to treat high blood pressure. Many are also used to prevent the heart-related chest pain or pressure associated with angina pectoris (a condition often occurring during exertion where too little blood reaches the heart). Atenolol, metoprolol, timolol, and propranolol are used to improve survival after a heart attack. Propranolol is used to treat heart rhythm problems, other special heart conditions, migraine headaches, and tremors. Beta blockers can be used for other conditions as determined by your doctor.

Beta blockers cannot cure these conditions. However, by blocking certain receptors in the body, beta blockers lower and regulate the heartbeat and lessen the heart's workload.

While taking beta blockers, it is important that you continue any diet and exercise program prescribed by your doctor, as these are often important parts of the therapy for the conditions being treated.

HOW TO TAKE BETA BLOCKERS

Beta blockers can be taken either with food or on an empty stomach.

If you are taking an extended-release product such as Inderal LA (propranolol), swallow it whole. Don't chew it or crush it in any way.

If you are taking the concentrated solution of propranolol, always use the dropper provided. You can mix the solution with water or any other beverage (or, if you prefer, pudding or applesauce). After taking a dose, rinse the glass with some liquid and drink that liquid as well to be sure that the entire dose is taken.

Be sure to take the right number of tablets or capsules for each dose. Taking your medicine at the same time each day will help you remember to take it regularly.

continues

continued

MEDICINE TIPS

Don't store medicines in the bathroom medicine cabinet. Heat and humidity may cause the medicine to lose its effectiveness. Keep all medicines, even those with child-resistant caps, out of the reach of children. Remember, the caps are child-resistant, not child-proof. Discard medicines that have reached the expiration date.

MISSED DOSES

Do not suddenly stop taking a beta blocker without first talking to your doctor. Your condition could worsen if you stop taking this medicine or miss many doses.

If you miss a dose, take it as soon as you remember. If you take the beta blocker once a day, you can take it up to eight hours before the next scheduled dose. If you take the medication more often than once a day, you can take it up to four hours before the next scheduled dose. Ask your doctor or pharmacist if you have questions.

Never take two doses at the same time. Always have enough of your beta blocker medicine to last over weekends, holiday periods, and when you travel.

RELIEF OF SYMPTOMS

For conditions such as high blood pressure, angina, heart rhythm disturbances, or tremors, some effects can be seen immediately and usually peak within a week. If treating migraine headaches, it may take up to six weeks before the full effects occur. For any of these conditions, the dosage of the beta blocker may need to be adjusted by your doctor when you first begin taking it. Also, the appropriate dosage can vary greatly among people, depending on individual response.

Since many of the conditions that beta blockers treat are chronic, you may have to take this medicine for the rest of your life.

SIDE EFFECTS AND RISKS

Common side effects include slowed heartbeat, tiredness, nausea, diarrhea, constipation, and decreased sexual ability. Other mild side effects can include difficulty sleeping or nightmares, headache, drowsiness, and numbness or tingling of the fingers, toes, or scalp. Also, if you have diabetes, beta blockers can obscure some of the signs of low blood sugar, such as tremors or rapid heartbeat. Check with your doctor if any of these side effects seem troublesome or if you have any questions.

continues

continued

More serious reactions can sometimes occur with beta blockers. These include the following:

- the beginning or worsening of heart failure (Symptoms of this include shortness of breath, especially on exertion; coughing; weakness; weight gain; and swelling of feet, ankles, or lower legs.)
- severe wheezing or difficulty breathing, especially in people who have or have had asthma, chronic bronchitis, emphysema, or other breathing conditions (Because beta blockers can trigger or worsen these conditions, make sure your doctor knows about them.)
- an extremely slow heartbeat (less than 50 beats per minute)
- cold hands and feet or blue fingernails, which could mean reduced circulation to these areas
- confusion, hallucinations, or depression

If any of these or other serious reactions occur, call your doctor immediately.

PRECAUTIONS AND WARNINGS

If you suddenly stop taking a beta blocker, you could worsen your condition and experience potentially dangerous side effects, such as chest pain, fast or irregular heartbeat, high blood pressure, and headaches. Always check with your doctor before discontinuing a beta blocker.

Learn how the medicine affects you. Don't drive or operate machines if this medicine makes you drowsy, dizzy, or light-headed. If you are taking labetalol, dizziness or light-headedness can occur when getting up from sitting or lying down. If this happens, sit up slowly, placing your legs over the side of the bed or couch, and stay there for a few minutes before trying to stand.

Before any surgery or dental work, tell the doctor or dentist that you are taking beta blockers. Tell your doctor if you are taking or considering taking any other prescription or nonprescription medication.

Drinking alcohol while on beta blockers can sometimes increase the chance of side effects such as dizziness or tiredness.

Source: *FDA Consumer*, 24:1, U.S. Food and Drug Administration, Rockville, Maryland, 1990.

Index